Pills-A-Go-Go

Pills-A-Go-Go
A Fiendish Investigation into Pill Marketing, Art, History and Consumption

Jim Hogshire

With contributions from Skylaire Alfvegren,
an109010@anon.penet.fi, Will Bleifuss, Edward M. Brecher,
Dorian, Adam Gorightly, Itchy DuPont, Melissa Hoffs,
Heidi Hogshire, Pollyanne Hornbeck, Tim Johnson,
David C. Morrison, Adam Parfrey, Phreex,
Sylvia Remora, Rhodium 980729,
and Michael Starks.

feral house

The publisher wishes to thank Jim Hogshire, Skylaire Alfvegren, Melissa Hoffs, Pollyanne Hornbeck, Sean Tejaratchi, Cake, Kim Seltzer, Chuck Shepherd and Billy Shire for their contributions, inspirations, labor and madness.

Design by Linda Hayashi

Feral House
P.O. Box 13067
Los Angeles, CA 90013

www.feralhouse.com

ISBN: 0-922915-53-9
10 9 8 7 6 5 4 3 2

Dedicated to Dr. Leo Sternbach and Dr. Gordon Alles

Contents

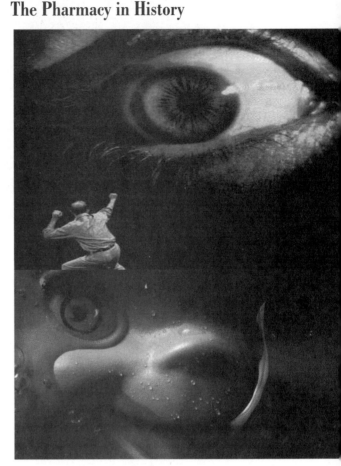

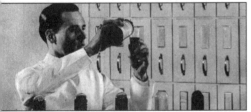

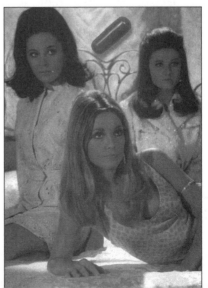

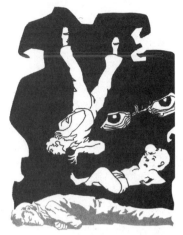

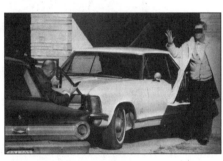

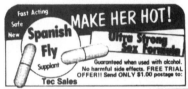

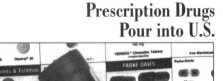

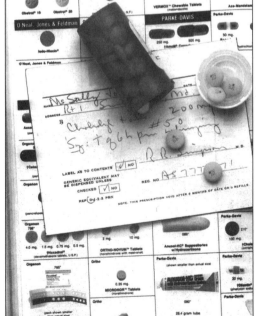

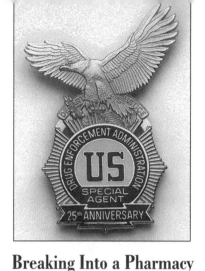

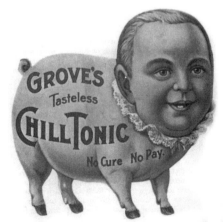

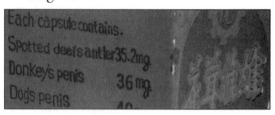

The pill is the quintessential icon of Western Civilization. One small tablet embodies our history, our world view, our vision of the future. It is the perfect, symbolic encapsulation of man's progress—from the ancient Phoenicians to the internet. Pills are integrated into our very being, even more than the car, the firearm, the written word . . . anything.

The beauty and perfection of pills is something readers know, instinctively or even subliminally from their own explorations. *Pills-A-Go-Go* is not a project we simply wanted to do; pilldom is a field that beckoned us, atom by atom, by its limitless molecular allure.

So here it is: *Pills-A-Go-Go,* the book. A cultural study of pills. Not medicine *per se* nor health nor pharmacology—just pills, all pills, any pills. Pills that drop from a purse and roll under a couch where they sit for years. Pills that get you stopped at the border. Pills that associate you with the rich and famous. And pills that link you to skid row.

Pharmaceutical products, so tightfistedly prescribed by the medical monopoly, so sternly monitored by tight-lipped authorities, and so scowlingly dispensed by white-smocked druggists, have been seen as the domain of the joyless, the authoritarian. But not any more.

When *Pills-A-Go-Go* emerged as a 'zine, its 22 issues forever ruptured the medical, government and corporate protocol. No book or 'zine ever examined the products of of megacorporate drug manufacturers from the point of view of unrepentant drug takers. Which pills worked, which pills didn't, and how they could be hacked so as not to ruin one's internal organs. And best yet, tips were provided on obtaining pills in a world in which dirty hardcore non-pharmaceutical drugs like heroin and crack have become far easier to obtain than an innocent sedative like Valium.

The book herein provides the best tidbits taken from the 'zine as well as further information, paraphernalia and inspiring graphics collected by yours truly and several other friends, when the 'zine went though a sabbatical. Read on for the many taboo, absurd, ignored and forgotten ways pills continue to shape our lives and provide so many of us with enjoyment.

"I like pills so much I can feel a warm glow in my body when I look at a Dristan ad in the subway . . ."
—ex-stewardess/pillhead quoted in *The Tranquilizing of America.*

—*Jim Hogshire,* APRIL 1999

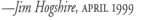

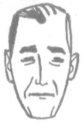
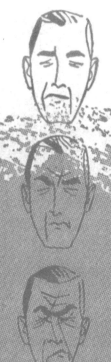

The Pillhead in Society
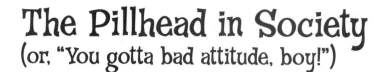
(or, "You gotta bad attitude, boy!")

In high school I had a friend who just loved pornography. Of course, I liked it too, but I lived out in the suburbs where hardcore porn wasn't available. Besides, I was too scared to buy the stuff. Not my friend; he would brazenly take a bus to the porno store and buy whatever he wanted. The magazines could get pretty pricey, but he financed his porn habit by doubling the price and reselling them to this pudgy guy who became incoherent when Gary pulled out the raunchiest, most explicit fuck books.

One day, the summer before I went to college, Gary came by my house with four grocery bags filled with porno.

"I'm giving this to you," he told me. "I've got a girlfriend now and I'm never gonna jack off again. Those days are over."

The porno was worth almost $2,000. It didn't matter that Gary was back in less than a week begging for some of his old collection (the girlfriend thing didn't pan out). I kept 'em. And of course I brought them with me to college.

It soon became known around the dorm that I had stacks and stacks of hardcore (and my own softcore stuff). The guys' initial reaction was to ridicule me as a pervert. "God, man, whaddya do—jack off alla time? I never seen so much porno!" they'd say, the whole group feigning disgust, shaking their heads and laughing.

One by one, though, they all found a reason to drop by my room and ask to look at the porn. And, "Hey, d'ya mind if I just borrow this one for awhile? Y'know, this is kinda interesting."

Soon I had to institute a lending policy and kept records like a library. My porn circulated all year through the dorm. Nevertheless, I was "the porno guy." Because the other

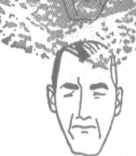

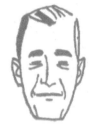

dudes only borrowed (and sometimes failed to return) my porno they felt detached from it—maybe even a little superior. After all, they didn't have the obvious perversion I had.

It's the same with being "the pill guy." Because I make no secret about my fascination with pills, keep large stocks of pills around and read everything I can about them, people have come to know me as some kind of a pill pervert.

Even people who smoke dope, snort cocaine or even (in some cases) shoot heroin, view pillheads as morally bankrupt.

Most pill references in popular culture are derogatory— "Mother's Little Helper," the confessions of Kitty Dukakis and Betty Ford, the movie *I'm Dancing as Fast as I Can* (in which Jill Clayburgh gets all mellowed out on Valium overdoses, then abruptly stops taking them, sending her into a manic anxiety jag). Part of their negative image comes from being viewed as the drug of the establishment. Pills are made by staid pharmaceutical companies, after all. When Mick Jagger sings about Valium, he's clearly jeering at this harried woman who seeks relief from the drudgery and pain in her life through a pill. The very fact that such an unenviable character as Sonny Bono took pills is bad enough. But when they get around to copping to their pill-love, it's usually in the midst of some kind of public purging of their "demon" pills.

Pills are also viewed as cheating. Using pills—even to deaden physical pain—is seen as the resort of a wimp, somebody who can't even take a little pain. Taking pills for relief of psychic pain or, God forbid, enhancement of mental faculties, is even more indicative of moral weakness.

Even people who take pills regularly feel compelled to condemn them—especially when they're used by somebody else and even more especially if they take them "for the wrong reasons." Of course, Mick Jagger has consumed plenty of mother's little helpers in his lifetime. So has everyone else. Even people who claim to "never" take pills, take pills. Just ask 'em what they do for a headache. Well, in that case, they take a pill, they'll tell you. If you press further and ask which pill, you'll find they often have a preference. Within moments of declaring they never take pills, you can coax most folks into admitting they like Advil better than Tylenol or aspirin.

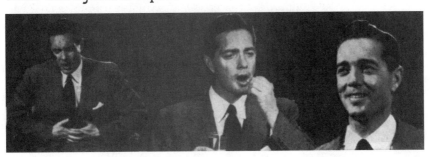

So much for their stoic freedom from devil pills. If you wanted, you could probably wheedle them for the other pills they take, but why embarrass them? Let 'em live in their fictional world where only the morally deficient depend on pills for help.

Except, of course, they don't stay in that fiction world. Like my porno-seeking friends, they sought out the pillhead to ask advice, or more frequently, pills. I won't say that it galls me, but I sometimes give them a little bit of the business, warning them of their imminent entry into the vortex of pilldom in all its degenerate squalor.

I've noticed, almost without exception, people who are introduced to the wonders of pills eventually come around to liking them. All my girlfriends, for instance, who have started out with a leery attitude toward pills, wondering with mild disgust how in the world I could look to a pill without a doctor's permission, eventually realize the truth: They work just fine without the sanction of an M.D. Pills work just fine for more things and in more ways than you're supposed to know.

Suddenly a new and taboo world opens up to them. Galaxies of pills, tools for better living become available—at least theoretically if not practically. Once the lure of a better life becomes apparent it is impossible to turn back. From that time on, another pillhead is added to the population. Of course, the new pillhead will go on to spread the word of pills and increase our numbers—even if some decide to remain "in the closet" and hide their pill-love.

Thus, the pillhead's relationship to society is almost by definition insidious. Promoting a practice so wrapped up in conflicting opinions means one must take a clear stand. Pills are good. Saying that pills make good sense and do good things is heretical in American society. Everyone uses pills to some degree, so it is socially retarded to absolutely argue against them with the vehemence a pillhead might argue for them. Pills have proven more useful, cheaper, and versatile than the scalpel in treating disease. To argue against pills would be lunacy. Yet actively promoting their use is considered just as loony.

Society cannot reconcile its ambivalence toward pills. Instead of attacking the healing creations of science, society launches its ridicule and torture upon the pillhead whose undisguised enjoyment of the pill tears paternalistic ritual and hypocrisy to bits. It's a sin to smile in church.

A Short History of Pills

UR WORD "PILL" COMES from the Latin *pillula*, meaning "little ball." In ancient times and for centuries that followed, pills had but one form— the little round ball. Even today, nitpickers cringe when they hear the term applied to any other sort of "solid oral dosage form," like, say, a *tablet* or a *capsule*. The pill's earliest ancestors emerged from ancient Egypt, where docs mixed active ingredients with clay or bread to form the little balls to concoct a standard dose and a convenient method of taking medicine.

Pill's ancestry is worth noting because ancient Egyptian medicine followed an entirely different methodology than contemporary medicine. According to Worth Estes, professor of pharmacology at the University of Boston and author of the book *Ancient Egyptian Medicine,* "about the only thing the two systems had in common was the view that disease existed and the goal was to make the patient well again."

Ancient Egyptian medical theory believed all bodily energy and health centered around invisible tubes running from the colon. They viewed the laxative as the most critical medication and shitting the most important bodily function. Drilling holes in the head or bloodletting and other Egyptian medical practices are alien to modern medicine. Only one thing from their medical arsenal survived the millennia—pills.

In modern times, pills symbolize the rational and scientific, though they are offered in a fun-loving variety of receptacles besides the coated and uncoated pills of yesteryear: scored tablets, medications with their famous "tiny time-pills" emanate from the larger mother pill, or slowly dissolving pills (inspired by jawbreaker hard candies) that release their fractions of a dose as each layer dissolves deep inside the body.

There are the familiar, brightly-colored capsules containing powders in their hard-gelatin shells, and the pastel tints of soft capsules encasing yummy, liquid centers. Some pills are little works of art made to swallow. Although produced at a rate of thousands per minute, pills display a kind of crisp intaglio printing on their flawless surfaces that is technically stunning even if they don't compete with craftsmanship of Faberge eggs or grains of rice inscribed with the Lord's prayer.

Some pills are made to dissolve under the tongue, the medication passing directly into the capillaries so close to the surface. Others (known as a "buccal" tablets) take advantage of the absorption characteristics found in the natural pocket between cheek and gum to best deliver their active ingredients.

The latest pill engineering feats promise even more exacting and exotic delivery systems. There is the robot pill that carries the medicine in a tiny, motorized vessel that recalls the ever-shrinking injectable submarine from *Fantastic Voyage.* Either through timing or by watching its course via radar-like equipment, the incorporeal submarine pill releases its cargo at just the right spot to achieve maximum benefit. Other futuristic pills include nearly microscopic bits of protein bound to a few molecules of medication, biologically "trained" to travel directly to the site of injury or disease, depositing exactly enough of the right medicine to do the job and no more.

Besides the many variations on the pill theme, drugstores' shelves are packed with an array of breathtaking marvels of pharmaceutical engineering: single-dose, disposable syringes, ointments, eye drops, nasal sprays, medicine-impregnated chewing gum and the ever-more-popular transdermal patch!

Pharmacy, with Doctor Selecting Drugs German School, 16th century. From this woodcut out of H. Brunschwig's *Buch der Chirurgia*, Strasburg, 1500, we get some idea of the interior of drug stores around 1500; and we also gather that the doctor often did not write out a prescription but went in person to select the ingredients.

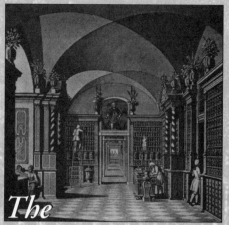

The
Pharmacy
in History

HE ORIGINS OF THE MODERN PILL stretch back beyond ancient Egypt when various concoctions were mashed up with bread or clay for easier ingestion. The Sumerians compounded medicines from such rustic ingredients as saltpeter and willow bark along the Tigris-Euphrates.

Greek physicians collected and prescribed the best drugs of older civilizations and passed them on to Rome, where detailed prescriptions first emerged.

The first apothecary appeared in Baghdad near the ninth century. While the master races of Europe were busy worshipping trees, Arabs were already training, licensing and inspecting pharmacists and pharmacies. Medicinal preparations were manufactured in the great cities of the Middle East and shipped out in caravans as far as sub-Saharan Africa. A hospital in Damascus was built in 1160, remaining in operation for hundreds of years.

Perhaps the surest sign that Europe had emerged from the Dark Ages was the appearance of the apothecary. Looking to Damian, the patron saint of drugstores, nuns and priests who had saved six centuries' worth of Arabian medical knowledge through Greek translations, abandoned their fear of heathen science and began to make and dispense medicines.

Even more information streamed into Europe from the Middle East, adding to the existing pharmacopoeia and spawning the codified study of medicine. Encyclopedias of drugs began to appear and by the twelfth century, pharmacies started to appear all over Europe, and the government of Venice started to "supervise" the drug trade—a sure sign that it was profitable.

Medieval drugstores were not much different than any other type of store at the time. Like other businesses, they were storefront operations that opened up directly onto the streets. Horizontal doors were fastened with hooks and pegs to form both a roof and a counter from which the pharmacist could sell his wares. Behind him, the apprentice was mixing and grinding or doing whatever other work the master decided he should do, including the laundry. Doing double-duty as a doctor, the pharmacist spent some of his time listening to complaints, peering down throats and inspecting a person's urine or feces for tell-tale signs of disease.

Emperor Federico II of Sicily was the first to recognize a conflict of interest between the two professions and in the 1230s forbade physicians to either own or operate pharmacies. He further ordered druggists to follow doctors instructions explicitly and not play around with the prescription.

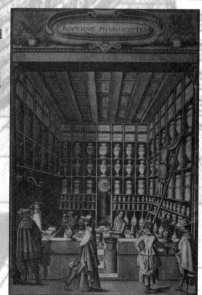

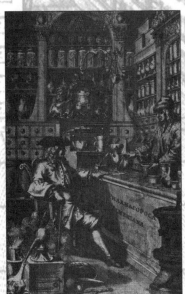

Medieval monks added their own folk remedies to the Greek and Roman instructions, equipping their monasteries with a hospital, physician and pharmacy. The growing number of Catholic hospitals continues this link between religion and medicine.

Renaissance was a time when pharmacies became a common business. Local pharmacopoeias were drawn up to help standardize medicines (no more "special recipes"), beginning with Nuremberg and the Dispensatorium of Valerius Cordus (1546). Pharmacy organizations sprouted. Apprenticeships gave way to academic study and formal training.

In Britain, apothecary shop owners were members of the Grocer's Company before they formed their own guild, selling medicines in open competition with doctors.

But things lagged behind in the Masonic frontier of America. People visited apothecary shops for medical advice as often as they went to doctors, and there was little difference between a physician and a druggist. Most doctors bought raw materials from a wholesale druggist and mixed their own compounds. The idea of separating doctor from pharmacist didn't come to the United States until one John Morgan studied medicine in Europe and then returned to the wild colonial territories in 1765.

Morgan thought overdrugging of patients seemed a big problem, too, but both patients and doctors disliked his idea of separating doc from drugs. Patients didn't want increased expense and inconvenience, and doctors weren't thrilled about handing over part of their livelihood to future pill-counters. Needless to say, Morgan won no popularity contests and died penniless in the gutter.

The making of medicines finally became pharmacist's domain after the War of 1812. Seduced by medical school, doctors began to illegibly write prescriptions rather than compound drugs. Gregory Higby notes in his essay, "From Compounding to Caring: An Abridged History of the American Pharmacy," "By the turn of the 19th century, the position of the pharmacist in the American health care system was firmly established. Physicians had agreed to dispense medicines only rarely and pharmacists reciprocated by limiting their diagnosing and prescribing to cases of minor ills and emergencies." Finally the merchant was the merchant and the doctor the doctor.

The Pill as Virgin/Whore

Every pill released to the masses goes through a "Therapeutic Life Cycle," a process that tracks the fluctuating level of public acceptance. "The Benzodiazepines," a 1981 article in *Pharmacy International,* tracks the acceptance level of pills—the line in the graphs starts fairly high, then climbs steeply before experiencing a sharp drop, leveling out somewhere between the initial rate of acceptance and its highest point. And indeed, this is the pattern of most drugs. When first introduced, the new medications are regarded with

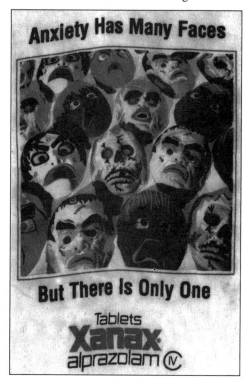

curiosity. As news spreads, faddism comes into play, and hope springs forth that a "miracle pill" has been discovered.

Then all possible side effects, most of which were known and announced at the very start, start cropping up in an ever-growing population of new users. Tabloid horror stories begin to appear, demonizing the pill while buck-chasing lawyers start advertising for victims of the satanic tablet. If lucky, an ambulance chaser will find a sensationally freakish victim to parade around in lurid videotapes shown on tabloid news programs, encouraging the FDA to pressure pharmaceutical firms into discontinuing the pill's manufacture. Or else laws are passed to make the newly demonic drug illegal, ensuring further growth of the prison industry by providing even more victims of the so-called Drug War, an unconstitutional, classist and racist program so unconscionably evil that even such cop and prison-loving, right-wing leaders like George Schultz and William F. Buckley, Jr. have voiced their opposition to it.

It should be pointed out, however, that most demonized pills are not withdrawn or made illegal when clinical use of the drug becomes more firmly established, and drawbacks are measured against the drug's therapeutic value. Following the initial controversy and government retests, the drug is transformed from being an imminent threat to a crashing media bore.

Prozac offers a perfect example of the process most pills undergo—glorification, demonization and normalization. Introduced as a "miracle drug," then skewered soon after as a "devil drug," Prozac finally became accepted as just another pill. Its demonizing period created so much press that Prozac finally became such a dull media cliché that the multitude of immediately published Prozac books can now be found in the Ed Hamilton remaindered book catalogue.

To see how pills lend themselves to quick and dirty "feature" articles we only need glance at weekly news magazines or "investigative" television news programs for the typical evil pill lead story. In its September 7, 1992 issue, the leftist weekly, *The Nation,* ran an exposé purporting to examine the dangers of Xanax. Little did the reader know that most of its anti-Xanax information came from a public relations agency whose client produced a competitor pill that had a lot to gain by Xanax's troubles. Mass market magazines and television news shows reveal their deficient investigations when they depend almost solely upon press releases to either tout or denounce any pill.

As a measure of how implicitly the American masses trust their news sources, consider the kinds of lawsuits filed against pills. While in the devil pill stage, both Prozac and Halcion were involved in some ludicrous claims by people who sought to blame their own stupidity or criminal actions on a pill. Between 1992 and 1993 these two pills were named in more than a hundred lawsuits alleging they had transformed an otherwise mellow Dr. Jekyll into a raging Mr. Hyde.

None of these claims turned out to be true, but the stories created such a fear of these pills that its detractors in the mainstream media no longer had to prove anything. Soon, anybody could be an expert.

The Nation once once again sneered at pills in William Styron's April 11, 1993 article entitled "Prozac Days, Halcion Nights," in which the author made a good case for himself as someone quite fearful of pills. Styron's bestselling autobiography, *Darkness Visible*, recounted a bout with depression, for which he made good money discussing on the lecture circuit. Even though Styron's speeches were often paid for by pharmaceutical firms marketing competitors to the drugs he was dissing, Styron claims his missionary zeal was motivated out of the "charitable impulse to tell others similarly afflicted not to give up hope." He thought his very presence as a survivor and his kind words of encouragement could be "life-saving" to audience members paying a high tariff.

Unlike his memoir, Styron's article in *The Nation* didn't discuss his depression, and instead took up anti-Prozac zeal, a drug he had never taken and ignorantly describes as "merely an improvement on an old formula." At least several paragraphs admit that he's seen evidence of Prozac helping the depressed, but alternately warns of its dangers, as told him by other depressed individuals who popped the drug.

Styron informs the depressed that they should never take tranquilizers. Even if plagued by

sleeplessness and anxiety, tranks "should be shunned like cyanide." And that's it. Like cyanide. As for Halcion, Styron writes that it made his depression worse. That's because for a time he was taking the pill to get to sleep. And during that time, he was depressed. Then he frankly admits Halcion couldn't have either caused his depression or suicidal thoughts.

Still, he calls Upjohn (Halcion's makers) the "crazy Eddie of the [pharmaceutical] industry."

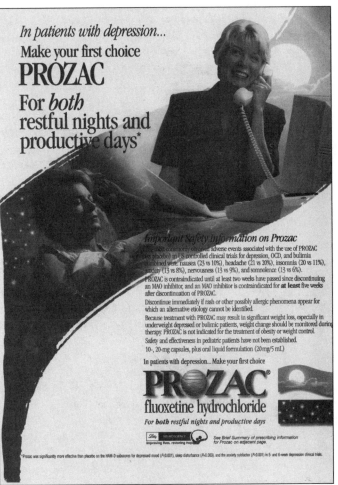

To provide an example of just how bad Halcion could make a person feel, he cites a character in a Philip Roth novel. The article proves that Styron is obviously prone to depression as well as hysteria. He recalls being so fraught with anxiety over an operation he visited a doctor to treat insomnia. The doc prescribed Halcion. Here's the kicker—while chewing his nails in sunny California, he says he thought of suicide.

While recovering in the hospital Styron complained to a doctor that he suffered from lack of sleep but was still taking Halcion. When the doctor switched him to another sleeping pill, he took that as a special sign that Halcion was evil.

Prozac and the Death of Tragedy

One of the best examples of a love/hate relationship with pills is Elizabeth Wurtzel's book, *Prozac Nation.* This tiresome, 300-plus page whine says Prozac saved her from a life of debilitating depression—unfortunately it failed to save her from yammering at the drop of a hat.

One of Wurtzel's biggest complaints about Prozac seems to be that other people take it, too. How would anyone know how special she is, if everybody's taking Prozac! Especially people didn't earn it like she did. Her comments are perfect examples of medical Calvinism—the belief that feeling bad is good and feeling good is bad, the belief that taking medication to improve mental state is cheating. She takes her attitude a step further when she exalts the pill to holy status she feels the drug is being profaned.

Consider the following excerpts:

"Maybe you find out that the guy who fixes your plumbing is on Prozac, that your gynecologist is on Prozac, that your boss is on Prozac, that your mother is on Prozac, maybe your grandmother too . . . "

"I never thought that this antidote to a disease as serious as depression—a malady that easily could have ended my life—would become a national joke."

Wurtzel is peeved. Prozac may have relieved she was suffering but it made the mushy dark swamp of her worst despair mundane. I mean, the cab driver takes it. She has no choice but to put these people, the Wurtzel wannabes, in their places.

"Every so often I find myself with the urge to make sure people know that I am not just on Prozac but on lithium too, that I am a real sicko, a depressive of a much higher order than all these happy-pill poppers with their low-level sorrow.

What can she do except moralize on the sheer wrongness of others taking Prozac to escape depression?

"But it seems to me that there's something wrong with a world where all these pills are circulating . . . I have no way to be certain of this, but my guess is that most of the people on Prozac haven't taken the circuitous path to this drug that I did. Many general practitioners give Prozac to patients without much thought . . ."

Unlike you, she paid her dues!

"Sometimes I find myself resenting the ease with which doctors now perform this bit of pharmacological prestidigitation. By the time I was put on Prozac they'd tried everything else possible, I'd had my brain fried and blunted with so many other drugs, I'd spent over a decade in a prolonged state of clinical despair. Nowadays, Prozac seems to be a panacea available for the asking."

Prozac as Some Kinda Nazi Drug

Of course Prozac has been implicated in sinister scenarios. It was once accused as being a part of a plot to sedate black youth. This theory mainly came from Dr. Peter Breggin, of Rockville, Maryland, who has devoted his career to fighting any and all psychotropic pills—especially anti-depressants. In his book, *Talking Back to Prozac,* he suggests that "giving anti-aggression drugs to inner city kids would be an excuse for continued neglect. "Indeed he says the mass-drugging of "inner-city kids" (code phrase) is the hidden agenda of a group called the Violence Initiative. Like others before him, he romanticizes mental illness as the only sane reaction to an insane world, maybe even a sign of genius. In his 1991 book, *Toxic Psychiatry,* he asks "How is it that some spiritually passionate people find themselves being treated as mental patients?" Instead of seeing mental illness for the anguished condition it is, he wants disturbed people to stay that way, at least without pharmaceutical treatment.

Thus the horror of "Soma," Huxley's *Brave New World,* is upon us. Relief from psychic pain is indeed an abomination.

The Pill as Holy Eucharist

The unrealistic view of pills is possible because of what we could call the "holy pill" syndrome. Pills are viewed by society as something holy, sort of a Eucharist.

In this analogy the pill—or host—is capable of miraculous things but only if it is treated in a certain ritualistic way. Thus, a high priest (your doctor) must first authorize its use in accordance with proper canon. It must be further consecrated by another level of priest (your pharmacist) who will place it into your outstretched hands from a counter three feet above your head.

You must not vary from the bottle's holy procedures. You must not transfer any of the pills in the bottle to another person or else something unspeakable may happen.

When pills are handled by lay people, they can become hideous things, instruments of death, sowers of discord. Drugs routinely used by psychiatrists in the U.S.A. to treat schizophrenics were the very ones used by the evil Soviets to "torture" patients in its mental hospitals. Mom's Darvon is good for mom only. If anyone else takes the pill consecrated for mother's use, they are abusing it. To give anyone else one of your sleeping pills is a heretical act. To act on your need for an antibiotic without prescription is also heretical. It is also irreligious, not to mention illegal, to manufacture your own medicine without proper license—tantamount to permission from the Bishop.

As long as a pill keeps its prescription status, it stays holy. Once it goes over-the-counter it is never viewed in quite the same light. That's why Benedryl was such a "powerful" pill before. Now its OTC competitors make fun of it. Once a pill passes into the land of the profane, it cannot go back. The only exception to this might be when an OTC remedy is banned outright by the government—thus achieving a low-grade "devil status."

But there is always hope for a banned pill.

The Grand Ju-Ju men of the FDA and DEA can rehabilitate an excommunicated pill. Thalidomide, once reviled as the archetypal satanic pill, has been quietly and very successfully used to treat leprosy and lupus for the last couple of decades, and has shown promise as an AIDS drug as well. In the public's mind, however, it remains locked in a world of untouchability.

Drugs as the Devil

In Ceremonial Chemistry: The Ritual Persecution of Drugs, Addicts, and Pushers, the brilliant social analyst and medical doctor, Thomas Szasz, may have been the first to notice the

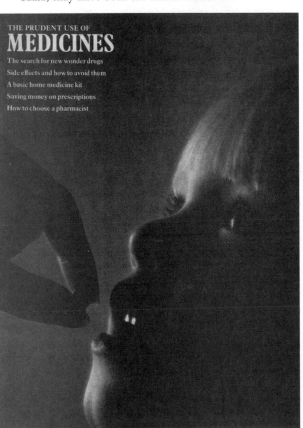

THE PRUDENT USE OF
MEDICINES
The search for new wonder drugs
Side effects and how to avoid them
A basic home medicine kit
Saving money on prescriptions
How to choose a pharmacist

similarities between pill culture and religious culture. In his book he makes this view of a "medical theocracy" quite clear.

First, he points out that the separation of Church and State may have looked good on paper, but man's need for organized religion will not go unsatisfied. Taking the Church out of politics is impossible—the two are so hopelessly entwined. Both organized religion and politics depend on shared illusions and ego-tripping—two psychic needs of all human beings. Any attempt to remove the pomp and magic from political life is doomed. People seem to need it.

Szasz also points out that individual autonomy is intolerable to a ruler. Authority cannot abide by any "subject" entity that considers itself a "non-subject," and will discipline the offending subjects until they behave. As Szasz puts it: "There is only one political sin: independence; and only one political virtue: obedience."

At the same time, the rulers provide an unassailable explanation for such deviant behavior: evil. During the late middle ages and well into the Renaissance, the Roman Catholic Church tirelessly sought out and punished the "heretics" who questioned authority or tried to reason for themselves. Such behavior was called "blasphemy." Its cause was always the same: Satan. No action was too extreme in the face of such a manifest evil. No punishment could be too excessive, let alone wrong.

The War against Satan was a constant in the hundreds of years of Inquisitional battle. Like the War on Drugs, this religious oppression sprang from seemingly innocent, well-intentioned plans. What began as a mere inquiry soon became a huge state-run enterprise of torture and fear. The harder the rulers sought to extinguish satanic thoughts, the more insidious they became. New heresies were being discovered all the time, some so subtle even the Church didn't recognize them right away. It wasn't long before the Inquisition discovered heresy in anything.

With this in mind it becomes clearer why we treat drugs the irrational way we do. Drug War rhetoric seems identical to the Inquisition. The use, possession, and, at times, even thought of them (and explanations how to procure them) are considered illegal. It follows that no reaction is too extreme to rid society of such an evil. Life in a hell behind bars is considered just punishment for anyone who comes into contact with the evil. Even from a public health point of view, sequestering contaminated people is a rational way to deal with a fearsome and contagious disease. Commitment to a mental institution because of heretical drug use is called "treatment," and considered compassionate even though it is compulsory.

This, according to Szasz, is part of the politics of scapegoating. With a scapegoat, all of a society's ills can be blamed on the witch, the foreigner, the social (or political) outcast, the schismatic, the "criminal." "Good" (obedient) citizens are weak and need guidance and control by the authorities. In return for recognizing this, good citizens are allowed to participate in the ritual persecution of scapegoating.

Earlier in human history the "scapegoat" was a real goat, symbolically loaded with a community's sins and chased into the desert. As time went on, things became considerably crueler. The Greeks used human beings instead of goats and began killing, instead of chasing, the "scapegoat."

Szasz gives us an eerie lesson in etymology when he traces the word pharmakos back to its earliest meaning of "scapegoat." Only after 600 B.C. did pharmakos come to mean "poison" or "drug," whence we take our word "pharmacy."

How Low We've Sunk

The War on Drugs reached and surpassed the limits of mere hysteria and superstition many years ago. It has now come to the point that a microscopic bit of cocaine (or heroin or whatever illegal thing) on a piece of paper currency can ritually (that is legally) "contaminate" its owner. It contaminates him so much that all the owner's property can be taken from him and his own body becomes subject to forfeiture and confinement (jail) and purification (physical punishment, incarceration, "treatment").

It has been almost ten years since Ronald Reagan officially and repeatedly declared drugs the nation's number one foe, even greater than the Soviet Union. These have been the very words used by Presidents, Attorney Generals, Customs Directors and nearly every other politician since then. Maniacs like former "Drug Czar" Bill Bennett have unashamedly called for the beheading of anyone who sells drugs. LAPD chief Daryl Gates declared that all drug users should be summarily executed ("taken out and shot"). One has to wonder why a call to mass murder by a city's police chief wasn't immediately denounced and Gates run out of town on a rail. But if people really believe in the diabolical nature of drugs . . . then murder doesn't seem so bad.

It should be recalled that one explanation for the beating of Rodney King was the possibility of his use of PCP, the magical substance that makes an ordinary human immune to pain and as strong as five or ten men. Yeah, that was it! There was PCP. Drugs!

As Szasz recounts it, all of our country's anti-drug laws have been concocted as responses to political problems, seeking to vilify and punish feared elements of society. The relentless hunting of communists, anarchists, Bolsheviks, drug pushers, kingpins, aliens, spies and plain old colored people is a theme that has been played out countless times in American history. And each time, drugs have been there to provide the evil talisman that justifies it all. The steady output of propaganda has created children so terrified by the mere sight of white powder that they call the police on their parents. I have seen a little kid become unnerved as we drove past what he must have considered the incarnation of his most terrifying nightmare—a DRUGstore!

The Latest from the Front

Drugs have proven themselves political tools more powerful than communism. Cocaine was the reason given the American public to justify the invasion of Panama, the kidnapping of its leader, and the killing of thousands and thousands of Central American citizens. Cocaine was ample justification to arrest a foreign citizen, on foreign soil, for a crime alleged to have been committed outside the United States. Cocaine has proven to be more heinous in the eyes of the U.S. government than Nazi war crimes.

That's outside the borders of the United States. Inside the country, the demonization of drugs has provided enemies of the Constitution their best weapon to undermine our rights. The U.S. army could not have been legally called in to help attack the Branch Davidians at Waco until Texas governor, Ann Richards, lied that there was a methamphetamine lab on the premises. That assertion was the magic phrase that made it all right to do what is otherwise considered reprehensible. Muttering the word "drug" is enough to allow a conviction for "conspiracy" even if the person is alone and does nothing more than talk about planning a drug crime.

More bizarre thinking is evident in the outlawing of imaginary things. A federal law known as the "Analogue Substances Act" prohibits the legal possession of chemicals that do not even currently exist, and never have. But if they are created sometime in future, their possession will require 20 years in prison. Maybe life.

It is possible to be prosecuted for simply planning to, or inventing, a brand new substance that has the ability to get people high.

On the flip side, the establishment sanctions some drugs as sacraments, their consumption being a symbol of acceptance and obedience. The same customs official who will gladly coerce, threaten and bribe people to inform on each other about heroin, knows he's made it to the top of his organization when his superior takes him out drinking.

This celebratory drink as totem recalls an incident involving then Vice-President George Bush, returning from a drug war stump speech in Miami Florida. Relaxing aboard Air Force Two with a few DEA agents, he invited them all for a drink. At least one agent declined, giving as his excuse that (among other things) he was on duty. Bush continued insisting, but the agent continued to just say "no." Finally, Bush told the agent, "Don't be such an asshole."

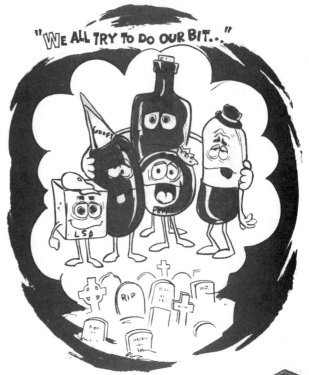

"WE ALL TRY TO DO OUR BIT..."

By not drinking, this agent had incurred the substantial wrath of the executive office. In effect, he was rejecting not just the drink, but a class of people—and apparently Bush himself.

State-Approved Religion

For Szasz, theocratic religion banned by the state was replaced by a Therapeutic Religion that currently holds sway. The medical government neatly replaces the traditional Church, in which the citizen is seen as a patient instead of a wayward soul in need of guidance. The therapeutic state views antisocial behavior as

The "Identification" Store Front.

WE HELP OTHERS TO HELP THEMSELVES

an illness that requires "treatment." The social illness is diagnosed to have grown so verifiably large that practically everyone is told they need "treatment". Nazi concentration camps are now explained as being the result of nationwide psychosis.

Pill Worship and pillfiend hatred can be viewed as the contemporary version of medieval Catholicism. But the anxiety-ridden public perception of pills also comes from a decidedly Protestant point of view.

The term for the Elizabeth Wurtzel scorn of pills, "Medical Calvinism," we derived from the phrase "pharmacological Calvinism,"

coined in 1970 by G. Klerman to explain resistance to the use of tranquilizers. Medical Calvinism simply widens the scope to all pills. It is a doctrine that sneers at too much dependence on the host for help.

This is why Princess Di attacked British doctors in a 1994 speech for prescribing "too many pills" to women. She didn't say which pills, but hinted at anti-depressants. Her message is one often repeated in America, too, where maintenance treatment of any mild mental disorder is frowned upon as encouraging weak behavior.

Anti-depressants are often dismissed as a panacea for a fake disease. Could Di have gotten away with saying the docs were handing out too many antibiotics? Maybe. How about too many diuretics or—hormones? Possibly. She could have taken issue with these drugs, but her audience wouldn't have taken her seriously. Her arguments were emotional, not medical.

Totally in character with the suffering Calvinist, Di's speech is all the more astonishing having been made after she recovered from a well-documented depression that saw her roaming about the castle making crank phone calls, barfing in a bulimic frenzy, bursting into tears and considering suicide. If she pulled through with pills, her hypocrisy is almost commendable in an English Protestant sort of way. If she recovered from the depression spontaneously, her pride in suffering is just as understandable. It's obvious "Di" didn't simply stand for "diazepam!"

Small Comfort : A History of the Minor Tranquilizers (1985) a fascinating social history by Dr. Mickey Smith devotes a chapter to the glorification and demonization of tranks, from its beginnings as "Wonder Drug of 1954" to a thing of criminal terror, more dangerous than heroin.

Using the drug Miltown as a benchmark, Dr. Smith, a professor at the University of Mississippi, exhaustively and entertainingly depicts the emperor's clothing worn by the lawgivers and "expert" writers.

Small Comfort

"Miltown" (meprobamate) introduced the era of the tranquilizer, a term that first appeared to describe the drug in 1957. Then came Librium, Valium and a cavalcade of "happy pills," including one with the unlikely name of "Darvo-Tran" marketed for a short time by Eli Lilly. Smith discusses the impact of these so-called minor tranquilizers on doctors, society, and medicine itself. Along the way, he launches into topics like the "medicalization" of social problems—something that hadn't been clearly examined since it was decided to restrict the use of opium in the early part of this century. Smith quotes arguments that say today's benzodiazepines serve the same function as opium for the stir-crazy housewife or benumbed factory worker. Others describe tranquilizers as "the psychiatrist's morphine" that helps deal with pain while the psychic fracture is set.

Smith also explains how medical Calvinism affects the use of tranquilizers. At first, "happy pills," "aspirin for the soul," and "don't give a damn pills." were widely seen a societal boon New Yorker cartoons confirmed their acceptance in the highest echelons of society. Farmers even began to add them to feed to produce mellower, fatter pigs!

The pills were seen as a cop-out. Emotional distress could be dealt with by moral fortitude and simply getting back to work.

Today, tranks are seen as just another type of medication, although their use is still freighted with social and quasi-moral ramifications. Small Comfort muses on the role of tranquilizers in society, from the doctor's office to everyday situations. Does the use of tranquilizers by a single person affect the people he associates with?

One of the best chapters deals with media coverage of the pills, with charts demonstrating the rise, decline, and leveling out of the minor tranquilizers.

Other chapters reveal the marketing strategies used by the various drug companies, aimed primarily at doctors. Smith painstakingly describes how doctors prescribed the pills over the years, and why. In the chapter called "Doctor's Dilemmas," Smith explores the degree to which physicians and patients play ridiculous cat-and-mouse games with these pills. Fear of "addiction" overcoming therapeutic

value is something Smith refers to as "cultural lag"—that is, technology's ability to outpace society's ability to cope with tranks. 🔴

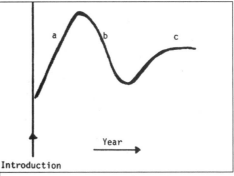

Representation of curve of acceptance for a new drug. (a), wild enthusiasm, cures everything, no side effects. (b), Nihilism, many side effects, don't use. (c), rational therapeutic use established. [From Marks, J., "The Benodiazepines—Use and Abuse: Current Status," Pharmacy International, Vol 2, pp 84–87 (1981).]

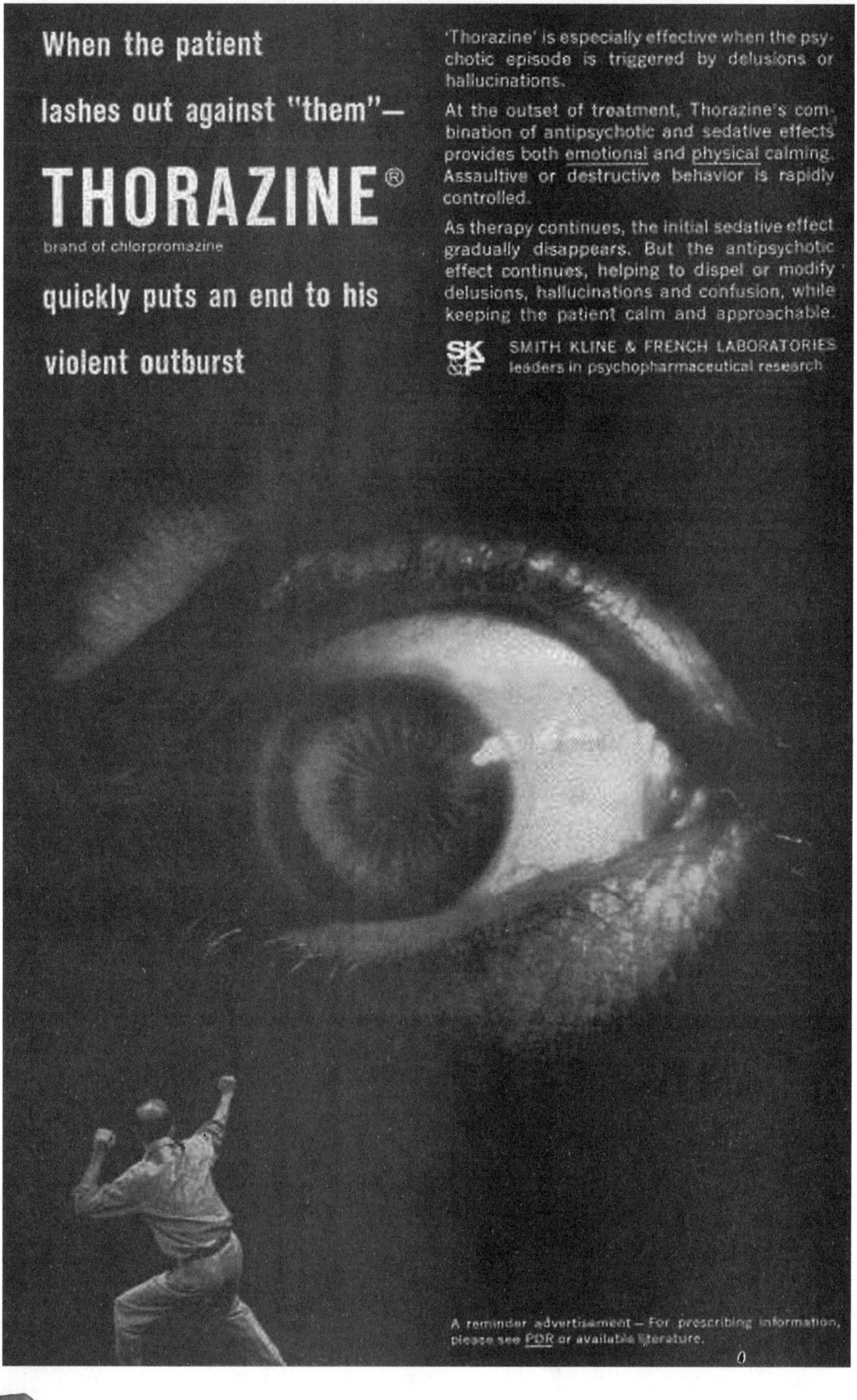

When the patient

lashes out against "them"—

THORAZINE®
brand of chlorpromazine

quickly puts an end to his

violent outburst

'Thorazine' is especially effective when the psychotic episode is triggered by delusions or hallucinations.

At the outset of treatment, Thorazine's combination of antipsychotic and sedative effects provides both emotional and physical calming. Assaultive or destructive behavior is rapidly controlled.

As therapy continues, the initial sedative effect gradually disappears. But the antipsychotic effect continues, helping to dispel or modify delusions, hallucinations and confusion, while keeping the patient calm and approachable.

SK&F SMITH KLINE & FRENCH LABORATORIES
leaders in psychopharmaceutical research

A reminder advertisement — For prescribing information, please see PDR or available literature.

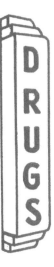

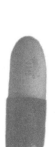

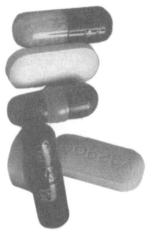

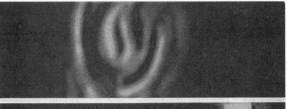

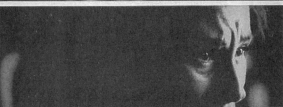

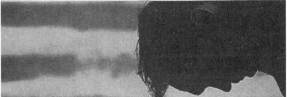

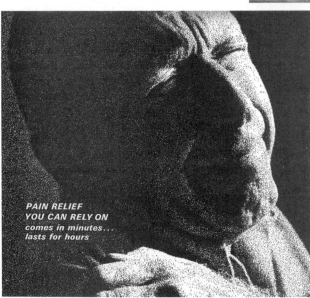

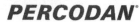
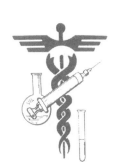

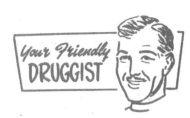

Your Friendly DRUGGIST

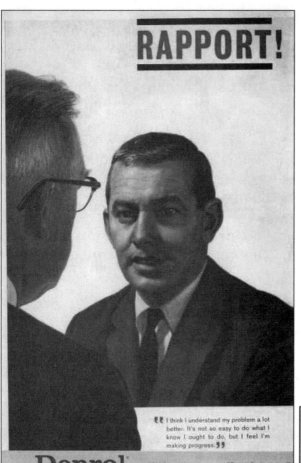

RAPPORT!

"I think I understand my problem a lot better. It's not so easy to do what I know I ought to do, but I feel I'm making progress."

Deprol® Effective...well tolerated

meprobamate 400 mg. + benactyzine hydrochloride 1 mg.

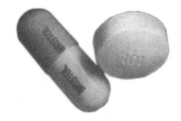

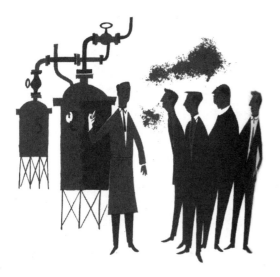

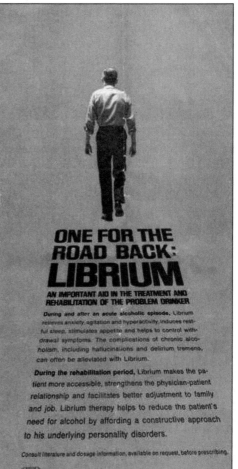

ONE FOR THE ROAD BACK: LIBRIUM

AN IMPORTANT AID IN THE TREATMENT AND REHABILITATION OF THE PROBLEM DRINKER

During and after an acute alcoholic episode, Librium relieves anxiety, agitation and hyperactivity, induces restful sleep, stimulates appetite and helps to control withdrawal symptoms. The complications of chronic alcoholism, including hallucinations and delirium tremens, can often be alleviated with Librium.

During the rehabilitation period, Librium makes the patient more accessible, strengthens the physician-patient relationship and facilitates better adjustment to family and job. Librium therapy helps to reduce the patient's need for alcohol by affording a constructive approach to his underlying personality disorders.

Consult literature and dosage information, available on request, before prescribing.

ROCHE

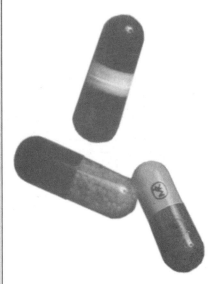

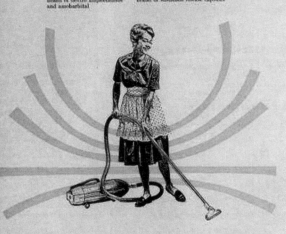

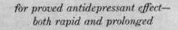

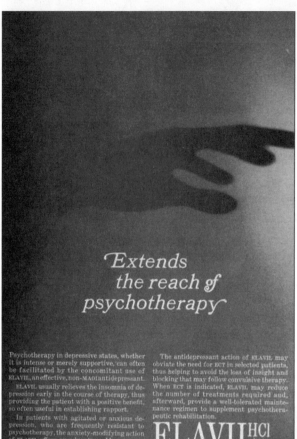

*Extends
the reach of
psychotherapy*

Psychotherapy in depressive states, whether it is intense or merely supportive, can often be facilitated by the concomitant use of ELAVIL, an effective, non-MAOI antidepressant.

ELAVIL usually relieves the insomnia of depression early in the course of therapy, thus providing the patient with a positive benefit, so often useful in establishing rapport.

In patients with agitated or anxious depression, who are frequently resistant to psychotherapy, the anxiety-modifying action of ELAVIL offers an advantage. If necessary, relaxation may be induced in most patients in 15 to 30 minutes with parenterally administered ELAVIL.

The antidepressant action of ELAVIL may obviate the need for ECT in selected patients, thus helping to avoid the loss of insight and blocking that may follow convulsive therapy. When ECT is indicated, ELAVIL may reduce the number of treatments required and, afterward, provide a well-tolerated maintenance regimen to supplement psychotherapeutic rehabilitation.

ELAVIL HCl
AMITRIPTYLINE HCl

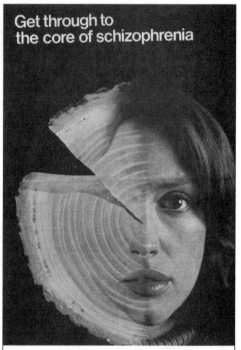

Get through to the core of schizophrenia

Serentil
(mesoridazine)
as the besylate

"..Remarkably low incidence of adverse reactions when compared with other phenothiazine compounds." *

Boehringer Ingelheim

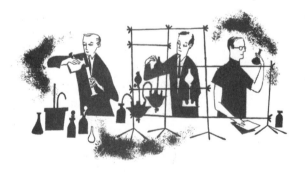

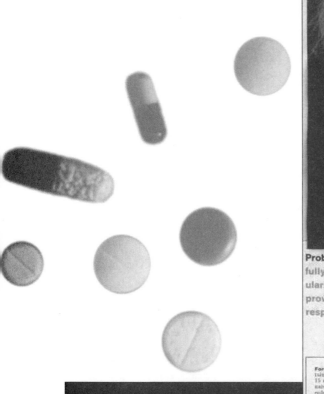

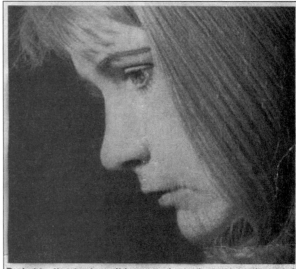

Probably the basic antidepressant...and certainly the most fully documented, is 'Dexedrine'. In depressive states, particularly those marked by lowered motivation, 'Dexedrine' helps provide rapid symptomatic relief. The patient is more alert, responds more favorably to her environment.

DEXEDRINE® SPANSULE®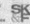

brand of dextro amphetamine sulfate sustained release capsules

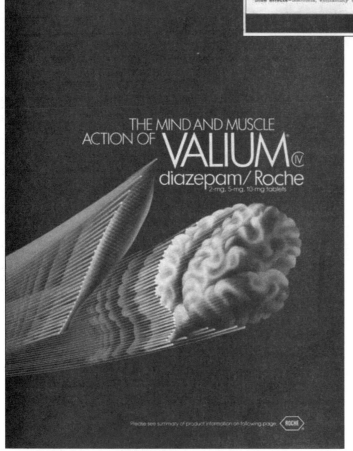

THE MIND AND MUSCLE ACTION OF VALIUM℞ diazepam/Roche 2-mg. 5-mg. 10-mg. tablets

Please see summary of product information on following page. ROCHE

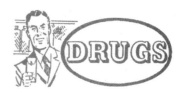

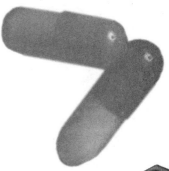

The choice is simple

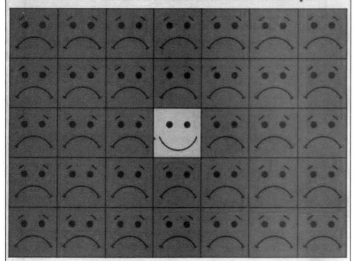

New LUSTRAL* offers a logical alternative treatment for a wide range of depressed patients,[1] young and old.[2,3] A highly selective serotonin re-uptake inhibitor,[4] LUSTRAL* is as effective as tricyclic agents[3,3] yet with a significantly different side-effect profile.[5]

For example, LUSTRAL* appears to be much less toxic in overdose,[1] does not potentiate the effects of alcohol,[6] and is most unlikely to induce convulsions[5] or adverse cardiovascular effects.[13] There is no evidence of dependence[8] after chronic use, and its once-daily dosage encourages compliance. LUSTRAL* simplifies the choice in antidepressant therapy.

New once-daily in depression
LUSTRAL ▼
sertraline

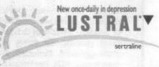

With bright prospects in mind

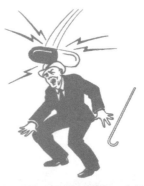

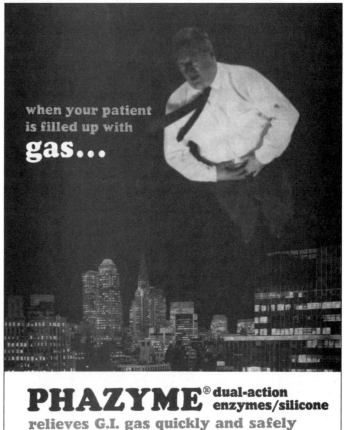

when your patient is filled up with
gas...

PHAZYME® dual-action enzymes/silicone
relieves G.I. gas quickly and safely

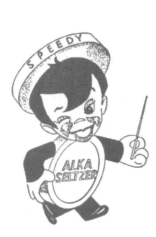

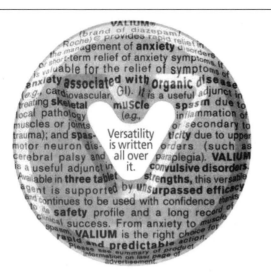

VALIUM®
(brand of diazepam/Roche)© provides rapid relief in the management of **anxiety** disorders. or short-term relief of anxiety symptoms. It is valuable for the relief of symptoms of **anxiety associated with organic disease** (e.g., cardiovascular, GI). It is a useful adjunct in treating **skeletal** **muscle** **spasm** due to local pathology (e.g., inflammation of muscles or joints) or secondary to trauma); and **spasticity** due to upper motor neuron disorders (such as cerebral palsy and paraplegia). **VALIUM** is a useful adjunct in **convulsive disorders.** Available in **three tablet strengths,** this versatile agent is supported by **unsurpassed efficacy** and continues to be used with confidence thanks to its **safety** profile and a long record of clinical success. From anxiety to muscle spasm, **VALIUM** is the right choice for **rapid and predictable action.** Please see summary of product information on last page of advertisement.

Versatility is written all over it.

UNDERWRITE YOUR CHOICE

Write "Do Not Substitute"

on all your prescriptions for VALIUM. By preventing substitution, you ensure that your patients receive the one you know best, from the company with the most experience in researching, manufacturing and answering physician inquiries about benzodiazepines.

With VALIUM, no substitution means no surprises for you or your patients—no surprises in color, no surprises in tablet design and no surprises in brand name.

As with any benzodiazepine, caution patients about driving, oper-

ating machinery and simultaneous ingestion of alcohol or other CNS depressant drugs. Advise patients to consult their physician before increasing the dose or discontinuing VALIUM.

VALIUM®
diazepam/Roche ℞

THE ONE YOU KNOW BEST

A13

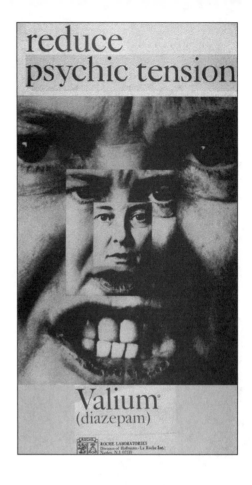
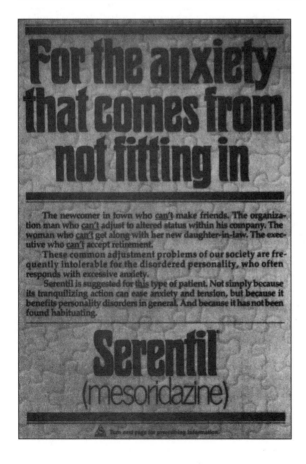
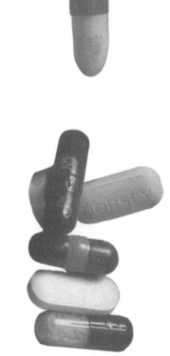

Pill Advertising and Marketing

There is a clear distinction among pills when it comes to marketing. There are those available to the public with little or no regulation (aka Over-The-Counter pills) and there are "ethical" drugs—pills that require a doctor's prescription. Methods of marketing these pills take into account very different audiences. OTC meds can be hawked without much in the way of seriousness or an overly technical language since they're geared toward the great unwashed who enjoy cutaway drawings of a man's sinus cavities adorned with bolts of pain or a relentless hammer pounding on an anvil.

Whimsy is inappropriate for ethical drugs since prescription pills are marketed to physicians or, lately, to those segments of the public likely to be bold enough to ask their doctors for a certain pill. (Holy protocol forbids a layman from even being so informed as to know the names of the components of pills!) The primary target of ethical drug advertising are doctors. Given the tremendous amount of money behind these ads, and the relatively small number of people for whom the ad is intended, ad-men have the luxury of tailor-making an ethical pill ad in a way they never could for, say, lip balm.

These ads are fascinating in what they say about the way doctors view their patients, particularly women. Women are the primary gender featured in tranquilizer ads, often as middle-aged, chronic complainers of a variety of problems. Relief for both doctor and patient might be found in a mild downer.

Other ads promise the one miracle a doctor needs from a pill—efficacy. Ad after ad promises the doctor that a pill is guaranteed to bring relief from the very first dose. This is an important guarantee for doctors, who were once thought to work miracles through their prescriptions, but patients are now jaded to penicillin. They just don't make miracle pills like they used to. And when they do, they don't stay miraculous for long.

Pharmaceutical science has begun to suffer from its own success. People now consider a pill substandard if it does not provide an instant cure. Ulcer surgery—painful, expensive and not-too-effective—is now extinct because of pills introduced in the late 1970s. Heart disease and the need for open heart surgery have both been greatly reduced by the introduction of pills to control diseases of the coronary-vascular system. Surrounded by little miracles that literally offer a new lease on life, the public is now largely concerned that they're being ripped off by drug companies.

Pill ads aimed at OTC consumers rely a lot on pounding a brand-name into the head of the ad's victim. Nuprin, for example, has developed what some think sounds like a mantra. "Nuprin. Little. Yellow. Different. Nuprin. Little. Yellow. Different."

Detail Men (and Their Gifts)

What distinguishes pill advertising from any other kind of campaign is its very elite demographic. Ads are aimed at doctors only, often categorized by type of practice, age, sex, or even previous prescribing habits. Enormous advertising budgets ensure reaching this target.

One of the most profitable industries in America, pharmaceutical corporations earn up to three times the profit margin of the average Fortune 500 company. But the products sold by this industry require a medical school education to be fully understood. Few industries face this particular dynamic to hawk their wares.

Such esoteric, niche products must focus its advertising at relatively puny audiences. But even if technically arcane Joe Consumer knows pills, and has developed expectations of the pills he consumes. He wants them strong. He wants them mysterious.

THE Nervous Woman
BESET BY FUNCTIONAL COMPLAINTS

fatigue
G.I. upset
headache
palpitations

Bellergal
Spacetabs

Doctors are the ones who must be convinced of a pill's worth. The real consumer of a pill is not the one who swallows it. The purchase decision is made by the doctor, who, convinced of a particular pill's worth, instructs his patient to buy and consume it.

Before 1985—when the FDA first permitted prescription drugs to be advertised in consumer publications—the only target of pill advertising was an MD or pharmacist.

Though direct to consumer advertising is also necessary, it is still the doctor who gets most of a drug firm's advertising attention. And competition is fierce. With all that money at stake, and with such a small group to pitch to, pill ads need to be innovative, extravagant and impressive. All pharmaceutical competitors have large advertising budgets competing for the same tiny, crucial market.

Spending millions on radio jingles is not enough. To ensure that pill buyers receive personal attention, pharmaceutical corporations send out swarms of employees to visit every doctor in the country.

About half of all pill advertising dollars are spent on armies of what used to be called "detail men." Today these guys are known as "pharmaceutical representatives" or simply "reps." Companies may employ one rep for every eight, 10 or 20 general physicians in the country! Men don't dominate the job anymore. Pill companies have begun to send out the pharmaceutical world's version of the Swedish Bikini Team. With as many as eight or 10 reps demanding just a few minutes of a doctor's time every day, a rep has to stand out somehow.

A rep's job is to hector a stable of doctors that can range from fewer than 35 to more than 150. He or she may also be responsible for dropping by certain hospitals and clinics as well as key pharmacies. Although definitely considered part of the "sales" sector, reps are not expected (and are prohibited by law anyway) to sell a single thing. Reps ply doctors with as much information and incentive as possible to encourage them to write prescriptions for their company's drugs. Often, a rep represents only a sliver of a company's pills, so their knowledge is specialized and extensive. In the past, Eli Lilly was required its reps to have degrees in pharmacy. Despite the appearance of

the exotic, erotic rep, they must be more than a friendly face or a pair of tits. Doctors are apt to ask complicated questions and the rep's got to answer them immediately.

To make sure this happens, drug companies employ information technology that helps them pinpoint the doctors to approach and the ways to they are best approached based on prescribing patterns.

A few years ago, a rep might drop by a number of local pharmacies, shooting the breeze with druggists about the prescribing habits of local doctors. Normally the pharmacist was given a little trinket of some kind to help cement the bond between the two. A good rep kept careful notes, applying the information to the field. Big coin is spent determining prescription habits, types of patient and the pharmacies the doctor's patients are likely to visit. Drug companies are very successful in gaining access to computerized records of the drugs a doctor prescribes. One clever way this is accomplished is by "donating" a computer and a program to a pharmacy for inventory control or tracking Medicaid payments. All the drug firm needs do to to get the pharmacy's valuable information is have the store access its website a weekly 15 minutes or so. Although patient's names and even doctor's names are supposedly not recorded, even raw data can give a precise picture of the sort of prescribing going on in a very small area.

Drug companies assiduously collect information on the doctor himself. Before a rep ever meets a doctor on his or her route, the rep knows the doctor's age, where he or she graduated from med school and the specialties of his or her practice. After each visit a rep might write up a short report (longer if necessary)

provides highly effective tranquilization, relieves agitation, apprehension, anxiety

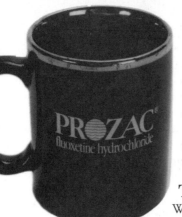

describing what went on and what was said during the meeting. Since today's drug rep is equipped with a laptop computer and modem, this information can be sent off to the home office from around the country each day to be compiled and scrutinized.

It says something about the intensity of the battle now that Eli Lilly no longer requires a pharmacy education for their reps. Now they prefer a candidate to have an MBA.

Trinkets

Wherever the drug rep goes, whether pharmacy, hospital, doctors' offices, anywhere, he leaves a trail of little gifts prominently displaying the name of the particular pill he's pushing. For quite some time, the coffee cup with the drug name enameled on the side was a favorite (and it's still a perennial giveaway). Other staples are the notepads, pens, diaries, rulers, calendars, clocks and even umbrellas—all with a bearing the name and slogan of a particular pill. In some cases, more expensive items are handed out to doctors—for instance detailed ceramic heart models, or a life-size take-apart model of a human brain may be left with a doctor as a visual aid when he or she (hopefully) prescribes the pills to patients.

Other useful artifacts available from reps are videotapes of gall bladder operations, stethoscopes, and stacks of information pamphlets to hand out to patients concerning diseases addressed by a company's drug. Reps are also a good source of reprints from medical journals which have run favorable articles about a rep's products. Reps can also give doctors reprints of articles unfavorable about a competitor's product.

Drug reps also show up with fairly enormous amounts of food for hospital and office staff, sometimes even baking trays of brownies in their own ovens the night before. Catering private parties is very much in the rep's job description. One hospital intern, who wanted to host a cook-out for his friends, was able to get a Kodak film rep to supply not only the food, but the beer. Kodak sells the highly sophisticated films needed for X-rays, CT scans and other medical imaging devices. Maybe that intern will someday be in a position to order film from Kodak. The cookout supplies would be a bargain.

Lately, a yen for novel ways to carry advertising into the houses of doctors has led to paper plates emblazoned with a drug's name and slogan, and microwave popcorn bearing a pill's name in such a way the doctor cannot help but see it. Even candy has appeared in wrappers printed up with a drug's name! In one case a bag of candy was also decorated with a Halloween theme, meant to be given out to trick-or-treating children.

Other prizes are socks, calculators, blood pressure cuffs, towelettes, phone cards, safety pins, coin purses, wall charts, magazine subscriptions, textbooks, key chains, puzzles, tickets to sporting events, T-shirts, handballs, tissues, Dixie cups, hats and other articles of clothing. The eye-catching gewgaws and trinkets a doctor gets from the reps are plenty enough to buy Manhattan from the Indians.

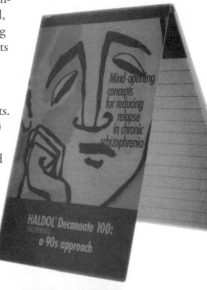

With their towering egos and framed degrees adorning the wall, doctors believe they are immune to petty bribery. One doctor at Johns Hopkins wrote the *New England Journal of Medicine* about how he had picked up a sales manual a rep had mistakenly left behind among the paperweights and penlights. In it the doctor found suggestions to provide doctors with "incentives." Ideas included cookies baked into the shapes and colors of particular pills, pizzas with a drug's initials spelled out in pepperoni, Easter baskets with eggs painted like pills and even festive baskets simply filled with samples of a particular drug. According to the manual, doctors "really enjoy them." The outraged doctor wrote that the drug company "obviously regard us as idiots who respond to Easter Baskets and italicized pizzas by prescribing more of their products."

"Could it be that they are right?" he asked.

Sure they're right. Drug companies simply would not spend the time and energy to hand out these door prizes if it did not bring results.

Doctors should keep abreast of the latest medical (and medicinal) advances, but most are simply too busy. General Practitioners, especially, with the range of conditions they treat, can hardly be expected to keep up with the avalanche of new drugs, and even entirely new classes of drugs that enter the doctor's lexicon each year.

As the expenditure of pill advertising dollars suggests, sales reps are at least as important as print or television ads.

Representatives provide most, if not all, of the information any doctor has about a particular drug—and sometimes a particular disease. A number of studies (including one at Harvard in 1982) have shown that doctors get most of their information about certain pills from advertising (including visiting reps). These studies also show (not surprisingly) that doctors think they have gotten their information elsewhere—from a journal or a colleague.

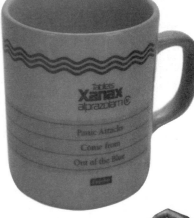

The rep is invaluable in convincing a doctor to prescribe a certain drug, and most companies train their reps to gain the respect and confidence of physicians they "sell" to. As they are likely to be a physician's primary source of information about a particular drug, it's crucial that the rep is believed by the doctor. Hiring pharmacists as reps and detail men was Eli Lilly's way to gain trust, but competition has forced the firm to widen its horizons. A voluptuous chick with a dazzling smile—and an MBA—is often more successful. Doctors are only human (even if they don't believe it) and advertising still seeks to activate the impulsive side of human personality.

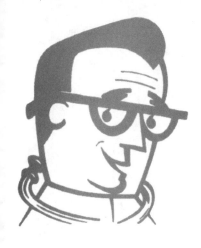

Doctors and Petty Bribery

One popular method of pill advertising is to outright reward a doctor for prescribing a certain pill. MDs seduced by pharmaceutical companies accept free trips, gifts, dinners, and even monetary kickbacks such as purchasing incentives.

Starting in 1986, Ayerst (a subsidiary of American Home Products) rewarded doctors who prescribed their hypertension drug, Inderal LA (propranolol), to a minimum of 50 patients by giving them a free airline ticket anywhere in the United States, or 1000 frequent flyer points on American Airlines for each patient prescribed. The more patients the doctor put on the drug, the more prizes he won.

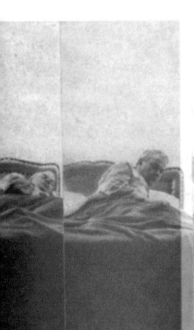

In 1988 Squibb required Canadian doctors to start just ten of their patients on Capoten (captopril) to receive a personal computer for use in a "study" of patients on captopril. Although Squibb nominally retained possession of the computer, participating doctors were allowed to keep them after the study was concluded. U.S. law permits most of these gifts as long as they can be argued to have "medicinal value." A coffee cup adorned with a pill's name and some factoid about it qualifies as having medicinal value. Socialized medicine has changed Canadian medicine in more than one way. Canada now bans sales reps from giving anything at all to doctors or other medical personnel. Not even coffee mugs.

But socialized medicine doesn't have to mean such austerity. Two years after the Canadian Capoten computer bonanza, Squibb offered French doctors who participated in a survey of a new drug free membership to a buying club where they could purchase everything from cars to toasters at a deep discount.

Free travel is a great incentive, even for doctors who make truckloads of money. Glaxo has paid for trips to Hawaii and CIBA-Geigy has sent docs (and their spouses) on all-expenses-paid trips to resorts in the Caribbean to attend lectures on Estraderm—a skin patch delivery system for estrogen.

Sometimes doctors who attended "symposia" on drugs are given "honoraria" for their trouble. Other companies hire doctors to go around the country extolling the efficacies of one or more of the company's pills. Nice work if you can get it. A respected MD can easily nail down a few thousand dollars per show, in addition to first-class airfare and hotel rooms.

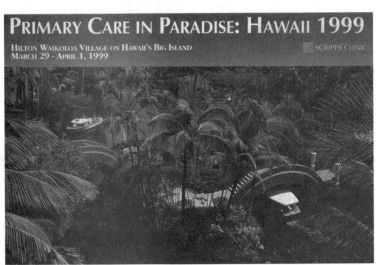

PRIMARY CARE IN PARADISE: HAWAII 1999

HILTON WAIKOLOA VILLAGE ON HAWAII'S BIG ISLAND
MARCH 29 - APRIL 1, 1999

SCRIPPS CLINIC

At times companies have resorted to giving cash money to doctors who put patients on certain drugs. For example, Roche paid docs $1200 for participating in a "study" which amounted to their having prescribed the antibiotic Rocephin for 20 patients.

This is no longer done in the U.S. today, but a form of it survives. Now doctors are made to choose a $100 gift from a special catalog as a way of compensating them for the hell of sitting through an expensive dinner with a rep, who need only mention the pill's name and say one or two sentences about it to qualify the dinner as a "meeting." The industry mag *Medical Marketing and Media* estimated in a 1990 issue that between 175,000 and 180,000 doctors are lavished with expensive promotional dinners. Pharmacists still have access to money, though, and can get as much as $35 if they convince a customer to switch brands.

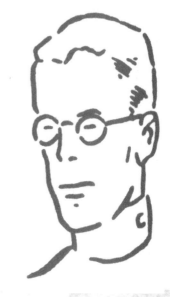

Yet another method of graft involves entering doctors in drawings to win everything from gourmet chocolates and travel to telescopes and exercise equipment. Searle offered pediatricians attending a conference in Brazil the chance to win bicycles, surfboards and skateboards as part of a promo for their anti-inflammatory med Benzitrat. Adverts described the pill as "balanced," so the prizes awarded had something to do with maintaining one's balance. Amazingly, everyone entered in these drawings tend to win a prize accompanied by literature and/or free samples of the drug is involved in the promotion.

The doctor who wondered if drug companies accurately pegged them as being influenced by coffee mugs and notepads need look no further than Upjohn's Anaprox. For one year the company dosed docs with exercise related prizes such as Walkman-type stereos, hand and ankle weights, jump ropes and fanny packs. At the end of the year Anaprox's market share for exercise-related injuries jumped from 33 to 43 percent. Even a single percentage point in a decent-sized market can mean hundreds of millions of dollars in sales to a drug company. Clearly the tactic works.

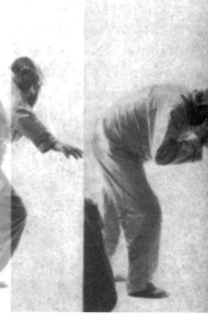

Another important item a rep distributes are thousands of dollars worth of free samples. The pills are given to the doctors who are asked to give them away to patients to whom the drug is prescribed. The ability to offer a patient a few hits of a fairly pricey pill is appreciated by doctors. It also helps forge a bond in the patient's mind between a pill and the inherent trust he has in the doctor. Free pills are often given out to office staff, family members and friends who cannot afford the pills themselves. Some doctors give the free pills to poorer patients, others use them as a marketing tool for their practices. Corrupt doctors simply sell them.

But wait! That's not all!

To make sure the doc gets the message about free medicine, many companies have a policy of giving "stock bottles" of 100 or more doses of any drug they make, as long as the doctor writes a prescription specifying brand name and—most importantly—signs on the "do not substitute" line at the bottom of the script. New doctors get "starter kits" with many bottles of a company's most widely prescribed pills.

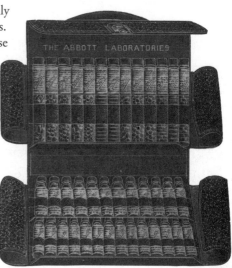

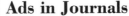
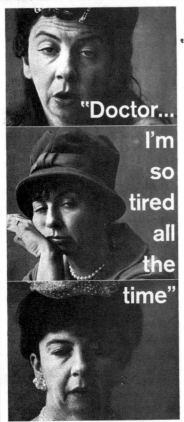
Ads in Journals

Pill advertising in medical journals differ very little from the fancy and slick advertising used to sell anything else. Apart from a few technical terms, these ads, like all others, sell moods, lifestyles and themes. They play upon the fears and hopes any human feels, while paying particular attention to the anxieties a doctor gets from standing on his pedestal all day.

The heyday of pill advertising that seemed to peak in the '50s and '60s. A look at these ads reveal the way a doctor pigeonholes his patients. Women are portrayed as insane or stubborn people to be dealt with by tranquilizers. And there are images of sensuous women who long for satisfaction, satisfaction the doctor can give (and get) by prescribing a certain pill. There is no significant difference in these ads from the "consume-this-to-have-sex" motif that pervades most advertising. All that's different is that the ad is pitched solely to the patient.

Ads in those classic days unashamedly showcased the pills themselves, emphasizing their beauty and the presumed efficacy that went with it. Best of all, there were no annoying fine print warnings to muck up the page. The ad artist started with a clean canvas. A pill advertisement was free to do what it was designed to do—sell pills, not give an in-depth education to the doctor who could presumably inform himself further, if he cared to.

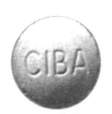

Planted Studies in Journals and Newspapers

As mentioned before, pharmaceutical companies sometimes host seminars in which doctors known to promote particular drugs are asked to speak on a more general topic of a class of diseases in which some of the therapies are discussed. Although consumer advocates and even some physicians profess to be so shocked that a seminar paid for and organized by, say, CIBA-Geigy would seek to promote CIBA-Geigy products, it's hard to believe anyone could fail to make the connection in advance. In any case, these seminars normally contain useful information about diseases and treatments and, because the speakers are legitimate researchers—not ad men—they are free to talk about experimental uses of a drug which have not yet gotten FDA approval.

This is how, for instance, doctors first learned that Abbott's pill, Depakote, which was only approved by the government as an anti-convulsant, was also useful in the treatment of manic depression—a seriously debilitating disease that is quite difficult to treat. Depakote, by the way, has now gained FDA approval. But luckily a lot of suffering people were afforded relief well before the government gave its official sanction.

Direct to Consumer

Direct-to-consumer ads have proliferated like mushrooms since the FDA permitted them in 1985. At the time, the FDA commissioner gleefully announced direct-to-consumer as the big marketing opportunity available to pharmaceutical corps that decade. Drug companies now spend about $100 million a month reaching out to pill takers, almost five times the amount spent three years ago. DTC advertising seems quite successful—a recent *Time* magazine survey found that "28% of the consumers polled would switch doctors in order to get a desired medication."

Pill poppers are now investigated to ask their doc directly for that breakthrough pill they read about or saw on TV. Restrictions in drug advertising make it difficult to discuss the drug in detail, but hints are given. Prescription drug ads found in mass market magazines are often dumbed-down versions of those directed at doctors, with an added visual gimmick consumers will associate with the medicine. Fireworks, fancy computer graphics and beaming former sufferers enjoying a leisure activity like golf, tennis or swimming are currently popular motifs.

Normally a drug company likes to advertise a drug to the great unwashed when it represents the only one in its class. That way the doctor has no choice but to prescribe their product. Since the patient already knows a drug exists, it's difficult to deny a request for treatment. Monoxidil is a good example of this.

For years, doctors had known about Monoxidil's ability to grow hair and dermatologists, especially, had been making a cream from the antihypertensive drug for just that purpose. But such individual drug compounding is hardly efficient and the huge potential market of balding men didn't have access to the cream.

So Monoxidil's makers, Upjohn, went through the expensive and time-consuming ordeal of having its drug approved for the purpose of growing hair. All the while, news of the coming drug spread among doctors and everyone else so that, by the time it got official approval, it was already well-known. At the time, it was the only drug approved to grow hair. Upjohn only had to run TV ads about the shame and horror of thinning hair, suggesting that there was a way to deal with it and urging viewers to see their doctor. Other promotions have given 800 numbers to call for more information, rebate certificates, videotapes and even lists of local doctors eager to prescribe. Sales were brisk, to say the least.

Cable's Lifetime Channel, programs its Sundays to run medical programs ostensibly oriented to doctors. All commercials are for prescription drugs and, while they contain plenty of technical language (it is almost absurd to see doctors changing in a locker room spieling off terms like "extrapyramidical" and "decarboxylase inhibition", there is none of the "fine print" revealing all the federally-mandated warnings. This is because the shows are permitted to wait until the end of the programming day when the fine print scrolls boringly up the screen to the strains of soporific orchestral music.

The people besides doctors who watch these programs are considered secondary targets to spread the word about drugs and wheedle the latest "breakthrough" from their own doctor. It's too bad the patient is put in a position to have to wheedle anything. It's too bad doctors are put in a position of having to satisfy their patients' manufactured desires in addition to providing medical care. This is not the fault of the drug companies. We should keep in mind the laws regulating and restraining a supposedly free market in medicines. Pill advertising is a good thing, however circumscribed it is now. As we've seen, advertisements are a doctor's main source of information for new drugs and pharmaceutical developments. If government functionaries stopped threatening prison to anyone who dared think for himself, and could self-prescribe, we could all—advertisers included—start treating doctors as physicians—instead of sources of pills.

Prescription drug advertising has a lot in common with the way children's products are pitched. The consumer is not in the position to simply go out and buy the stuff. An authority figure must be convinced to allow or make the purchase.

Doctors would prefer not to have it spread around, but the mighty demi-gods of the modern world are quite vulnerable to a nagging patient. They are sometimes impressed by forceful behavior. If a patient is intrepid enough to break the taboo against requesting a certain drug, the doctor will often give it to them. If he balks, he's going to get complaints and hostility. Doctors are not taught, either in school or by peers, to tell patients to fuck off.

On a business level, the doctor knows that the patient is ultimately his customer, his bread and butter. Turn away the patient just because you don't want to give him a lousy pill and no doubt they'll lose the steady income the patient's follow-up visits will bring in. If all the patient wants is an unscheduled medication that has few side effects and no legal ramifications, well, why not? Write a prescription with one refill and the patient is good for six visits per year.

A new kind of pill advertising, the phony news item, first appeared about 25 years ago and is still one of the best ways to push a new pill.

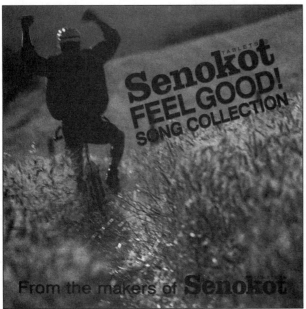

Laxative tablets have never felt or sounded better than in a CD with toilet inspiring tunes by Reo Speedwagon, Toto, Eddie Money and Cheap Trick.

When the new ulcer drug Tagamet was introduced in 1976, it was all over the news shows. A pill that could cure ulcers, halt the pain and make ulcer surgery obsolete was a newsworthy item! Sales were phenomenal and Tagamet's status as a news feature functioned as advertising. Light bulbs went on over the heads of pharmaceutical ad men everywhere. When pills are featured as news in the mass media, it's possible not only to escape FTC restrictions on claims made about a drug, further talk about the drug is promoted. Even if the speculation contains some negative information, it's still advertising. Tylenol sales soon grew larger even after it became associated with random poisonings. Apparently the mere repetition of its name stimulated sales. Since serendipitous discovery of news promos by Tagamet, newspapers, magazines, television shows, and other media receive plenty of press kits heralding the arrival of one or another pill.

When Eli Lilly introduced their new anti-inflammatory pill aimed at arthritis in 1982, the company sent out 6,500 press kits to reporters around the country. Six weeks later, a half-million people had prescriptions for Oroflex.

Another way of advertising a pill is to get a celebrity to start talking about it. That's what CIBA-Geigy did in 1988 when it wanted to promote its NSAID Voltaren. To help spread the word they took the same approach as Wheaties cereal. They hired baseball star Mickey Mantle to go on NBC's Today Show and crow about how the pill was the best thing for his arthritis. Nobody ever mentioned Mantle was a paid spokesman. Upjohn was a little more open about its funding of football star Earl Campbell's 1992 nationwide tour discussing his troubles with panic disorder. At the time, Upjohn's Xanax was the only pill with an official FDA indication to treat this problem.

Similar televised benefits accrued to Ortho pharmaceuticals when its Retin-A became the talk of morning chat shows after it was found to have anti-wrinkle properties. Collagen Corp., which manufactures injectable collagen to make bee-stung lips, must have loved it when lip augmentation was performed on The Oprah Winfrey Show and when Geraldo Rivera had his forehead wrinkles removed on live television.

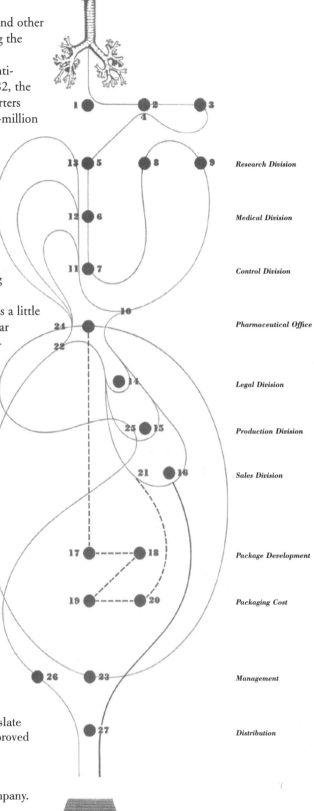

Research Division

Medical Division

Control Division

Pharmaceutical Office

Legal Division

Production Division

Sales Division

Package Development

Packaging Cost

Management

Distribution

"*Orthoxine*" The story of a tablet and of a typical drug development.

The argument: 27 steps of a highly co-ordinated pharmaceutical effort—whose complexities are diagrammed here—translate an unsolved medical problem into an improved drug for chronic asthma relief.

The cast: scientists, management, and specialized personnel of The Upjohn Company.

The time: 1935, when research began, to 1949, when the tablet was first marketed.

PHARMACEUTICAL FANTASIA
The Art and Poetry of Selling Pills to Doctors
BY MELISSA HOFFS

The fact that man thinks he grasps phenomena is an hallucination. Once hallucinations are sufficiently rooted, they become what we call myths, and cease to have outside limits.

History is the story of man's various hallucinations; once we think about some of the influential personages in the story—the devil, Venus, Christ, for example—it is plain that they in part owe their existence as historical personages to having been pictured by men with a gift for graphic hallucinations.

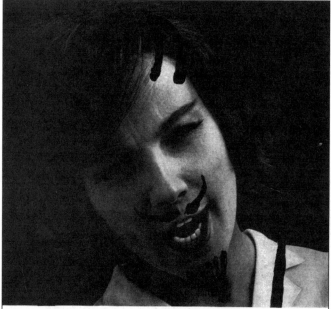

Premenstrual tension?

Premenstrual tension with edema can cause many and diffuse psychic and somatic symptoms. It can complicate diagnosis and treatment of other disorders. Yet, all too frequently, women accept these difficulties as inevitable. Fortunately, premenstrual tension is not inevitable. Once identified, it can often be helped with CYCLEX. CYCLEX relieves symptoms, but does not interfere with hormonal balance. The effects are direct...excess fluid is eliminated by the action of hydrochlorothiazide; the psychic component is minimized by meprobamate. CYCLEX may be given from the onset of premenstrual symptoms until the end of the menses.
INDICATIONS: Premenstrual tension with edema; hypertension; congestive heart failure.
CONTRAINDICATIONS: Hydrochlorothiazide: Anuria. Meprobamate: History of allergic reaction to meprobamate.
PRECAUTIONS: Hydrochlorothiazide: Reduce dosage of coadministered antihypertensive agents by at least 50 percent. Use caution during intensive or prolonged diuresis, in dietary inadequacy or salt restriction, impaired renal function, hepatic disease, rising level of BUN, hyperuricemia or history of gout, patients receiving other antihypertensive agents, surgical patients. Avoid hypokalemia especially during digitalis administration and in myocardial ischemia. Meprobamate: Use only in recommended dosage to minimize habituation or addiction potential.

SIDE EFFECTS: Hydrochlorothiazide: Electrolyte imbalance with hypokalemia or hypochloremic alkalosis may occur. A low-salt syndrome may be precipitated. Other possible reactions: hepatic coma, azotemia, decreased glucose tolerance, hyperuricemia and gout, blood dyscrasias, nausea, vomiting, diarrhea, dizziness, paresthesias, rash, photosensitivity. Meprobamate: Possible side effects include drowsiness, fatigue, allergic reactions (death reported), blood dyscrasias (death reported), visual disturbances, hypotensive crises, withdrawal symptoms. Large or suicidal doses may result in cardiovascular and respiratory collapse, shock, absent reflexes, coma, and death. Tolerance to alcohol may be reduced. Tendency to convulsions may be increased. Grand-mal seizures may be precipitated.
Before prescribing or administering, read product circular with package or available on request.
SUPPLIED: Tablets, bottles of 100. Each tablet contains 25 mg. of hydrochlorothiazide and 200 mg. of meprobamate.

CYCLEX DIURETIC-TRANQUILIZER
MERCK SHARP & DOHME | where today's theory is tomorrow's therapy

The risk in the power to create hallucinations is that they could be exploited by established authority for its own purposes, the way the Church, for instance, uses images to enslave its members. . . . But nowadays science knows very well how to test everything, it is once again permissible to create hallucinations, science can always prevent them from becoming tyrannical—except the scientific hallucination.

—Matta, "Hellucinations," 1948

Pharmaceutical advertising exemplifies the fact that science cannot—or will not—prevent hallucinations from becoming tyrannical. Scientific ideas about health and sickness, and about male and female bodies and sexuality, conform to a larger hallucinatory milieu, which is shaped by historical, art historical, economic and political factors.

The history of medicine is as much a history of evolving metaphors as a chronology of research and scientific breakthroughs. Darwin's and Freud's sciences were informed by the same myths and presumptions as the other belief systems operating during their times. In the 1990s, discussions of mental illness revolve around the theory that such problems are caused by genetics and chemical imbalances. Fresh metaphors are created to accommodate this view of the mind, and to explain how new psychotropic drugs can address the problems of the newly-reconceived sufferer. As science continues to pursue its current theories and their attendant metaphors, it is crucial that the process of metaphor-making be acknowledged—and examined.

So I reiterate: Doctors are people—above and beyond all, human beings. They have the same emotions, the same likes and dislikes, the same fed-uppishness with what they are doing. They like variety, diversion, entertainment. Through the mail they receive ten times more advertising material than the average person, only to relegate it to the same place as the average person—the waste basket. Unless, let me quickly say, it is such literature as catches the eye and snares the heart. A novel booklet or leaflet, die-cut in a curious shape—the kind of thing kids go for . . . Or a blotter that sympathetically takes them for a ride.

—"Doctors Are People Even as You and I,"
Printer's Ink, May, 1934

. . . Medical men are subject to the same kinds of stress, the same emotional influences as affect the layman. Physicians have, as part of their self-image, a determined feeling that they are rational and logical, particularly in their choice of pharmaceuticals. The advertiser must appeal to this rational self-image, and at the same time make a deeper appeal to the emotional factors which really influence sales.

—*Principles of Pharmaceutical Marketing,* 1962

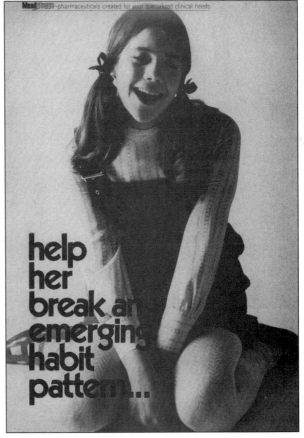

Mead Johnson—pharmaceuticals created for your specialized clinical needs

help her break an emerging habit pattern...

One simple and popular visual means for making this "deeper appeal" in pharmaceutical advertisements is to reconfigure the body to lend itself to a metaphor to which the advertiser hopes the physician will respond. Treatment may be determined by the advertiser's success in superimposing an interpretation onto the pictured subject which resonates with contemporary medical—and layman—attitudes toward that subject. Another factor in an ad's effectiveness is its success in delivering a comfortably simple view of both the particular disease and the action of the drug which addresses it. The process of metaphorization helps to separate the doctor from the realm of the patient; dehumanization of the patient is advantageous to the advertiser especially when his goal is to convince a doctor to prescribe psychotropic drugs.

An advertisement which at first glance seems simply bizarre can, with further study, reveal itself as the locus of an intricate matrix of outdated, fanciful, and disturbingly tenacious medical notions. The ad for Gynorest appears to show a pubescent girl masturbating. The tag line "help her break an emerging habit pattern" implies the drug will halt the girl's propensity to masturbate.

But the ad's copy discusses Gynorest as treatment for dysmenorrhea (menstrual pain), asking us to interpret the menstrual pain as the unwanted habit pattern. How can pain constitute a "habit pattern?" It can if the pain is psychologically generated, as this subject's is believed to be; her dysmenorrhea is described as "non-organic." A gynecology textbook published in 1971, the year after the ad appeared, advises that problems associated with menstruation were "generally a symptom of a personality disorder." In diagnosing many conditions, such as sterility, low back and pelvic pain, and menopause and menstrual difficulties, the same book counsels doctors to gather a personality profile of the patient, with the most important consideration being, "Does the patient accept herself as a woman?" Similarly, a 1972 gynecology textbook states that nausea in pregnancy "may indicate resentment, ambivalence and inadequacy in women ill-prepared for motherhood."

In the advertisement for Gynorest, the message to the doctor seems to be derived from 19th century ideas about the function and influence of the ovaries: as indicated by the photograph, the "habit pattern"— the disease to be cured—is sexuality. The prescribed cure is related to the 19th century practice of ovariotomy (surgical removal of the ovaries) as a treatment for masturbation and nymphomania: treat the reproductive organs themselves. (It seems illogical to believe that hormone therapy would address the problem if the pain is indeed non-organic; this paradox is not acknowledged.) In the milieu of this advertisement, masturbation and menstrual pain are both "symptoms" of the girl's emerging sexuality; the ad implies that either condition warrants a doctor's attention and should be "treated."

The doctor's need for a feeling of dominance over uncontrollable forces is a popular target for pharmaceutical advertisers. Fears of insignificance, impotence and mortality are perhaps more pervasive in the doctor's sphere than in the world outside his office; they may have contributed to making the doctor role appealing in the first place, and could in turn be exacerbated by the challenges of that role. Advertisers attempt to bolster the prospective consumer's sense of control by presenting images of the physician (discreetly endowed with the extra healing powers of the advertiser's wares) as God. Variations on this theme proliferate in the ad pages of medical journals, with larger-than-life hands frequently employed as metonyms. Felix Marti-Ibanex, founder of MD magazine and as such a kind of de Medici of pharmaceutical advertising, personally rallied healers to transcend their apprehensions in his lofty December, 1961, *Editor's Essay,* "The Legacy of St. Luke":

As Paracelsus said, the physician springs from God. He should therefore cultivate the relationship of faith with the patient in which resided the key to the healing miracle, which was accomplished through the physician's voice and hands and the patient's faith. For these are the things that ultimately direct the healing drug, the mending scalpel, or the reassuring psychotherapy.

The physician cannot simply break his patient down into cells and atoms in his laboratory. He must, with his perceptive mind, consider both the patient's life history and his spirit. Healing is a sacred act, requiring pure hands and as pure a heart. The physician must be an artist in his science, for his alliance with art will open within him a fount of healing forces for the good of his patients and for his own good.

Mutant Mascot
The Obnoxious *Speedy* Alka-Seltzer

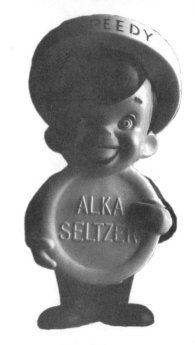

The world's most insipid drug mascot—Speedy Alka-Seltzer—
was developed to improve the pill's image after it got its ass
kicked by the FTC. For decades, Miles Labs and an assort-
ment of comic strip characters had claimed that drinking Alka-Seltzer
would equalize "systemic acidity" and thus cure a host of problems
from rheumatism to domestic disputes.

Sample ad from the 1930s:

> They've had a terrible fight. He snapped at her and left. It's all lovely now
> . . . what caused it? Too much acidity in the body. Be wise—Alkalize
> with Alka-Seltzer!

By the end of WWII, the company abandoned this method of
hawking the fizzy pills. Miles Labs admen wanted an Alka-Seltzer
ambassador. What they came up with was a twisted, red-headed
"sprite" who wore a giant Alka-Seltzer on his head and whose body
was, in fact, just a giant Alka-Seltzer. In one hand (at the end of an
absurdly long arm) he held a magic wand with which he cured stomach problems. Original named "Sparky," he was re-christened
"Speedy" to coincide with that year's ad campaign ("Speedy Relief").

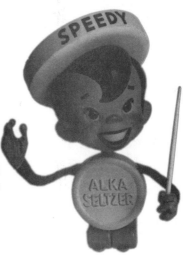

At first, Speedy appeared mostly in doctors' magazines. Then
the hideous mutant mascot went on the radio and became famous
among the general population. But Speedy was to find his true place
on television.

Miles sponsored a nationwide talent search for a suitable voice, and
found it in squealy little Richard Beals. Beals wasn't a little kid, he was
a full-grown adult who happened to be really short and looked and
sounded like a ten-year-old. Speedy made his television debut in 1954,
and Beals supplied Speedy's voice in 212 TV spots over the next decade.
(He recounts this exciting time in his self-published autobiography,
Think Big.)

In 1955, one could purchase their own limited-edition Speedy
doll. The bastard was even a hit in Latin America where he was
known as "Prontito!"

Although Speedy was mercifully killed off by Consumer Products
Group head Bob Wallace ("Speedy may have somewhat overstayed his
time," he said,) the half-pill, half-boy was resurrected for the 1976
Bicentennial.

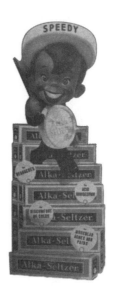

He was also scheduled for a comeback during the 1980 Olympics,
competing in winter sports alongside Sammy Davis Jr., but those ads
were pulled when President Carter canceled U.S.
participation in the games.

"Down, down down, the stomach through,
Round, round, round the system too,
With Alka-Seltzer you're sure to say,
Relief is just a swallow away!"

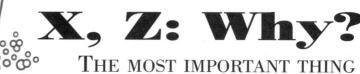

X, Z: Why?

THE MOST IMPORTANT THING
ABOUT A PILL—at least to
the marketing department—
is not its color or its shape.
It's not whether it's a capsule
or a tablet. And it's certainly not the
formula of the drug itself.

The most important thing about a pill is its name. Just as certain pills' appearances have made them stand out over the decades, the names of various pills have an important impact on the market, and on culture as well. It stands to reason that names have to be chosen very carefully. Recently, a group of pharmaceutical companies admitted, at a symposium at Harvard Business School, that if forced to choose between owning the patent or the trade name of a successful pill, the execs said they would take the name.

This was not always the case. In the good old days, pill crafters, like car makers, picked the name of their product almost as an afterthought. Pills were whimsically named. Miltown was simply the name of a nearby Jersey burg where the first minor tranquilizer was invented. Streptomycin is named for the microorganism from which it comes, Streptomyces. Both heroin and aspirin are trade names for headache remedies made by Bayer. These trademarks are no longer enforced.

But nowadays pharmaceutical companies spend up to half a million bucks for a single, memorable name! If that investment gives their pill only a few percentage points over any competitor, then the investment will be worth it. Once a formula goes generic, it can mean all the difference; it's hard to compete with something one-tenth your price, and it's unsound business practice to drop the price too much.

Consider Darvocet, a narcotic analgesic. Darvocet costs twice as much as generic propoxyphene, yet Darvocet continues to claim a large chunk of the pain-killer market. Why? Because for 20 years, doctors have been scrawling out something that seems to start with a D and they're not going to start scrawling "propoxyphene napsylate" now. This not only takes more time and effort, it can result in errors in prescribing and dispensing.

No doubt an Eli Lilly rep just showed up at the doctor's office again and dropped off a load of doughnuts, imprinted little flashlights, paperweights and coffee mugs. The doc knows better than to stop prescribing Darvocet.

What's wrong with that? Patients have ample opportunity to request generics from their doctors and most states provide for automatic substitution unless the

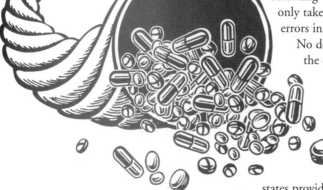

doctor specifically forbids it. We all know how most doctors frown upon patients who request a medication by name.

Since pill companies market to doctors, it stands to reason they care about what doctors think of names. Prescription pills aimed to appeal to doctors, not patients—that's why prescription drugs have serious-sounding names. Doctors seem to respond to pills whose names reflect a mysterious sophistication. As one professional namer put it, a prescription drug for life-threatening kidney problems won't be called "Renal-Rite." Such frankly descriptive names are bestowed upon pills aimed at consumers (One-A-Day, Nytol).

Xanax is a great example of a modern pill name. It is very distinctive—important in the fiercely competitive and teeming marketplace. And quite distinctive to a person who actually writes it out. The tactile prompt will further distinguish it.

The current trend for the z and x sound exist because they connote power in the mind of the physician and represent the comforts of space age technology in the mind of Joe Consumer. (Chances are you're familiar with Xanax, Zovirax, Zoloft, Zocor, Prozac and Zestril.) With Xanax, its visual, tactile, and auditory prompts imprint the product in the prescriber's brain. A very successful marketing strategy.

The palidromic name "Xanax" is also very easy to remember. Recall is key. An exotic or memorable name can make a pill stick in the mind, even when nothing else is known about it. The more people hear a pill's name, the more likely they are to use it. Marketing 101. Product identification, brand recognition. Even "bad" publicity further distinguishes a certain product. Each time some maniac went around dosing Tylenol with cyanide, sales rose to record levels after an initial dip. Tylenol is perhaps the only way regular Joes know how to say "acetaminophen."

It may seem odd that Stuart ICI copyrighted the name "Zestril" before having a drug to go with it, but the storing of names in advance is necessary. Drug companies employ teams of creative people to sit around boardrooms drinking coffee and barking out names they think sound good. They come up with thousands, and almost all of them are no good—unpronounceable, already in use, or else too close to another drug's name.

Not long ago, Merck Sharp & Dohme paid good money for the wonderful name Losec (for a pill that LOwered SECretion of gastric acid). It was quite a success. Unfortunately, doctors' handwriting resulted in too many dispensing errors of a diuretic called Lasix. Now, MSD calls the product Prilosec, risking a lot in the marketplace by changing the name of a successful drug.

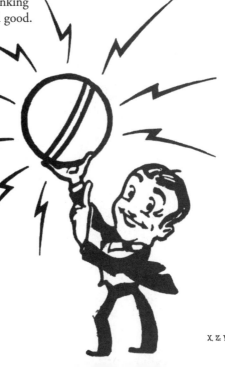

Scientists have long recognized the beauty of

pills and have never stopped trying to adapt this

eminently convenient form to every type of

medicine. Indeed, anything a person could

ingest is a potential candidate for pillification.

PILLS OF THE FUTURE

Now high technology has made possible the introduction of mechanical "smart pills" that travel the human body like mini-submarines before discharging medicine at a specific place.

Dr. Jerome Schentag of New York State University in Buffalo has developed a polycarbonate-coated pill less than one inch long that contains a tiny radio transmitter, power source and propulsion system along with a drug chamber that can withstand the rigors of normal digestion through the human body. A tiny computer and antenna worn in the patient's vest tracks the pill's progress and when it reaches the site, tells the pill to release the medication. Then you just excrete the spent pill.

"It can take chemotherapy right down to the site of a tumor or disease in the bowel and drop it right on top of it—just like a toxic bullet!" says Shentag.

Another design breakthrough—the amazing expanding pill—comes from a team of researchers at Duke University headed by Dr. Kinam Park. After being swallowed, the pill grows to ten times its original size and stays in the stomach for as long as a week, releasing medication before the hydrogel coating is finally totally digested.

So far, the pill has only been tested on dogs since it's still too big to be comfortably swallowed by people. Right now, the prototype is bigger than the size of a large fiber pill.

"We want the new pill to be something that can be easily taken by children and the elderly," says Park. "We want to get it down to where it's just a little larger than a standard aspirin pill."

Bayer, Heroin and Aspirin

The Aspirin Wars, a 1991 book by Charles C. Mann and Mark L. Plummer, devotes hundreds of pages to the history of this most famous over-the-counter pain remedy. All aspects of pill-hawking are covered, especially the awesome advertising campaigns and titanic lawsuits between competing drug firms and the government.

During the 1940s, the lengths aspirin makers went to sell their pills are truly amazing. Trucks loaded with equipment to set up an outdoor theater drove high into the mountains, stopping at impoverished Indian villages in South America to show newsreels and then sell little packets of three aspirins. In Buenos Aires, another company feverishly spent its time catching stray dogs, painting their brand's name on them and letting them go.

Preposterous as they may seem, the ads were important because of the staggering amounts of money involved in the aspirin business—even among the world's poorest people.

It's one thing to say Americans consume so many tons of aspirin per year and another to realize that all these tons of aspirin are consumed in chunks of less than a third of a gram each. The profit margin on a single aspirin tablet is small. But the number of tablets is almost incomprehensible, a blizzard of powdery white pills.

The patent was successfully challenged in Britain but in America, it was sustained. Aspirin (a trademark name for acetylsalicylic acid) was first synthesized by a French chemist named Charles Frederic Gerhardt in 1853. Bayer obtained the patent for aspirin in the United States in about 1900 and nowhere else but England. In fall 1916, just before the patent was due to expire, Bayer took out an ad in U.S. newspapers advertising simply: "The Bayer Cross on every package and on every tablet of genuine Bayer Aspirin protects you against all counterfeits and substitutes."

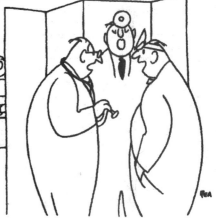

"Aspirin." "Aspirin." "Aspirin."

This guarantee against counterfeiting was an important issue. Bayer had sent out detectives to buy aspirin all over the country and discovered some 27 percent of aspirin being sold in its name was, indeed, fake. It wasn't such an outrageous claim. Still, the AMA threw a fit. Right away it published an editorial on the subject complaining of 17 years of Bayer hegemony of acetylsalicylic acid: "Not content with the iron-bound monpoly which had been granted though our patent laws, the company attempted further to clinch its exclusive rights by giving the preparation a fancy name, 'aspirin,' and getting a trademark on this name."

The AMA further advised doctors not to prescribe "aspirin" to anyone, using instead its chemical name—acetylsalicylic acid.

This may seem bizarre in today's medical world, where patents and trademarks are everything and many doctors don't even remember the chemical names for the pills they prescribe. But the idea of protecting, let alone promoting, a brand name, was alien to doctors at the turn of the century, who saw it as unseemly. At that time drug manufacturers were still very content to invent drugs, obtain patents and then supply

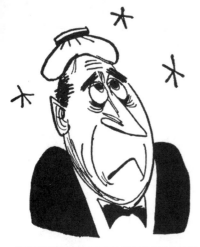

them to pharmacies, without ever bothering to name them—an inconceivable idea today.

Just as inconceivable was the way in which drugs were investigated and invented in those times. Before the appearance of the FDA and other regulatory agencies, drugs were either discovered accidently, or, as in the case of Bayer, deliberately sought out within their enormous drug laboratory. Even though drugs were specifically looked for, scientists often didn't (and couldn't) target a particular disease. Using a shotgun approach, they mixed up thousands of different concoctions, testing them afterward to see what they did. Meticulous notes were kept through the whole process and every now and then, something turned up. Heroin appeared the next year.

One of the first businessmen to understand how teams of scientists could worry at a problem like a dog with a bone, Duisberg kept stuffing workers into Bayer's crude, overcrowded research quarters. Lab tables were scattered everywhere in the facilities, with foul-smelling experiments being conducted in corridors, bathrooms, and an abandoned woodworking shop. Lucky researchers had access to sinks; unlucky ones worked outdoors, in the river fog [at Leverkusen, Germany]. They wore clogs because the muddy ground was full of harmless-looking puddles capable of disintegrating leather shoes. They had no chemical storeroom, no

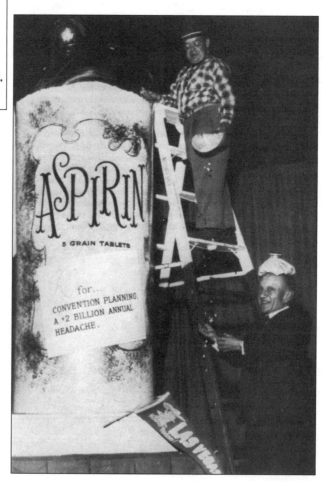

The 2 million aspirin tablets in this giant jar—a promotional exhibit at a Las Vegas exposition—represent less than one-third of the aspirin consumed by Americans every hour of every day.

technical library, and little equipment—nothing but a platoon of boys who cleaned retors and vials. By 1890, the company was ready to build a three-story, 1.5 million mark research laboratory. Within four years, Duisberg [head of Bayer] had crammed it with ninety full-time chemists—six times as many as had been at the company in 1881—and was looking for more. When it was snowing or raining, a thick trail of workers' footsteps could be seen in blue, yellow, violet, or green, leading right up to the middle of town.

. . . A photograph of some chemists at the time shows a dog lying under one of the lab's tables. It was one of many dogs that roamed the place at will . . . —from the *Aspirin Wars*

The Bayer name, along with its enormous state-of-the-art chemical and drug factory by the Hudson river in New Jersey, was confiscated by the U.S. government in 1915, then sold in 1918 to the highest bidder by "alien property custodian" Mitchell Palmer (who would later lead the anti-foreigner "Palmer Raids" during the 1920s). By the time Bayer was sold, fighting against Germany in World War I had completely stopped, and was in ruins.

What is Aspirin Good For?

Aspirin is good for so many things, it would easily qualify as some kind of quack medicine if it listed its scientifically-proven uses on the label. Luckily, aspirin has been around nearly 100 years now and the FDA has no real power to restrict its use—the backlash from the public would be too intense. Besides, its 100-year, worldwide history of use has proven the stuff to be incredibly safe although it can have a bad effect on the stomach lining.

The standard aspirin tablet contains 325 mgs of active ingredient plus whatever binders, buffers or coatings the manufacturer has added. Sometimes pill-makers add some caffeine, as this has been shown to potentiate the analgesic effects of aspirin.

But small doses, as little as 35 mgs (one tenth of a tablet), have been shown to prevent blood clots, heart attacks, strokes, and "mini-strokes." Slightly larger doses, say a single aspirin every other day, reduces a person's chances of having heart attacks, migraine headaches, and cancers of the colon and rectum.

In high doses, as many as 20 tablets a day, aspirin can greatly reduce the pain and inflammation of rheuma-toid arthritis, gout, and rheumatic fever. But watch out, as this much aspirin can do a number on your stomach, burning a hole through the stomach lining and causing an ulcer. Also, smaller doses of aspirin have the paradoxi cal effect of worsening gout conditions, so take large doses of aspirin only after obtaining proper medical advice.

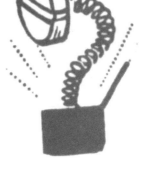

PLACEBO (Latin for "I Please")

Anti-pharmaceutical ingrates believe the "placebo effect" is certain proof that disorders don't really exist and could be corrected if the patient stops whining and gets some exercise for a change!

The "placebo effect" remains fairly unresearched. Who wants to research a medication that, by definition, does nothing? And how would placebos be marketed? Would a doctor be required to lie to the patient? If a placebo were ever approved for use, would the FDA require labeling to disclose truth about the unpill and ruin its required effectiveness? Or would the FDA require the printing of false information, violating labeling law?

Leaving aside commercial considerations, would it even be possible to market placebos outright? Probably not. Since placebos sometimes cause more side effects than the actual drugs they're compared to, the FDA would never allow such a dangerous medication to be sold to the general public!

Studies have shown that the mere presence of Valium in a person's pocket has a calming effect. In fact, most people who are prescribed Valium (and the like) take less than they are prescribed. It seems the idea of possible relief is a powerful remedy in itself. This same phenomenon is seen in post-operative patients who are allowed to self-administer pain medication. They take less medicine than is available to them. There are pharmacological reasons for this, but I suspect the feeling of control a patient gets from such an arrangement has a lot to do with it, too.

Research conducted on placebos have turned up some neat little tidbits about the way people view pills, and the importance of color, shape, taste, and other perceptual things that contribute to any pill's efficacy.

Capsules are widely perceived to be stronger than tablets. If the pill is taken in another form, say tablets, research shows bigger is regarded as better. Large pills produce even better results if they are brown or purple. Small pills, however, can increase their perceived effectiveness if they're colored either bright yellow, or bright red. It's probably not much of a surprise that people tend to believe two pills are stronger than one —no matter what's in them. And all medicines, including pills, are considered stronger if they don't taste too good. Sweet pills come off as weaklings.

"Hey, psychosomatic works for me!"

—anonymous pillhead waving off criticism of his latest pill combo

Just about everything contributes to the placebo effect. A drug's cost influences perceived effectiveness—the greater the expense, the better the pill seems to work. The attitudes of the person prescribing or dispensing the pill are especially crucial. Subjects can be primed to rate a pill favorably or unfavorably depending on whether the dispenser shows respect for the medication. Due to this, a placebo effect occurs without even using placebos. What the patient believes can overcome the effects of low doses of truly active drugs. College student test subjects receiving either 5 mgs of Valium or 5 mgs of Dexedrine reported effects that conformed to what they were told they were taking, regardless of the drug actually taken. This effect, however, disappeared when the dosage was increased.

Dosage also affects perception of placebos, and all pills, for that matter. For maximum effectiveness, dosing shouldn't be too simple, especially when instructions are given by a doctor. A three-times-a-day placebo generally produces better results than a placebo taken just once a day. And, naturally, prescription pills are always considered stronger than OTC products.

Last but certainly not least, a placebo's success depends on the type of person taking it, and what effect he or she expects from it. The unfortunate bias against placebos doesn't do much for insomniacs or anxiety sufferers, who almost always report better results from placebos than "control groups." This can lead to the unsupported conclusion that the person was not really suffering.

While the discovery by Edmunds Dimond of the University of Kansas Medical Center that the surgical ligation of an artery for treating angina pectoris was less beneficial than simply making an incision in the chest—as a placebo—led to the abandonment of the surgical technique. Pill scientists are paying more attention than before to the "placebo effect," and experiments using the most advanced brain scanning technology show definite physiological changes after a patient is given a dose of an "inert" medication.

Whatever scientists may be doing, pill-makers have long paid attention to the placebo effect. Marketing studies probably consist of the majority of data collected on the subject. This is exactly the kind of information pill companies put to use.

Consider two brands of ibuprofen —Advil and Nuprin. As they are the same medication they compete with one another. Nuprin takes advantage of what is already known about pill size and color ("little, yellow, different"), and is an almost literal textbook case in marketing. Advil, on the other hand, makes it known that you need only take one pill to equal the power of two pills. But you can take two, you know . . . .

The perceived power of capsules over tablets may be why MacNeil waited until a second wave of Extra-Strength Tylenol poisonings came about before they abandoned the capsule format. MacNeil quickly invented the "gel-cap"—a tablet painted to look like a capsule!

Back when prescriptions were written entirely in Latin (in large part as a measure to keep the patient in the dark about medicine), placebos were explicit and pharmacists played along. Until prescriptions came under government scrutiny, pharmacists filling a prescription for a placebo were taught to prevaricate. If asked what was in the medicine, pharmacists were instructed to tell the patient that it was the medication his doctor recommended. And yes, pharmacists would say, the medicine is of the highest potency. That's why it's by prescription only.

Doctors still use "placebos" by prescribing lower-strength medications than they could, or else pills are prescribed with little known effect. I say "known" because, as much as we proclaim our dedication to science and the exploration of the unknown, it is the status quo to believe our current knowledge is based on nothing but the soundest reasoning and correct conclusions.

Probably the most astonishing "placebo effect" is the unshakable faith they inspire in precisely those people who you'd think most immune to such an old trick: those engaged in drug research. It goes without saying that no company wastes much R&D money trying to develop a more effective placebo. Even if they have a high response rate, placebos are assumed to have no effect.

Consider the illustration of the scientist investigating the efficacy of a weight-loss medication against a placebo, and a weight-reducing diet regimen.

If results show 40% of those taking the new medication lose weight, 45% weight loss in the placebo group, and only 15% weight loss among those using a pill-free diet, the researcher might well conclude the experimental medicine is a failure—but the diet works a little. This conclusion wouldn't be irrational given the official doctrine of a placebo.

Because the medication was measured against a placebo and results were nearly equal, this is usually construed as *prima facie* evidence the new drug does nothing at all. That's because placebos are known to have no real effects. But the non-pill diet treatment, m e a s u r e d against the ineffective placebo and the now-discredited drug, gets full credit for any success and is regarded as most effective of the three—despite having the worst results of all.

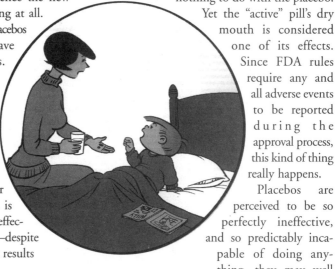

It's no wonder so many good drugs have been shelved almost immediately upon being invented. All it takes is one slip-up against the lowly placebo or some other failure in a "known" test, to overlook another contribution to the world of pills.

Blind faith in a placebo's ineffectiveness is evident when testing for a "real"

"One pill is for your sore throat; the other is for your ear ache."

"How do the pills know where to go?"

pill's side effects. If 4% of those taking a medication report dry mouth, and 8% of the placebo group reports the same thing—it is likely the new medicine will include "dry mouth" as a possible side effect. The placebo pill's higher incidence of dry mouth is assumed to have nothing to do with the placebo. Yet the "active" pill's dry mouth is considered one of its effects. Since FDA rules require any and all adverse events to be reported d u r i n g t h e approval process, this kind of thing really happens.

Placebos are perceived to be so perfectly ineffective, and so predictably incapable of doing anything, they may well come close to being the perfect pill. One of a pill company's favorite claims is that its latest product has a side effect profile "comparable to a placebo." Yet, if placebos have no effect, why mention them at all? Wouldn't it be more correct to say the new pill has no side effects on its own, without comparing it to the placebo?

Sure, the big pill-makers might put a lot of dough into the names they give their pills, but that doesn't mean they aren't humorous in a Beavis & Butthead way, like Asacol, Doryx, Bonine.

Some require a loose pronunciation: Effexor, Eulexin, Asbron.

Some names seem to be a kind of greeting—Halotex, Hylorel, Haloperon.

Some are just stupid: HemaWipe, Amen, Buf-Puf Medicated Acne Pads or are inherently funny—BumbEx, Ceptaz. Some could be phrases, like: Diagen, Dimacol, Cinalone.

Others seem more like anagrams—Insulatard, Ergamisol.

In our opinion, here are a few of the best-sounding names for pills and other medications. In no particular order, we have:

Asmalix, Hismanol, Nudol, Pentasa, Di-Spaz, Anaspaz, Android-5 Ascomp, Azdone, Kenalog, Bonamine, Elixicon, Diphenacen, Diosuccin, Gentafair, Aut, Bilagog, Beesix, Beepen VK, Gonak, Grorm, Fungizone, Gee Gee, Balminil, Climacteron, Creamalin, Clindex, Comazol, Iophen, Compal, C-Lexin, Bronkelixer, Lixolin, Geopen, Largactil, Largon, Licon, Dexitac, Lomanate, Barbidonna, Barbita, Anabolin, Chardonna-2, Crystamine, Jenamicin, Kaylixir, Lectopam, Benuryl, BenzaShave, Bisac-Evac, Bleph-10, Baldex, Cycoflex, Deficol, Buf-Bar, Dopamet, Cytospaz, Doak Oil, Eurax, Butyn, Carbodec, Cardec-S, Cortenema, Astramorph, Jumex, Hip-Rex, Chooz, Diar-Aid, Evac-U-Lax, Insta-Char, Koffex, Dixarit, Keneject, Glo-Sel, Fluorodex, Cleocin, Cotrim, Duralone, Efudex, Kasof, Humorsol, Duradyne, Endur-Acin, Duadacin, Levsin, Gas-Is-Gon, Kiddy Koff.

COOL DRUG NAMES

Please Don't Blame the Pill

Many people believe that doctors routinely shove pills down their patients' throats, thus forcing us into a destructive pill culture, but this is a simplistic view. Doctors are reacting to a variety of influences when they write a prescription—not the least among them being that a patient expects one. A prescription is tangible proof of an office visit, of medical care. Many physicians have told me that patients, especially senior citizens, will feel cheated and become hostile, if a prescription or bagful of free samples from the doctor's bounty, are not offered. Doctors are also asked by patients to provide results —pronto!—much faster than the body is able to heal itself. Drugs yield results more quickly, efficiently, and often more cheaply than anything else.

The root of the "pill problem" is really a failure of both doctors and patients. Doctors are naturally defensive, since they've set themselves up as the mini-Gods of our society. So they end up practicing defensive medicine. CYA— Cover Your Ass—is often bandied about medical institutions as reasons for questionable medications or procedures. Prescriptions mollify patients that "something decisive has been done." And since medication is indicated for damn near anything —malpractice suits can also be avoided.

This Medical Mantra: CYA, CYA, CYA . . . shouldn't it be http—Heal The Patient, Heal The Patient, Heal The Patient?

Pharmaceutical manufacturers are frequently seen in the news whenever their profits are particularly high. Then comes the implication that they are gouging and maybe even responsible for the current "crisis in medicine." But the truth is that just 7% of U.S. healthcare costs are from pills. Yet pills do the lion's share of the "work." Pills such as H2 antagonists have practically eliminated ulcer surgery. New oral antibiotics can cost $5 per dose, but obviate the need for hospitalization or IV antibiotics (which themselves require someone to administrator them, and a host of other difficulties). Yes, each pill is expensive, but as compared to what? To the disease? To an idealized world where everything is free?

Pharmaceutical companies make a persuasive argument about the amount

LIFE

DOCTORS AND THE Rx SCANDAL

How some M.D.s short-cut ethics and profit from their own prescriptions

Pills like these cure illness. But some doctors seize the chance to make money from them

JUNE 24 · 1966 · 35¢

of money expended in researching a single drug (the average is something like $230 million). For this, they find that only one in 10,000 compounds ever make it to market, and the normal course of FDA testing requires 10 of the 17 years a company can retain exclusivity on a drug patent. This does not include the inevitable onslaught of me-too drugs that follow a new pill's debut, further eroding the market share of the debuting drug.

After a patent expires, the price drops dramatically as other companies begin to manufacture and sell the compound. In the pharmaceutical marketplace, the key to success is recouping the money invested in the drug as quickly as possible, which usually means charging the highest price possible initially, with periodic changes (read: increases) in the price. Sometimes, the price of a drug might be increased four to six times a year, and then remain at the highest price for a year. Then the company uses this as a marketing tool: they will put ads in *USA Today*, and info sheets at your pharmacy, explaining how they haven't increased the price of their drug, unlike some other companies, for an entire year. Of course, they do not mention their activities the previous year, but they still get sympathy votes from the clueless.

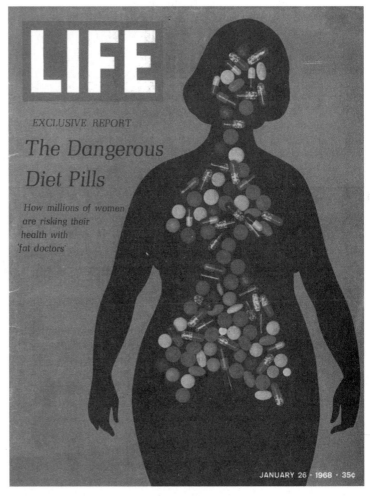

"That is a good company," says the consumer. "They must care about the average American and understand that we cannot continue paying from our own pockets for these expensive drugs."

Some of the sympathetic, and deluded, patients will ask their doctors to switch them to the so reasonably-priced med on the next office visit. What was first a questionable practice of repeatedly increasing prices and then holding steady becomes a successful marketing tool for that same drug.

What is wrong with our pill-taking society is not the fault of pills. It's the fault of all the humans involved in the process—the doctor, the patient, the insurer, the manufacturer, the legislature, the special interests, the media. Nor do the answers lie in further control of a drug (banning it, giving people more, making it more difficult to prescribe, requiring exhaustive paperwork, etc.). This simply makes a drug less available to people for its true purpose. A blame-the-pill mentality presupposes that both the doctor and the patient are such jerks when it comes to medical treatment that lawmakers must step in and exert authority.

The Mystical Art of Making Pills

Pill technology has been an important part of pill culture since William Erasmus Upjohn started his "Pill & Granule Co." featuring his fabulous invention, the "friable" pill, which could be easily crushed into a powder beneath the thumb. When the patent expired in 1921, everyone rushed to copy the friable pill, and Upjohn still boasted of its invention in its company logo.

Modern pills are normally the products of high-tech machines, whipping the tiny dosage units at vision-blurring speeds within a complex labyrinth of pure pill production. Spinning and zooming in single-file they halt long enough to get doused in a coat of carnauba wax or dry off a layer of enteric coating in a puff of hot air, before the pills disappear in a whir, off to the next station. Mega-contraptions used by pharmaceutical houses crank out thousands of pills per hour, each pill indistinguishable from the other, depositing them neatly in triple-sealed bottles ready to be shipped to pharmacies around the nation, where they wait on shelves to be plinked out on counting trays for you, the beaming pillhead.

But the fine art of pillmaking is still practiced by modern-day pillmakers—mainly in those few "compounding pharmacies" where small batches of specially-ordered medicines are made one-by-one on hand-operated presses. The process is slower but the product is just as uniform and defect-free. This is what the pharmacist strives for even today: complete uniformity and error-free work. It requires attention to detail and resistance to boredom that goes beyond anal-retentive. To help keep the modern pharmacist from going insane avoiding mistakes in his main task of counting pills,

expensive pill-counting machines promise 99.7% accuracy in every batch it counts.

Not every innovation in pill-production is high-tech, however. Nor does every operation require a skilled craftsman. One novel improvement in pill production goes beyond fancy machinery to solve the problem of human error caused by boredom and fatigue but makes no use of ultra modern technology. To prevent deformed pills from contaminating the pill world, pills whisked down conveyor belts pass by vigilant inspectors who scoop up the sub-standard pills. It's not the most exciting job in the world, but it's important enough not to entrust to an electric eye and a solenoid. True creativity in pill manufacture was evident in a photograph I once saw of a pigeon whose "job" it was to stare down a band of traveling capsules and literally peck out the defectives. Seems like perfect work for a pigeon; my only hope was that he didn't replace a human worker. It's one thing to be replaced by a machine, but imagine being replaced by a pigeon. Perhaps it is the knowledge that he could be replaced by a pigeon that erodes a pharmacist's self-esteem to the point that they are more than three times as likely to commit suicide than the general public.

Today's pageant of pills of every shape and type sport two-tones, vibrant colors, gel caps, fancy logos and inlaid patterns, yet pill manufacturing has changed very little since the old days. Although some methods are new, the biggest difference is a matter of scale.

All pills have common elements. They are all mixtures of active and inactive ingredients. Because the real size of a proper dose is often very small (measured in milligrams and even

UPJOHN'S FRIABLE PILLS

REDUCED TO A POWDER UNDER THE THUMB

fractions of milligrams), a pill that's nothing but medicine would just be too small. A filler or binder is added to hold it together; a "disintegrator," like corn starch, is included to ensure the pill will break open when it comes in contact with digestive juices. Other substances are thrown in to add color and geometry.

Although pills vary in size in comparison to each other, they are all within a certain narrow range. The smallest pill rarely has a length or diameter of less than a quarter inch. The largest pill doesn't exceed three quarters of an inch.

Lined up pill to capsule, a variety of pills look pretty different from each other—a trend in pill design that continues to grow ever since it started sometime in the early '60s. One might expect that pills look different so people don't confuse them and take the wrong medicine. But, as with all things, money enters into the equation. In Japan, where pills are sold primarily by doctors loyal to a particular pharmaceutical company, most pills seem to be round, coated tablets colored either white or red, generally lacking distinguishing marks or imprints.

Historically, Western pills tended to look alike and ordinary—that is to say, round and white, until fairly recently.

In the '60s, pill makers started to make greater use of dye and shape. Capsules got a makeover too, and began sporting festive colors not only on the outside but inside to be shown off through clear gelatin (think Contac's "tiny time pills"). Gelatin melts at body temperature, and is the perfect vessel for holding together powders that can't be compressed into tabs. Gel caps can be tinted to one of some 80,000 color combinations, which serve as identification or help to guard the contents from deterioration.

Some pills are reminiscent of bundt cakes or Twinkies with creamy white fillings. Others are flecked with bright colors, and some are adorned with miniature works of art—such as the tiny horseman on some Burroughs-Wellcome pills.

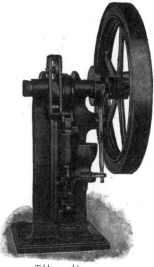

Tablet machine

Although the early '60s *PDR* lacked the color photos so popular with present day pill connoisseurs, such an index can be found in virtually every contemporary pill book.

Today, pill design not only reflects science, but art as well. Faceted edges, arched surfaces, and colors ranging from pastel to carnival-like rainbows all attempt to ensure the consumer that the pill will do the job it's intended to. New antibiotics tend to be fiery shades of red or purple to suggest strength, while anxiolytics (anti-anxiety drugs) are more likely to have soft shapes and pastel colors. Some, like Valium, have a rounded V-shaped hole cut in the middle. This change was made the same year the drug went off patent and generic diazepam began to compete with its parent pill for market share. Valium's characteristic V not only made it easier to identify Valium as "the real thing" but made the pill far more beautiful than any generic competitor. The choice of a heart-shaped V makes one smile just to see the thing.

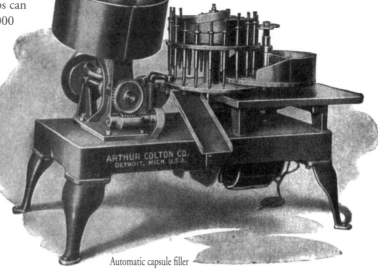

Automatic capsule filler

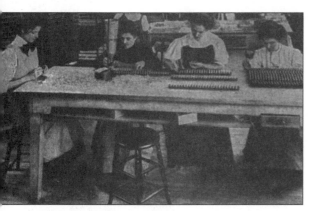
Filling and scaling soft capsules.

A Pill, A Pulvule

Ancient Romans identified ointments and other medicinal substances by marks imprinted into the soft material with the engraved end of a rod. These days pill markings tell the consumer the company that made the pill and what the pill contains. Colors and shapes further serve to identify a pill, but pill design goes further, helping to establish a relationship between the pill and its consumers, including the doctor and pharmacist along with the patient. This kind of identification is worth as much to a pharmaceutical manufacturer as the pill's name or chemical patent.

Pills are not only protected by patents on their ingredients and formulas, and trademarks on their names, shapes and colors—they are also protected by their particular form. For example, Eli Lilly does not sell anything in capsules. The company has instead trademarked their own bullet-shaped capsule they call a "pulvule." I don't know of any real difference between an ordinary gelatin capsule and an Eli Lilly "pulvule"—besides the distinctive bullet-shaped end. A pulvule works the same exact way as an ordinary gelatin capsule. Abbot sells coated-tablets known as "film-tabs," scented with the comforting and familiar smell of baked cookie. These and other pills are time-released—their contents are absorbed incrementally through the stomach. Stomach juice is acidic enough to strip zinc off roofing nails—so it can surely destroy drugs that aren't properly protected.

Enteric-coatings allow pills to pass through the stomach and into the milder environment of the intestines before the drug is released and absorbed into the body. This is also the true function of tiny time pills, which are nothing more than bits of a drug slathered with various densities of coatings so that the pill dissolves over time (the SmithKline pill scientist who invented this "time-released" dosage form says he got his inspiration from jawbreaker candies!) I say "nothing more," but some pills are made up of multiple layers of coating and ingredient. The coating formula changes among the layers, depending on what it is called upon to do. Or not do.

A pill's coating is often its most complex element. Some tablets require as many as 100 successive coatings before they are finished—some for taste, others to protect the medicine, and still others for identification. Each coating must be applied evenly and allowed to set before the next can be applied. This application process can take up to 20 days to complete no matter how swiftly the conveyor belts move.

A happy coincidence in pill manufacturing styles and current therapeutic ideas occurred in the 1960s when pills commonly contained two, three or more different drugs, formulated to work together in concert or in series.

One of the cleverest examples of this multi-tasking pill was a Canadian pill that made extensive use of time-release coatings to guide a person through the night as he slept. The first layer released amyl barbital to rapidly bring on

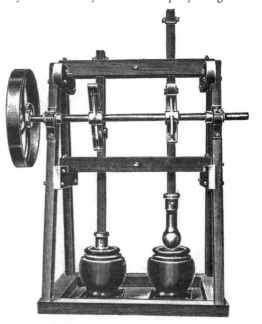
Mechanical mortar.

sleep. Later, the pill let loose a dose of phenobarbital to keep the person sleeping once the
first barbiturate wore off. Next, (hopefully
toward morning) the pill's final coating
dissolved and amphetamines were released
into the system to help the patient wake up.

Pills aren't ready for market once coatings
are applied. They must still be polished and,
using engraving wheels, delicately imprinted
with identifying marks. Then comes another
inspection.

Since the invention of precision, high-speed
production equipment, barrels of pills can
be turned out every hour. This is also true
of less complicated pill designs, like stamped
tablets, even those made with special dyes that
cut designs into pills like Valium or Haldol.

The mass production pill machines of today
are essentially sleek, scaled-up versions of the
clunky machines of yesteryear. Long ago, pharmacists used manual pill-making machines to
form a long rod of intimately mixed drug and
filler. Rolled in a groove on the machine's
surface, this rod (something like a thin roll of
cookie dough) was known as "the pill pipe."
From this standard diameter pipe, the com-
pounder cuts like-sized sections and forms
them into pills between two spatula blades.
Coatings are applied in rotating drums that

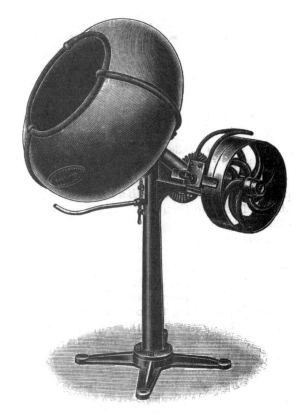

Pill coating pan.

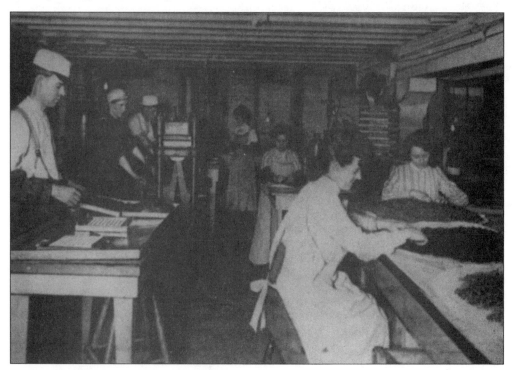

Manufacturing soft gelatin capsules at the turn of the century.

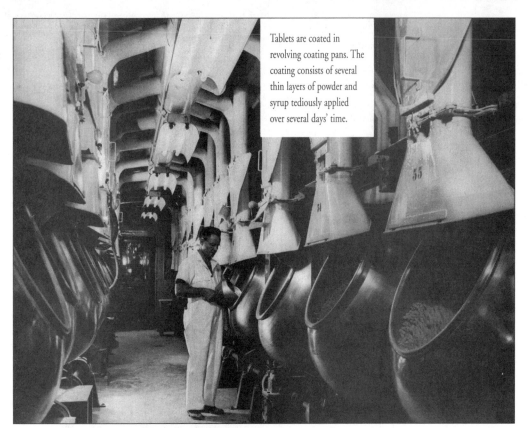

Tablets are coated in revolving coating pans. The coating consists of several thin layers of powder and syrup tediously applied over several days' time.

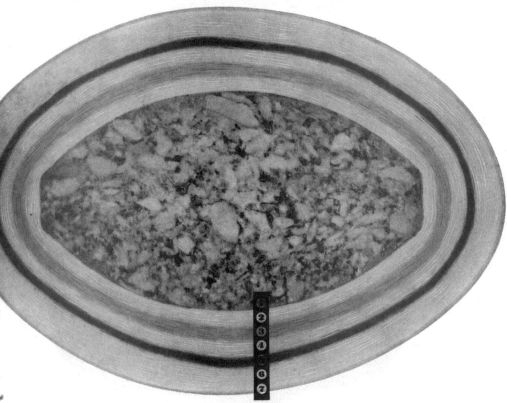

1 Core containing Ferrous Gluconate, Ribo-
   flavin, Nicotinamide, Folic Acid
2·4·6 Protective coatings
3 Layer containing Thiamine Hydrochloride,
   Pyridoxine Hydrochloride, Ascorbic Acid
5 Layer containing vitamin B_{12}
7 Outer coating

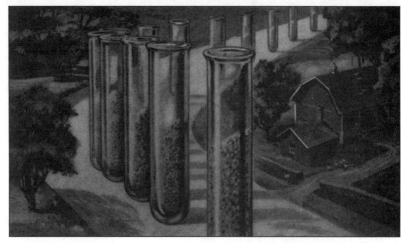

can be as small as a hat or nearly as large as a cement mixer.

Modern pill machines can also make tablets by taking dry granules of active ingredients mixed with binders and, under pressures of four tons or more, squeeze them into hard shapes that will not easily crumble with normal handling, yet still dissolve in the stomach. Such machines can either be hand-operated or switched over to faster, electric automation. Once the operator gets the hang of a pill machine, it's easy to produce thousands of pills an hour. Dye punches in the machine can both score the tablets and imprint letters or numbers into the tablet as it is pressed. Such a machine is small enough to fit in a coat closet.

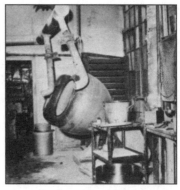

A pill coating machine.

Pill-making machines are difficult to come by today, and their owners must register with the DEA. The DEA has also contemplated restricting the sale of capsule-filling machines, but since such a "machine" can be improvised from a two by four with some holes drilled into it (to hold the capsules while filling) there's not much chance of any serious crackdown, and they continue to be sold in health food stores and by mail order vitamin companies. However, the only empty gelatin capsules a regular citizen is permitted to purchase without government permission are clear. For colors, you need a license.

At one time, pill-making was something of an artisan's craft, and pharmacists took pride in their skills. The mixtures had to be absolutely correct and each pill as nearly identical to the other as possible. Even today some pharmacy schools require pharmacists to learn how to make not only pills, but syrups, elixirs and other dosage forms—although they will probably never have use for them.

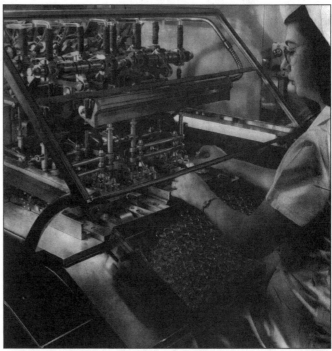

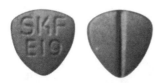

Sterile vials filled and sealed.

The Strange Case of George Bush and Eli Lilly

Bush was practically a secret employee of Eli Lilly while both Vice-President and President, and very obviously did specific work on Lilly's behalf. Lilly tried to deny all of this (including Bush's stint on their Board of Directors) when *Pills-a-Go-Go* researched the matter. Alexander Cockburn cited *PaGG* articles on this and other subjects in his *Nation* column, "Beat the Devil."

In March of 1992, President Bush suddenly announced that the $4 billion genetic-engineering industry could grow to $50 billion by the end of the decade "if we let it." To help "let it," the administration proposed speeding the FDA's approval process for biotech drugs only.

But since biotech drugs don't grind through the approval system any more slowly than other pharmaceuticals, why should the president single them out?

The answer is easy! The administration's move is a payoff to an old friend —Eli Lilly. It is not the first time the President put himself on the line for the Indianapolis drug manufacturer—George Bush and Eli Lilly worked together for two decades, perhaps even longer, depending on when you figure Bush's career there really began.

Lilly has had a special relationship with the backroom aspects of government ever since it obtained the rights to manufacture and market methadone, the synthetic narcotic invented by the Germans during World War II. Essentially war spoils, Lilly continues as the country's largest producer of methadone (brand name Dolophine) for use in hospitals, junkie clinics, and where ever else federal money flows in as funding.

In 1953, when LSD's inventor Albert Hoffman would not supply the CIA with his new compound for use in their mind experiments, Lilly began making acid for the agency. It even devised a method to mass produce the stuff and seriously discussed the possibility of manufacturing it by the ton, for use as a battlefield weapon.

Given this kind of coziness with spooks and the military it's not surprising that in 1977, after Jimmy Carter fired Bush as head of the CIA, Lilly promptly put him on their board of directors. Although Bush had no experience in pharmaceuticals and, indeed, no particular business expertise beyond running CIA front company, Zapata Oil, he "worked" for Lilly for the next two years.

Bush fails to include this in his official biography. Lilly, too, seems to want to forget the whole thing. According to the corporation's librarian, Bush has never worked there! Eventually one spokesman for Lilly admitted Bush had been on the payroll, but refused further comment. The matter, for all practical purposes, remains secret.

George Bush conveniently forgot about his job at Eli Lilly in 1979 when he began running for President the first time. He sought to cover his Lilly assets by omitting them on his financial disclosure form, thus concealing more than $80,000 worth of stock he had in the company. He even went so far as to claim he had divested himself of all Lilly stock in 1978. When he got caught in the lie, his lawyer regretted the "factual inaccuracy" and Bush pressed on as Lilly's secret employee—by now in the guise of Vice-President of the United States. He used this position to lobby the government to lower taxes on Lilly's Puerto Rican investments. At that very same time the IRS was getting aggressive with Lilly in seeking hundreds of millions of dollars it said the company had avoided paying by pretending those profits had been generated in tax-sheltered Puerto Rico. Bush eventually made such a pest of himself, hectoring the state department, that the Supreme Court issued an order to him to abandon his lobbying efforts, as they were illegal.

As luck would have it, Bush's actions may have been illegal but the law specifically exempts both the President and the Vice President from prosecution in such conflict-of-interest cases. In the end, Bush kept his job and Lilly kept the tax shelter. The grateful company continued its heavy financing of the Republican party. It also helped finance Dan Quayle, who had "come from nowhere" to serve as Bush's second in command when Bush became President in 1988. One of Quayle's aides on the Vice President's Competitiveness Council also owns a sizable chunk of Lilly stock.

So it's not surprising that Quayle's Council should recommend certain alterations in the FDA drug approval process—especially in ways that were sure to benefit Eli Lilly in particular. Just to be positive it all worked out though, Lilly executives did conduct a secret meeting with the Council just before the Vice President emerged with his new recommendations to relax pollution controls on one of Indiana's largest polluters (Lilly) and to make crucial changes in the FDA handling of biotech drugs.

Bush and Quayle might not otherwise have stuck their necks out so far for Lilly if it weren't that the company was in the midst of a massive shift in direction to save itself from an ever-bleaker future. Lilly knew if things didn't get better in the early '90s, the company could have found itself in serious trouble.

For one thing, Lilly had no new drugs "in the pipeline." While other pharmaceutical companies were introducing new drugs at an unprecedented rate, Lilly still had only Prozac, which accounted for an enormous percentage of the company's entire earnings. Competitors to Prozac were already coming over the walls, and Prozac was dealing with some 60 lawsuits and the negative publicity they caused. The Church of Scientology launched a ferocious and effective media attack on the pill and Prozac was in trouble.

For another thing, the FDA had inspected Lilly at least nine times in the preceding three years and cited the company for improper manufacturing practices, failure to file timely reports with the government and—contamination problems in its cherished Puerto Rico facilities. The company's stock was falling hard. In May of '92 *Barron's* went so far as to advise its readers to avoid Lilly stock, even though it promoted optimistic investment in a number of other pharmaceutical companies.

To save the company, Lilly had begun to buy up impoverished biotech firms with promising but under-funded projects while dumping its more traditional moneymakers. For instance, in exchange for its worldwide capsule manufacturing operation (Qualicaps) Lilly got the rights to sell its human insulin in Japan. Quite an interesting trade for a "conservative" company.

It began to invest in a small North Carolina research firm to research a biotech drug delivery system. Lilly money is even behind the ultra-cool "Shaman Pharmaceuticals," which makes its money by stealing the recipes of South American medicine men and working out patents for them.

Kickbacks Sometimes Kick Back

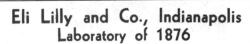

Like any industry, pharmaceutical corporations pay off people who push their wares with giveaways, paraphernalia, even vacations. But it seems the pharmaceutical corporations do it with remarkable panache. All those rubber character dolls, pens, clocks, CDs, not to mention those cabinets full of free medication and trips even as far away as Antarctica so that doctors can do their "professional homework."

Eli Lilly came under fire in April, 1993, for a three to four million dollar advertising blitz encouraging the public to seek professional help for depression. Half-a-million went to a Virginia nonprofit organization to conduct a nine-month public education campaign to identify potential candidates for treatment. The "public service" campaign was seen as a way to gain new patients for the world's bestselling antidepressant, Prozac, which, in case you forgot, is manufactured by Lilly.

The FDA accused Genetech, in its charitable, nonprofit Human Growth Foundation, of conducting a bogus health program in which they screened children in public schools for potential shortness to drum up business for the growth hormone, Protropin.

Hoffman La-Roche agreed to pay the government $450,000 as a settlement against allegations it paid kickbacks to physicians through the use of bogus "research grants." The grants, which ranged from $500 to $2,500, were nice payoffs to doctors who prescribed the intravenous antibiotic Rocephin.

The Massachusetts Attorney General accused the pharm firm Rugby Group, Inc. for offering a variety of travel packages, including a four day, three night "Vacation Celebration" to Disneyland and Las Vegas once $6,000 worth of pills were purchased. Rugby Group was fined a few grand.

Eli Lilly and Co., Indianapolis
Laboratory of 1876

"On May 10, 1876, with cash capital amounting to seven hundred dollars and goods . . amounting to six hundred dollars, Colonel Lilly [having operated drugstores before and after the Civil War] opened a small laboratory on an Indianapolis side street . . . The laboratory equipment was very simple . . . A small engine that had seen service on a little steam ferry boat, furnished the power." (*Tile and Till*, 12: 30, 1926.)

The effective and selfless part played by Eli Lilly in the development of insulin from a test tube product to a reliable and marketable preparation will always remain one of the outstanding deeds of American pharmaceutical industry.

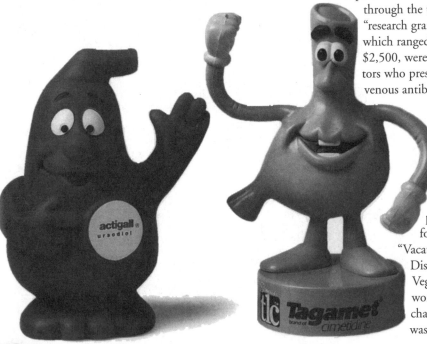

CIBA-Gygy paid out $200,000 and agreed to donate free pills to welfare programs when they were nabbed for another sort of kickback scheme.

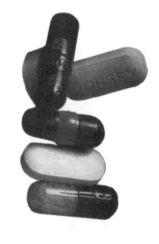

The "Me, Too" Pills

Commercials make them seem like America's No. 1 complaint. The commercials. The remedies. Headaches are at once common and inscrutable. There's no way to clinically prove they even happen, but they are real. Some headaches might not even exist as "problems" until we learn to see them that way. Some pills for headaches are taken as a response to something that is psychically painful but not headache-producing—stress. In the end, stress is the condition most often portrayed on headache remedy ads. These ads don't show someone bumping their head on a car door, or dealing with a mighty hangover. They depict people in stressful situations—a car full of screaming kids, a demanding boss, a flat tire—situations where a headache is hardly unavoidable.

When speaking of headaches and pills, this would be as good a place as any to remark on the enormous government bureaucracy that governs pills—and the headaches it creates for all of us. Government control over pill-making has resulted in a colossal waste of energy and brainpower. Scientists, chemists, and businesspeople divert too much energy to spend time trying to copy some other company's formula without violating the patent (producing what is known as a "me too" drug) or in creative marketing, finding ways to make a pill more profitable by issuing it as several different pills for a variety of ailments—thereby possibly extending a patent or receiving government money for "orphan drug" research. This is known as "salami slicing."

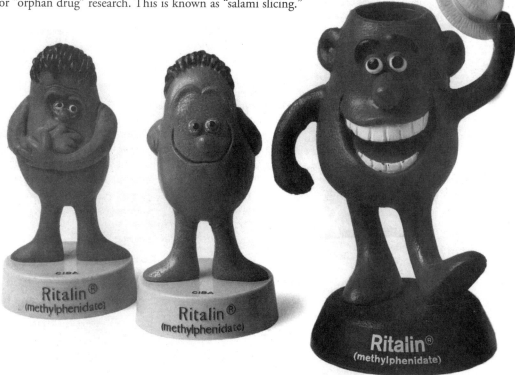

The pill world's law-ridden atmosphere has caused companies to "invent" more than 82 types of benzodiazepines to compete with Valium and all its variants. Ibuprofen, now just a ho-hum pill found in supermarkets has spawned a good 50 or so imitating NSAIDs. There are 57 varieties of penicillin and 42 kinds of cephalosporin antibiotics either on the market now or under development. This kind of research results in an enormous duplication of effort but does have a payoff—however minimal.

For instance, the introduction of SmithKline's Tagamet—the H2 antagonist that revolutionized ulcer treatment and quickly became the country's number-one selling pill—caused other companies to hurry and whip up their own brands. From this research came Zantac, which proved to be not only more powerful, milligram for milligram, but did not interfere nearly as much with the absorption of other drugs the way Tagamet can. Merck then introduced Pepcid, which turned out to be even stronger and so lacking in side effects, it was the first to be sold over-the-counter. On the other hand, Eli Lilly's me-too version of Zantac (called Axid) was simply sold at a lower price to get its small slice of the H2 antagonist market, even a sliver of which is worth an armada of Brinks trucks stuffed with gold bullion. Recently the price of Axid has risen, as intensive marketing by a small consortium of drug companies (including Roche and Glaxo) gained the pill a larger following.

Another slight good caused by this enormous investigation and development of new classes of compounds is the way it serves to broaden the clinical knowledge of any one of them. When a pill spawns a few dozen clones, the compound is in effect being tested many times more than would otherwise be the case. Research like this may turn up slight differences which could matter a whole lot to some patients, even if those groups are small. As we all know when you are the person who needs relief, no effort is really too great to provide it.

Still, government patent laws and overly stringent FDA testing requirements tend to hinder vigorous research into and development of new pills. The invention of a new "blockbuster" drug is the dream of every pharmaceutical company, but it is not without costs. Even though the successful development of such a pill can just blow away the competition in a particular therapeutic market (thus securing big profits for the company that makes it), there is only a limited amount of time to recoup the cost.

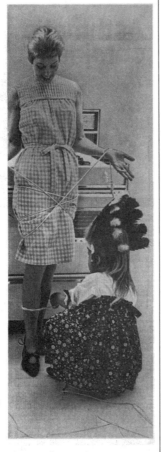

Since the U.S. government, and governments of other countries around the world typically require patents to be filed early in the development process of creating a drug, problems arise. Patents generally don't last more than 20 years, and a company may find it has only eight or 10 years to profit on its investment, an investment that is said to average a quarter of a billion dollars. Developing a new drug is wildly expensive, it entails a lot of false starts (the search for Tagamet involved the extensive development and testing of more than 10,000 substances). And there is no guarantee it will pay off.

The next danger is "poaching." As soon as a patent is filed, other companies are able to use the now public information to begin their own copycat research. A lot of work has been done for them by this time and they might just beat the originators of an idea to the lucrative punch. If nothing else, a competing company can see what their rivals are up to and, if they happen to be working in the same areas, the technical information gathered from a patent can save loads of research time and effort.

It is not surprising that pharmaceutical companies don't typically spend much on progressive R&D into new, virgin areas. It's too risky. Innovative research is simply not as profitable as short-sighted investigations into copycat drugs. For a pharmaceutical company it makes far more sense to duke it out in the pain-relief or estrogen replacement markets with a marginally different pill sporting a new and improved label. Miracle pills just don't pay off. Potential winnings are just as great as the lottery, but the odds aren't as bad.

Even for breakthrough drugs, it is ironic how often and how close

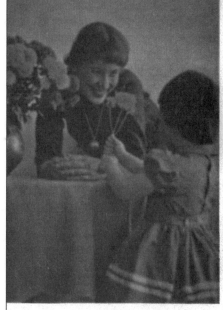

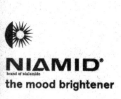

NIAMID
brand of nialamide
the mood brightener

Now you can treat the underlying cause of many imaginary ills

When ills turn out to be imaginary, depression usually is the cause of annoying symptoms. In many such instances, NIAMID can raise the patient's spirits, free her from the doldrums of imaginary disease, and renew her interest in friends and family.

NIAMID treats the underlying cause of many depressive syndromes, occurring alone or complicating a physical disorder. This effect appears to be achieved by restoring neurohormone balance. Response to the gradual, gentle action of NIAMID begins within a few days in some patients, and in most other patients within two or three weeks.

An exceptionally well tolerated antidepressant—more than 500,000 prescriptions in many clinical conditions—more than 90 published papers.

NIAMID is supplied as 25 and 100 mg. scored tablets. A Professional Information Booklet is available on request from the Medical Department, Pfizer Laboratories, Div., Chas. Pfizer & Co., Inc., Brooklyn 6, New York.

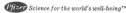 *Pfizer Science for the world's well-being™*

blockbuster pills come to being killed off. Sometimes, funding death for miracle pills have been scheduled just a few months before their successful completion. This is precisely the case with Tagamet, and its inventor, James Black.

Dr. James Black first made a name for himself when he invented the beta blocker propanalol for ICI (now Zeneca). Black's propanalol project came within weeks of having its funding cut off before Black was able to prove his then-revolutionary theories in drug development. The drug soon became a gold standard in anti-hypertensives. And the theories behind its development promised more of the same

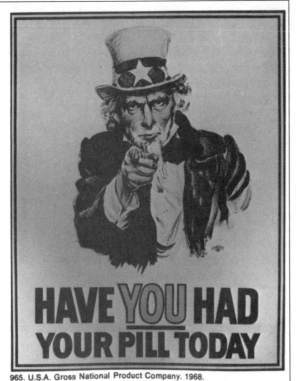

HAVE **YOU** HAD YOUR PILL TODAY

965. U.S.A. Gross National Product Company. 1968.

kind of blockbuster pill. Naturally Black was eager to use his techniques to go after other types of drugs to treat other medical conditions. But ICI, happy to have its breakthrough propanalol, wanted Black to develop yet another beta blocker—in effect creating their own "me-too" drug to compete with the ones they knew were sure to follow. While this made economic sense, it had little allure for a scientist like Black, who promptly accepted an offer by SmithKline to come work on an ulcer drug for them.

SmithKline planned to axe Black's funding for his new drug research because it soaked up "too much money." Luckily, Black had been careful with his budget, got in under the wire and discovered cimetidine (Tagamet) just weeks before the money ran out. ⬤▬

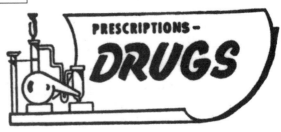

PRESCRIPTIONS – **DRUGS**

tense, anxious, jittery, emotionally "bushed"

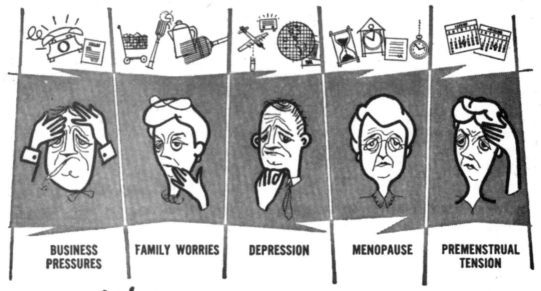

| BUSINESS PRESSURES | FAMILY WORRIES | DEPRESSION | MENOPAUSE | PREMENSTRUAL TENSION |

USE safe, modern, relaxant-sedative

According to the Pharmaceutical Manufacturer's Association, 48 drugs were introduced between 1962 and 1984 that were later found to have an additional 82 indications which won eventual approval from the FDA. Forty-eight pills with 130 uses. This statistic hints at the number of uses for a pill that the FDA does not officially sanction, but which doctors nonetheless use to treat their patients.

Still, the AMA is worried about a recent FDA policy to "get tough" on drugs prescribed for unapproved uses. At least 400 million of the 1.6 billion prescriptions written by U.S. doctors every year are for treatments that lack FDA approval. So far, this is perfectly legal. Not all companies can afford the expensive process for getting FDA approval for every "claim" a drug can make. Still, the word gets out, and this is what the FDA has vowed to prevent. Unapproved uses for a pill have now become unapproved information.

We know, from our own pharmacopeia, that many drugs can do more than one thing. Vasopressin, for instance, helps with diabetes and memory loss. Aspirin, as we now recognize, not only relieves pain, it prevents heart attacks, strokes, and colon cancer. What else can it do? Oh yeah, it can lower fevers. Anything else?

The government's policy of restricting information about all the things for which a particular drug can be used means you, the pillhound, may have to inform your own doctor. Here are a few pills that do more than one thing.

- Propanolol lowers blood pressures, halts "stage fright" and can prevent some migraine headaches.

- Phenytoin is useful for both epileptic convulsions and OCD. This last discovery was made decades ago and a whole foundation devoted to researching the stuff was endowed by a millionaire who also wrote a book about Dilantin called *A Remarkable Drug Has Been Overlooked.*

- Clonidine lowers blood pressures and diminishes narcotic withdrawal symptoms.

- Ritalin works as an anti-depressant, treats narcolepsy, attention deficit disorder, and is useful for Alzheimer's patients.

- Imodium AD, an over-the-counter diarrhea medicine is another pill that halts the pain of heroin withdrawal and is far, far cheaper than methadone. It is also far, far less abusable. It also has some analgesic effects.

- A mixture of a B vitamin and doxylamine succinate (the ingredient in the OTC sleeping pill, Unisom) are the same ingredients as the banned pill Benedictin. Benedictin was developed as a safe medication for pregnant women to take to stave off the persistent nausea that can go along with growing a fetus. But as it turns out, Benedictin was banned based on fake experiments by the same guy (Australian doc William McBride) who discovered Thalidomide's horrific effects. The doc turned to fraud "in the broader interests of humanity," he said.

Pills That Do More Than One Thing

- Thalidomide, on the other hand, is seeing a rebirth of therapeutic use as it shows remarkable effectiveness in diseases from lupus to leprosy.

- Quinine pills stave off malaria and relieve leg cramps. Too bad they're banned now. According to the FDA quinine doesn't really relieve leg cramps.

- Amitryptaline relieves depression and enhances the effects of analgesics.

Caffeine gets you going, makes you score better on intelligence tests, and is a diuretic. It can also halt migraine headaches.

Monoxidil lowers blood pressure and grows hair.

Nitroglycerin relieves angina pain and is a high explosive convenient for demolishing buildings or certain kinds of mining. Mixed with clay, it's dynamite!

Aspirin does everything. Good for headaches, colon cancer, heart attacks, it keeps cut flowers fresh a day longer, reduces a woman's risk of developing pregnancy-induced hypertension by 65%, reduces the risk of delivering severely low weight babies by 44% and it, too, can be made into an explosive.

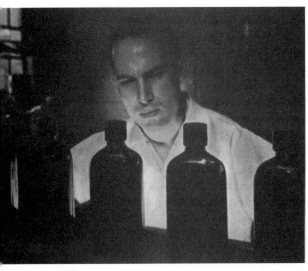

Vitamin C improves body tissues, fights colds, is a potent antioxidant and is also a diuretic. In fact, all vitamins do more than one thing.

Ex Lax's active ingredient, phenopthalein, is now banned, but for years it was a popular brand of laxative. Now it's back to its other use: the color-changing chemical in litmus paper that indicates the pH of things.

Codeine stops pain, coughs, and narcolepsy.

Benedryl is used to treat hay fever, Parkinson's, and insomnia.

Phenobarbital is a sedative and anti-convulsant.

Dexedrine makes you lose weight, treats Parkinsonism, head injury and other trauma to the nervous system.

Klonapin (clonazapam) treats convulsions, anxiety, and greatly enhances the effects of heroin.

Colchicine is a treatment for gout and for causing genetic mutations in plants, it can't be beat!

Depakote (valproic acid) is the only drug besides Lithium carbonate deemed suitable as a treatment for bi-polar disease (manic depression). It is also a preventive for migraine headaches.

Claritin is a non-sedating anti-histamine that's also been approved as a treatment for hives.

Ibuprofen, an OTC NSAID analgesic, seems to help Alzheimer's patients.

Mellaril is another do-anything drug. It stops hiccups. It stops raging schizophrenia. It can make you feel less sad when you break up with your girlfriend or boyfriend.

Cyclosporine, a fine immunosuppressant, anti-rejection drug used by organ transplant recipients, is also good for treating severe psoriasis.

The combination of two pills—misoprostol, (an ulcer medication known as Cytotek), and methotrexate (an anti-cancer hormone drug) causes an abortion in eight out of ten women. It is even possible to use misoprostol alone, especially if the pill is placed directly into the uterus.

Birth control pills not only prevent conception, but can cause an abortion as long as

72 hours after the deed has been done. Abortion is effected when a woman takes a two tablet dose twice, 12 hours apart. This is information that is especially suppressed by the authorities.

● Estrogen was proven to reduce heart disease by 40% in a group of 46,000 post-menopausal women studied for 10 years.

● RU-486 is not just an "abortion pill," it could also be called the "healthy uterus pill," since a small study of 12 women in France showed a marked reduction in uterine fibroid tumors. Other researchers think it could be used to treat at least two kinds of cancer. The pill also has the potential to become a once-a-month birth control pill.

● The ulcer medication, Tagamet (cimetidine), is now a therapy for warts. Docs think the pill's tendency to strengthen the body's immune system is what makes it effective against the virus that causes warts: human papillomavirus (HPV).

● The anti-herpes pill, Zovirax, is a good pill for chicken pox, healing it a day or so faster and with less fever, itchiness, and fewer pox. Zovirax is helpful in treating spinal meningitis and appears to double the survival rates of AIDS patients being treated with AZT.

● The anti-depressant Wellbutrin, also marketed under the name Zyban, can help people stop smoking.

● Buproprion is an amphetamine and has many effects. One of them is to increase libido—more so in women than men. In women the pill appears to enhance frequency and intensity of orgasms, too.

● Is Valium a miracle pill or what? Like a lot of drugs, Valium is now considered useful for ailments the makers never dreamed of. Valium accomplished something no other drug has even come close to—bringing a man out of an eight-year-long coma.

After a car accident ten years earlier, a Wisconsin man (a former airline pilot) remained unconscious for three long months before he began to stir. Although his family undoubtedly prayed this was a sign he was getting better, he degenerated into a persistent vegetative state. This condition was much like a coma except that the person continued to go through waking and sleeping cycles, make facial expressions, move limbs, and occasionally "utter words." Maddeningly, all these seemingly conscious gestures were unrelated to the world around the person. They were simply random reflexes or movements. Vegetative states are considered by many doctors to be grounds for removing life support systems as the person is for all intents and purposes, dead. They do not see, speak, hear.

But something remarkable happened to the 45-year-old (still unidentified) motorist on March 12, 1990 when, sedating him for a routine dental operation, docs injected the man with liquid Valium. He soon fell asleep and stayed asleep for five minutes. Suddenly he awakened. But instead of being a vegetable, he shocked those around him by being able to say his name, read, write, do math problems and carry on intelligent conversations. He could even walk with assistance!

Then he lapsed back into his coma.

Another shot brought him around again. This time he remained lucid for 90 minutes, discussing his family, his former workplace, and for the first time in years, he was feeding himself. Then it was back to oblivion as the Valium wore off.

Doctors continued experimenting with Valium and other, longer-lasting benzodiazepines until the man remained awake and clear-headed for as much as 10–12 hours at a time.

No more information about this man has appeared in the press since April, 1990 when it was first reported at the University Hospital and clinics in Madison, Wisconsin.

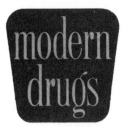

modern drugs

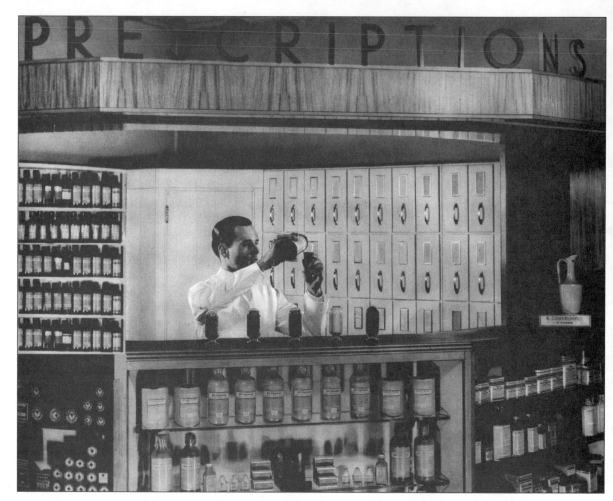

The Tormented Mind
of the Pharmacist

"You know, I hate pharmacists. Doctors are just dumb. If they write, they're dumb for believing your story. If they don't write they're dumb for not believing your story. But pharmacists are evil. They have a special ability to see right through a dope fiend. They can tell instantly, just by looking at a prescription, whether it was written in response to a story you concocted. They give you these withering looks . . . . If I ever get off narcotics I'm never going to speak to a pharmacist as long as I live."

—Eric Detzer, former junkie, in his book, *Poppies.*

Pillhounds are not only the ones who hate the pharmacist. Practically everybody else hates the pharmacist, too. In turn, he hates everyone back and, for that brief moment when he is in charge of your medical treatment, will jack you around out of pure spite.

He challenges your prescription, he makes you wait an extra half-hour, he makes you talk out loud about your medical problems. He makes you sit up and beg.

A pharmacist shuffling papers behind his altar-like counter won't even look up when you arrive. He won't even grunt before he's good and ready to peer down at you and acknowledge your existence.

And then, no double-talk, he wants to see that prescription. Hmm, you got the clap don'tcha? Prozac, eh? Don't look depressed to me. Isn't it a little early for you to be refilling this codeine? In fact, I'm not sure you should have any more codeine.

Once they've got the script, they can make you grovel.

How did the pharmacist become so odious? Does pharmacy simply attract people who like to seethe with inner malice while maintaining a stony facade? Are they born this way or does something happen to them?

There is no evidence that pharmacists have a genetic problem. Like sadistic prison guards, pharmacists are largely creations of their surroundings. Something about the job does it to them.

To understand what you and your measly prescription look like to the pharmacist, it's crucial to have an understanding of his constant anger; the anger born of being hoodwinked and conned, soaked and hung out to dry—with only his gullibility to blame.

A pharmacist's soul is a hundred times more embarrassed than any sap taken to the cleaner's in Vegas. His self-esteem is more acutely wounded than a town full of jilted lovers. All the land sold in Florida cannot have caused the pain a single pharmacist feels by the time you see him there among the pills.

The Big Scam

It probably doesn't take more than one day on the job to show a newly-minted pharmacist that he or she has been tricked. Pharmacy school is rough—you can't get through it without advanced calculus, chemistry and super dedication. Pharmacy school lasts five years. And it costs a lot.

No one would endure pharmacy school for the chance to count pills, let alone to be hated by customers and held in contempt by doctors. So, to make students cram pharmacokinetics (which they will never use on the job), the school outright lies to them. It promises that they will be liked. This is the opposite of reality, of course, which just makes the hoax crueler. Here are students who want to be liked and valued by the community, and slave away for respectability and honor they will never get.

Pharmacy schools promise an esteemed position in medicine, in society even. Students are told again and again about the high degree of trust placed upon pharmacists by patients and doctors. They see pictures of kindly people in smooth coats holding up test-tubes or being beamed at by reassured old ladies. They are shown photocopies of a folklorish survey rating how certain professions are trusted. As they are told, pharmacists are only a notch or two below Supreme Court Justice—and far above a doctor.

As a pharmacist, they learn, "You Are Trusted."

The Sucker Punch

Of course, the reality of pharmacy is that it is a service industry, not much different than a dry cleaner. Pharmacists are not pillars of the community, they are pill-counters and stock boys. And respect? Please.

Instead of being part of a benevolent triangle of medical care, the pharmacist finds himself at the raw end of an abusive process nobody likes.

Here's where you, the consumer, come in.

Customers arrive at the pharmacy because they have been hurt or are sick. They have already made the trek to the doctor's office, lost a day of work, been kept waiting and charged a hundred bucks to spend three minutes with a doctor who hands them a piece of paper. Now they have taken the bus to the drugstore and are about to be appalled by the money they are going to shell out to a grump behind a counter so high it makes them feel like a three-year-old.

Pharmacy customers are not happy to be there. They aren't happy, period. Nothing the pharmacist does is going to make them happy. But, too bad, the pharmacist isn't all that content himself. He's been swindled so badly he's never going to trust anyone again. Since old people take the most medicine, the majority of his customers are old people—cranky old people who complain about prices and ask the same stupid questions a thousand times a day. This is just more gravel in the pharmacist's shoes.

The collision between a sick, ripped-off patient and a tired, ripped-off pharmacist is as predictable, and mean, as a cockfight. The customer grumbles at the pharmacist and asks some ridiculous question. The phone is ringing. People standing in line start clearing their throats. The pharmacist slows down, shoots a few withering looks, then doles out the pills. Sufficiently abased, customers begin to limp home—finally. The pharmacist counts pills and waits for more abuse.

There are no test-tubes in sight. No mortar and pestles, no hand-in-hand work with the doctor. In fact, there are no real prescriptions anymore. A clerk in a pizza joint has a more complex job than a pharmacist.

Doctors prescribe ready-made medicines, often by brand name. Doctors decide if a generic can be substituted. The pharmacist just gets the right bottle of pills and starts counting. A pigeon could do the pharmacist's job. There is no pharmacological expertise going on in a pharmacy. All those nights of midnight oil, learning absorption rates of alkenes into mucous membranes means nothing now. That was just the price for a pill-selling license. The pharmacy school didn't breathe a word of this.

Neither did the pharmacy school teach practical skills the pharmacist actually needs. They don't teach how to run a cash register or catch shoplifters or even things related to pills. Pill identification for example. Pharmacy students can draw the molecular structure of a drug, but cannot visually ID or even name the top 20 or 100 drugs they will sell.

Of course, as years grind by under fluorescent lights, behind a silly counter, the pharmacist eventually learns all this. But it's all on-the-job and self-taught.

Then there's pill-counting—the most obvious part of pharmacy drudgery. Just how much organic chemistry is necessary to count pills? This is even more humiliating since the number of pills in a bottle are often counted by mechanical devices; and if they're not, it's a job a pigeon could do quite well. It's also something the old bag snapping about high prices can and will check.

Pharmacists are not taught to read doctor handwriting, which really and truly is bad. Despite the jokes, inability to read doctors' handwriting can lead to serious mistakes. People have been killed by script fuck-ups and pharmacists commonly misdispense drugs because of errors in reading the prescription. Then they get sued and kicked out of the business forever.

Calling the doctor's office for clarification of a prescription just makes the pharmacist a pest. The receptionist treats him as an irritant. The doctor treats him as an idiot. Should the pharmacist have any other "problems" with a prescription, he comes dangerously close to questioning the doctor's wisdom. It's bad enough to be an idiot, it's even worse to be a loathsome pipsqueak. The brittle ego of a pharmacist cannot risk calling a doctor every time he thinks there's something wrong with a script.

On the other hand, the drudgery of pharmacy makes catching fake scripts practically the only "fun" thing about being a pharmacist. Other "fun" things open to a pharmacist are diverting drugs, selling stolen drugs and dealing controlled substances illegally. These guys still keep a sharp eye out for fake scripts—but, according to whim, they just might not call the cops if they see one.

Then again, as law enforcement begins paying attention to pharmacists, enlisting their help in the war on drugs, the police may be the only source of feelgood a pharmacist has. But in their broken little hearts, most pharmacists know it is futile to call the cops on a single guy and won't even bother. Hell, they might just fill the damn thing.

Minor Superpowers of The Pharmacist

Pharmacists in many states have the power to self-prescribe. In practice this means the pharmacist ends up prescribing to family and friends, so for whatever it's worth, a pharmacist is allowed to decide if he should take an antibiotic or not.

Although severely restricted compared to a couple decades ago, pharmacists still retain vestiges of a right to refill a prescription without contacting a doctor. Before 1970, refills were still the province of the patient and pharmacist. A doctor merely prescribed a medication and a regime. It was up to the patient to comply. One prescription was essentially good for life.

Of course, if a doctor complains to proper authorities, the pharmacist gets suspended and fined. This happens almost exclusively when little old hunchbacked ladies come in to get more heart pills and the pharmacist goes ahead and refills the damn thing, knowing she's gonna be on that med the rest of her life. When the doctor discovers this, he may get insulted and retaliate against the pharmacist.

A pharmacist may have the statutory right to prescribe certain medications to the public at large. In practice, this is almost never done because of the severity of punishment should some authority be brought down to investigate.

In a sick kind of way, the very fact that pharmacists ever get busted for selling medicines to people who have convinced them they need a certain drug betrays their essential soft-heartedness. Instead of being seen as a positive trait, this trace of mercy in their souls makes them perfect targets.

Just to torment pharmacists some more, *60 Minutes* once sent a team of middle-aged, well-dressed and well-spoken women with out-of-town IDs to pharmacies around Washington, DC, and had them beg the pharmacist to give them just a few days' supply of Valium since they had forgotten their's back home.

Lo and behold, some pharmacists went so far as to dispense a few days' worth of the (at-the-time) number one selling drug to a person who, from all outward appearances, was not only a typical patient for Valium, but verging on hysteria. A believable story and supporting identification clinched it.

60 Minutes sent their women all over town and managed to collect a stock of Valium which they dramatically poured into a little pile in front of the camera declaring with shock an outrage that such a "haul" was possible.

Why didn't they send in scrungy men with three-day beards and no coherent story to get the pills? Why didn't they try for a more controlled drug or one that was less popular? Because tabloid news needed to torment a tormented mind even a bit further.

Rude Pharmacists

One of those Smug, Jr. detective pharmacists finally got his ass fired for constantly challenging customers' prescriptions. Now he's using the police to force his old employer to give his job back.

Because Salt Lake City pill-counter, Jim Ryan, was getting paid $27.85 an hour, the store manager didn't think it was cool for him to waste so much time on the phone double-checking nearly every pre-scription. Besides lollygagging on the phone, he was rude to customers who took offense at his mean behavior.

"When you have a low-volume store," said the manager, "you can't afford to lose any customers at all."

Despite Ryan's antics he only managed to help police catch no more than five script forgers in two years.

But cops love him. "Jim Ryan was just following the law and he gets fired for it," one of them griped.

Ryan, who was fired else-where for rude treatment of customers, had another angle on the problem.

"There hasn't been a phar-macy robbery in years." he mewled, "because people know they can call or steal a pad from the doctor and bring it into the pharmacy . . . that's how critical this problem is."

Huh? A lack of crime proves how "critical" the situation is?

The American Pharmacist's Professional Oath:

At this time, I vow to devote my professional life to the serv-ice of mankind through the profession of pharmacy. I will consider the welfare of human-ity and relief of human suffer-ing my primary concerns. I will use my knowledge and skills to the best of my ability in serv-ing the public and other health professionals. I will do my best to keep abreast of develop-ments and maintain profes-sional competency in my pro-fession of pharmacy. I will obey the laws governing the practice of pharmacy and will support enforcement of such laws. I will maintain the highest stan-dards of moral and ethical con-duct. I take these vows volun-tarily with the full realization of the trust and responsibility with which I am empowered by the public.

common *Pharmacist* errors

Typing errors
Wrong quantity
Wrong drug
Wrong strength/dosage form
Wrong dosage calculated
Wrong directions
Intellectual errors
Deteriorated drug
Monitoring errors
Compliance

—from U.S. Pharmacist-NABP State Boards, 1994, Eckerd Drug Co., Prescription Error Prevention

Gray's Prescriptionist

❧ REVISED ❧

℞

CONTAINS fac-simile copies of Physicians' odd, unique and obscure prescriptions, with methods of procedure to properly compound the same; Tables of abbreviations, Latin directions, weights and measures, metric prescriptions, doses, poisons and antidotes, etc; Short, concise directions for making ointments, cerates, pills, suppositories, emulsions, etc. A

Hand Book

for prescription clerks, being designed for and specially needed by those who have not had a college course and city experience in dispensing. Bound in cloth. Sent postpaid on receipt of

$1.50

M. M. Gray & Company, Publishers,

P. O. Box 593...CHICAGO, ILL.

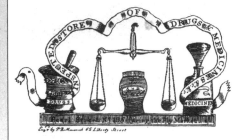

This engraving, now the Seal of the American Institute of the History of Pharmacy, was done about 1800 by the renowned American artist Peter Ruston Maverick (1755–1811), for Jacob Schieffelin, ancestor of William J. Schieffelin, Jr., President of Schieffelin & Company, wholesale druggist, New York City.

Bad Pharmacist Stories Online

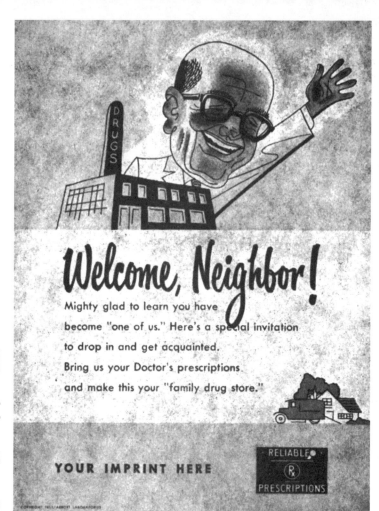

Welcome, Neighbor!

Mighty glad to learn you have become "one of us." Here's a special invitation to drop in and get acquainted. Bring us your Doctor's prescriptions and make this your "family drug store."

YOUR IMPRINT HERE

RELIABLE PRESCRIPTIONS

> I have used it for my own refills. The ones that do have refills, no prob, unless it's too soon since the last refill. If there aren't any refills left, then they have to call the doc. It's in their computer system. Been there, done that.

> The Pharmacist at my local Walgreens is very skeptical of me anyway. My dentist left it blank for refills for 20 Lorcets and I being a newbie . . . filled it in with 3 refills and got BUSTED by the Pharmacist. I had just left the dentist after having some major stuff done and could barely talk. So I cried a bit and he said, as he wadded up the script and threw it at me, "I should call the cops." Scared the shit outta me. Haven't been back there since. I straightened out the wadded up script and wrote over the 3, a big Zero and took it to K-Mart and got it filled there. Live and learn.

> What an asshole! Just reading about that pharmacist pisses me off. Something similar happened to me. I was using my insurance with too many different pharmacies, and when I called for a refill of Valium, Walgreens noticed that I had Lorcet from from another doc and ratted me out. They called the doc who was giving me the vals and he refused the refill coming to me. They also notified all the other pharmacies in the area. Evidently, they didn't call the Lorcet doc or he didn't care, because he still gives me scripts.

> When I went to another pharmacy to get a Lorcet script filled, the pharmacist who was always friendly with me, showed me an insurance form that said on it something like, "watch this individual." I'll never go back to that Walgreens. Righteous Nazi fucks. **—posts from pain-killers@egroups.com**

r.required quantites and mail
(FAX) entire sheet to:
AP Inc., P.O. Box 42510, Cincinnati OH 45242

SEE OTHER STYLES ON REVERSE

TOLL FREE
PHONE (800) 366-7135   FAX (800) 788-2377

1195

WE CAN SUPPLY ALL PHARMEX LABELS
- EVEN THOSE NOT SHOWN -

Copyright 1995 COVAP Inc.

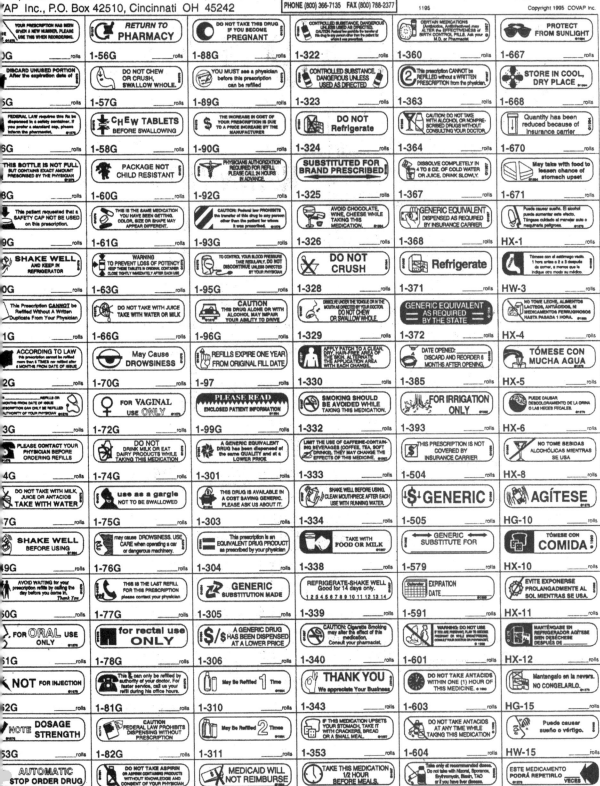

What's that Pill's Name?

Time and again pill buffs are frustrated by the media's refusal to go into detail about the pills that shape our lives—and indeed, history. Jeffrey Dahmer, the Milwaukee serial killer, used pills to drug his victims before killing, dismembering and eating them. While the stories go into gruesome detail about the stench of his apartment, the reader is left shouting at the newspaper, "WHAT pills!?"

Same thing with George Bush. When he was Vice-President and President, he was taking a number of different medications. It was not enough to say he took a "pain pill" every night to help him sleep, and "powerful" medications for his thyroid and heart conditions. It was not enough to say "medication has stabilized him." At least one of the medications in question is known to "slow down mental processes" and cause "confusion."

Bush seemed to be on at least three different medications, including "baby aspirin," Synthroid to replace the hormones from his defunct thyroid gland, and procainamide—which affects thinking. He was also believed to have been on a "blood thinner" as well as a "hormone." It's hard to speculate which "blood thinner," but "hormone" can be a synonym for "steroid." Perhaps the Prez wanted to avoid a potential image problem there. And when Bush barfed on the Japanese Prime Minister, he was taking a prescription anti-nausea medication known as Tigan. (Compazine, Tigan's main prescription competition, could have made good use of this in an ad campaign. "If he'd used Comapzine, he'd still be President").

The names of the Bush pills were not generally reported. The exception was the sleeping aid Halcion which was "reported" at every turn.

The media reported that Jeffrey Dahmer used "sedatives" prescribed to him, or perhaps another drug prescribed to his grandmother, and a bottle of chloroform was found in his lair.

Only when the *New York Times* paid a janitor $200 to steal documents from a Milwaukee prosecutor's desk (the *NYT* denies this) did the public discover that Dahmer used Bush's favorite pill, Halcion to knock out a 13-year-old boy in 1988. Traces of unspecified benzodiazepines were found in two of the corpses recovered from the notorious apartment along with an unfilled prescription for the benzodiazepine Lorazepam.

Halcion and alcohol seem like a great combo for rendering someone unconscious. Yvonne Culmsee of North Dallas, known as a leading "Mickey Finn artist," went on a robbery spree of some 24 people and seems to have used just such a formula to knock her victims out.

In those rare cases when a specific pill is being touted or lambasted (Prozac or Halcion, for example), pills are relegated to an ethereal and secretive world—which leads to misunderstandings with potentially horrific consequences. Consider how often one reads that a person has committed suicide by an overdosing with "sleeping pills" or "tranquilizers." Does this mean you can kill yourself with Sominex? Is this what duped Robert MacFarlane into thinking he could kill himself with Valium? And what about Liz Taylor? How come she and all her other Hollywood buddies don't ever say what pills they're popping?

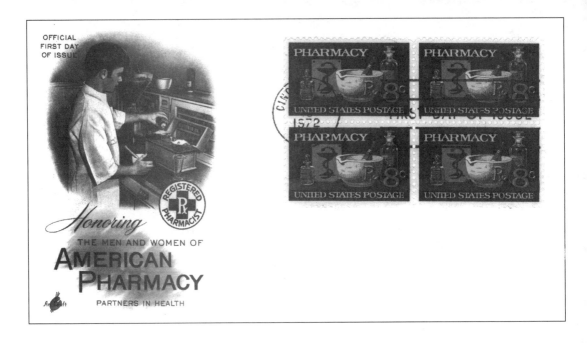

GREAT PHARMACIST AUTHORS
Six great writers who started their career as pharmacists:

Norwegian dramatist Henrik Ibsen (1828–1906)

English poet John Keats (1795–1821)

German poet/novelist Theodore Fontane (1819–1898)

Austrian poet Georg Trakl (1887–1914)

American master of the short story, O. Henry,
   whose real name was William S. Porter (1862-1910)

John Uri Lloyd, with Harvey Wickes Felter, was one of the
   co-authors of the 2172 page pharmacological encyclopedia,
   King's American Dispensatory, first published in 1880. Lloyd
   went on to write *Etidorpha* (the backward spelling of Aphrodite),
   one of the first psychedelic science fiction novels ever written.

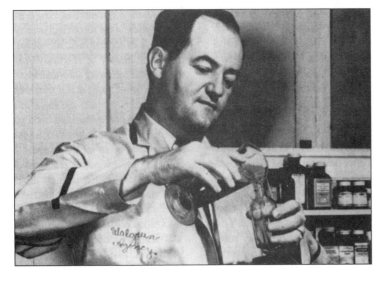

Hubert Humphrey, taking time off from the United States Senate in 1949, helps out in his family's South Dakota drugstore, where he was a partner and licensed pharmacist. Humphrey often debated politics with customers. He met his future wife in the store, when she dropped by one day for a soda.

Pills in literature, pills in film, pills in songs, pills in TV shows . . . Pills in our culture are so ubiquitous, so integral to our reality, they cannot help but be present in all our human works. Sometimes pills provide the motive force for a whole story as in *Drugstore Cowboy,* where the characters spend all of their time breaking into pharmacies, stealing and taking drugs and planning ways to keep the cycle going. Pill-popping is a running theme in the flick *Dead Ringer.* Sometimes a single pill is either an arch-villain (Valium in the movie *I'm Dancing as Fast as I Can*) or a hero (the bottle of nitroglycerin tablets just out of reach of the kindly old man, or L-Dopa in *Awakenings*). *The Simpsons* have made references to Prozac while Valium is referred to as "V" in Jay McInnery's novel of urban yuppiedom, *Bright Lights, Big City.*

In *Valley of the Dolls* (1967), pills are the stars and their female fans the supporting players. Originally "doll" or "dollie" was slang for dolophine or methadone, but over time the word came to mean nearly any pill, especially the barbiturates the character Neely loved so much. *Valley of the Dolls* advertising credits included "Seconal pills" along with starlets Patty Duke, Barbara Perkins and Sharon Tate, who commits suicide with the help of barbiturates in the movie. Russ Meyer's softcore sequel *Beyond the Valley of the Dolls* (1970) likewise exhibited pills along with everything and everybody else in reach.

A superhero (played by Wally Cox) in *Mr. Terrific,* depended on a pill to give him superpowers. Three years earlier, Cox began providing the voice of Underdog, a cartoon canine who is transformed from a mild-mannered Shoeshine Boy into a superhero after a dash into a phone booth and a revitalizing "Super Vitamin Pill" stashed in a secret compartment in his ring.

Pills can show up as instruments of a morality lesson—to be used for good or evil. And of course, lots of anti-drug movies focus on pills as a symbol of drug abuse just as the popular symbol for modern medicine is a handful of pills. In one way or another, pills are symbolic for nearly everyone—though emotional reactions to them range from evil to holy to indifferent.

This ambiguous cultural meaning of pills sometimes makes it necessary to alter their physical appearance. Pills employed in the arsenal of the good guys in popular media are sometimes disguised as something else.

Pills
in Popular
Culture

Much of the material ahead, describing Pills in Films, is excerpted, with permission, from Michael Starks' book, *Cocaine Fiends and Reefer Madness—An Illustrated History of Drugs in the Movies* (1982).

Popeye was chowing down spinach, yet it's clear his leafy greens were mean steroids. Similarly, the "spice" in Frank Herbert's futuristic *Dune* series can only represent drugs. The characters never use this "spice" as a condiment, only for its chemical effects. Still, the future is a comfortable place for pills. The Jetsons take 'em instead of meals and David Bowie's Major Tom swallows them while waiting for lift-off. In fact, in the world of science fiction, food and pills are nearly interchangeable.

Pills also show up in the media as unconscious props because a world without pills would be truly unfathomable. What bathroom has no medicine cabinet? What medicine cabinet has no pills? Who does not take a pill for a headache? What does anyone expect out of a visit to the doctor? If the prognosis isn't immediate surgery—expect a prescription.

The fact that the word "pills" rhymes with "thrills," "kills," "ills," and so many other catchy words makes singing about pills a favorite from John Cougar Mellencamp to The Nail. Ten years ago, the New Wave band 20/20 scored a hit with *My Yellow Pills*; Steppenwolf proves a drug-user's credentials by saying he "smoked a lotta grass" and "popped a lot of pills" before Goddamning "The Pusher."

Occasionally, a certain pill will capture the hearts of rock stars far and wide; around 1977, everyone from the Sex Pistols to Motorhead sung the praises of little blue pills. Some bands have fashioned whole albums around pills both brazenly, like the Happy Mondays' opus, *Pills 'n' Thrills 'n' Bellyaches,* and somewhat slyly, like the Bay City Rollers' Elevator. Electronic bands seem especially fond of pharmaceutical motifs in their album art. A bootleg recording of The Orb was released as *Space Pills*.

Some bands honor their favorite pharmaceutical as well as trendy fads, by naming themselves Codeine, Morphine, Ephedrine, Halcion, and Xanax-25 (which could be an erudite reference to LSD, too). Then there are the imaginary pharmaceutical namesakes: Wonderdrug and Placebo. The L.A. punk band, the Angry Samoans, called themselves The Queer Pills when releasing a seven-inch record.

A Philadelphia punk band was threatened with legal action by Smith Kline Beecham after they named themselves after the company's famous anti-psychotic Thorazine (chlorpromazine). The band said they simply couldn't change their name, as they'd already invested close to $1000 in T-shirts and stickers to promote their debut disc, *Coffee, Tea or Thorazine.* They couldn't have bought better promotion. One way to make rock and roll history—get sued for naming your band after a famous pill.

Barbiturates were introduced into the practice of medicine in 1903 and it was not long before sleeping powders made their appearance in films. Barbiturate addicts and sedative overdoses steadily increased in number and frequency, but it was not until after World War II when barbies became almost universally available.

Barbiturates are most commonly portrayed in movies as THE pharmaceutical tool to commit suicide or murder. A man kills his mistress with an overdose of sleeping pills in the German film *Die Nacht der Zwoelf* (1945). Few references to barbs occur in the next decade, and though barbiturates had been used as long as they had been around, it was only in the 1960s that they became dramatized as destructive implements. A modernized version of the Greek classic *Phaedra* (1962) has Melina Mercouri committing suicide with barbiturates, and Rex Harrison murders Susan Hayward with reds in the U.S.-British-Italian production, *The Honey Pot* (1967). Aspiring actress Kim Stanley winds up with reds and whiskey rather than fame and fortune in *The Goddess* (1958). *The Slender Thread* (1965) is the telephone line over which Sidney Portier attempts to locate an overdosed Anne Bancroft. Warhol's *Lupe* (1966) starring Edie Sedgwick, faithfully describes Lupe Velez's fatal overdose of sleeping pills. John Cassavetes' *Faces* (1968) has a troubled wife attempting suicide with sleeping pills. The film adaption of Joan Didion's portrayal of Nihilist pill-popping, *Play It As It Lays*, starring Tuesday Weld and Tony Perkins as vacant, strung-out Los Angeles residents forever driving its freeways and never getting anywhere,

There was a virtual epidemic of ups and downs in postwar Japan, and many films reflect this. *Bushido—Samurai Sage* (1963) has a modern episode in a long family history in which a woman commits suicide with barbiturates.

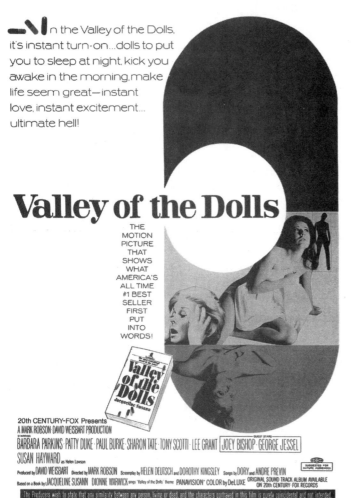

In the Valley of the Dolls, it's instant turn-on...dolls to put you to sleep at night, kick you awake in the morning, make life seem great—instant love, instant excitement... ultimate hell!

Manji (1964) has a similar theme. *Waterfront Blues* (1970), *Law of the Outlaw* (1971), and *Resurrection of the Beast* (1969) likewise depict sleeping pills as the modern alternative to cliff leaping for distraught women. Interestingly, men are seldom shown using downers for an easy demise in films, though they often do so in reality.

Suburban Roulette (1968) promised sex and swapping but delivered only dull dialogue and a barbiturate overdose. Someone forgot to tell them that sex would be more fun if they took off their swimming suits. Sophia Loren is a rock-and-roll singer who becomes enamored of priest Marcello Mastroianni and, driven to distraction by the impossibility of the liason, she attempts to terminate her misery with reliable old downers in *The Priest's Wife* (1970). Anne Baxter has her

Talent, Ambition, Jealousy and Self-destruction

second near-fatal cinematic bout with pills in *The Late Liz* (1972). The film was based on the autobiography of heiress Gert Behanna, whose religion forbade the use of alcohol.

Ann-Margret gobbles reds in *Carnal Knowledge* (1971), and Maude (Ruth Gordon) shuffles off this mortal coil and a youthful admirer in *Harold and Maude* (1971) with the help of pills. Joanne Woodward has a flash of her pill-popping mother gobbling handfuls of reds in *Rachel, Rachel* (1968). Barbiturates and tranquilizers are not used for murder or suicide but to keep a mental patient imprisoned in a hospital in the French-Italian film *To Die of Love* (1970). Turnabout is fair play and it is a mental patient who gives barbiturates to schoolchildren in *The Silent Playground* (1963).

Barbiturates mix with drugs, sex, and violence in the cycle saga *Black Angels* (1970). Rival gangs indulge in internecine rumbles after the blacks get the honkies loaded on reds. *Tribes* (1970) shows a Marine Corps recruit using downers to cope with the rigors of basic training. Army psychiatrist Gregory Peck gives "flack juice" (sodium pentothol—the so-called "truth serum") to his patients for therapeutic purposes, with modest results— one leaps off a tower—in *Captain Newman, M.D.* (1964). Another doctor administers barbiturates (Veronal) with untoward results in *House of Wax* (1953). Another health-oriented flick, *The Devil's Sleep* (1951), makes a woman's health spa do double-duty as a front for a sleeping pill racket run by the head of an illegal drug ring.

A few films even use barbiturates for comic relief. New Yorkers drop a few in the inferior Doris Day comedy *Where Were You When the Lights Went Out?* (1968), and disappointed groupies submerge their sorrows with buckets of barbies in Frank Zappa's wonderful madness *200 Motels* (1971). We end this rather depressing area of the cinematic pharmacopoeia with a bright scene from an otherwise dismal Bob Hope comedy—*Global Affair* (1964). Hope has some business with a cop whom he tells to hurry because he's taken some sleeping pills. Hope says he's taken Nembutals whereupon the cop opines, "I like Seconals better—pop a couple in the morning and stay groggy all day."

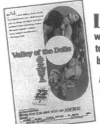

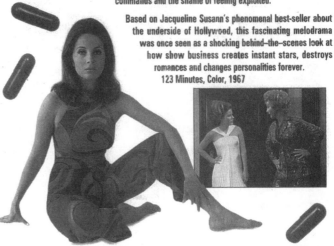

Lured by their dreams of fame and fortune, three ambitious young women enter the world of show business and discover how easy it is to sink into a celebrity nightmare of ego, alcohol and "pills."– the beloved "dolls."

A prim New Englander (BARBARA PARKINS) unexpectedly skyrockets from her job as secretary in a talent agency to a glamorous TV model. A determined singer (PATTY DUKE) finds that Hollywood success can also spell self-destruction. And a beautiful sex symbol (SHARON TATE) is torn between the money she commands and the shame of feeling exploited.

Based on Jacqueline Susann's phenomenal best-seller about the underside of Hollywood, this fascinating melodrama was once seen as a shocking behind–the–scenes look at how show business creates instant stars, destroys romances and changes personalities forever.
123 Minutes, Color, 1967

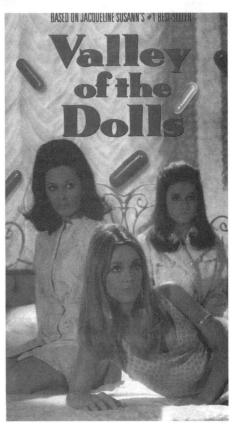

BASED ON JACQUELINE SUSANN'S #1 BEST-SELLER

Valley of the Dolls

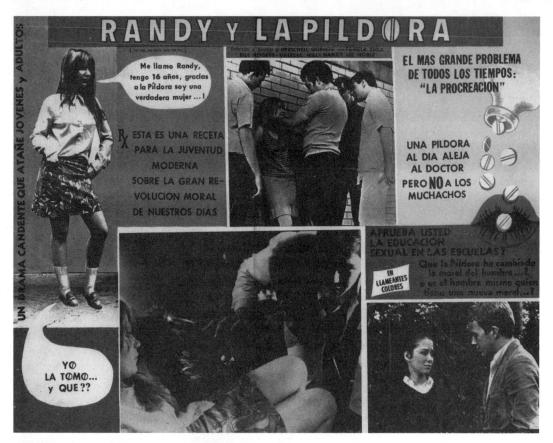

Mexican lobby card for Hershell Gordon
Lewis' *The Girl, The Body and The Pill*.

Speed is of the Essence

Although silent films often made use of accelerating potions and pills
(probably modeled on cocaine) for comic relief, amphetamines were
first introduced into medicine for their stimulant effects in 1935, and
the general public gained awareness of them only after WWII. Within
a decade amphetamines were used and abused all over the world and
Dexedrine had become part of the truck driver's standard equipment
along with his six-pack and radio. Seeing its opening, Hollywood
churned out *Death in Small Doses* (1957) with Chuck "Rifleman"
Connors as a pill-popping truck driver. An investigation begins when
some truckers consume so many Dexies that they sail their rigs across
fields and through buildings. Although Chuck grinds his teeth for
over an hour before his fatal climactic crash, most viewers will probably
need more than pep pills to stay awake through the dull melodrama.

A cycle racer strung out on speed buzzed through a few scenes of
Alice's Restaurant (1969) and the eminently forgettable pornie *Gutter
Trash* (1969) used ups to help them get down. "Pope" Ondine (Bob
Oivio) injects methedrine while receiving "penitents" in Warhol's
Chelsea Girls (1966), while Edie Sedgwick, another Warhol superstar,
is the speed queen whose downhill slide is documented in Palmer and
Weissman's *Ciao! Manhattan* (1970).

The title stud uses uppers, downers, inners, and outers while
balling his aimless way through college in *The Magic Garden of
Stanley Sweetheart* (1970), and a redneck is provoked to murder
when a cynical hippy addict gives his daughter an overdose of
methedrine in *Joe* (1970). Sally Kellerman plays charged-up speed
freak Kitty Kopetzky in *Slither* (1973), Cisco's friend Jesse is strung
out on speed and heroin in *Cisco Pike* (1972).

Inevitably, Hell's Angels types gulp "whites" in a few flicks. Both the *Black Angels* (1971) and their white antagonists do uppers prior to slaughtering one another, and in *Vanishing Point* (1971) Barry Newman bets the owner of a Hell's Angels hangout he can make it from Denver to San Francisco in record time with the help of "bennies" (he loses). This brings to mind *Drive, He Said* (1971) wherein Gabriel attempts to flunk his draft physical with a sleepless pill-popping marathon. Speed is one of many mind alterants incidental to (or integral with) the documentary action in *Medicine Ball Caravan* (1971).

Speed was the star of another 1971 film, *Believe in Me,* originally entitled *Speed is of the Essence.* Michael Sarrazin is an intern doing drug-abuse research with the help of his meth-head neighbor. He and his girlfriend Jacqueline Bisset are soon eating, snorting and shooting large amounts of the "non-addictive" substance. Although the insane life of a house full of speed freaks has potential for a good film, this one doesn't live up to it.

A Face in the Crowd, writer Budd Schulberg and snitch director Elia Kazan's 1957 take on vulgar redneck sales superstardom, has Andy Griffith making an OTC caffeinated-cruncher named "Vitajex" into a huge mass market success. In Roger Corman's, *Night Call Nurses* (1972), Kyle—a young, amphetamine-dependent truck driver crashes in the hospital and Nurse Janis helps him through his withdrawal hallucinations.

The Erotic Circus (1969), perhaps the only pornographic methedrine movie ever made, is appropriately bizarre. A family of nuts, including a rapidly aging methedrine dealer and assorted sadists and masochists, gathers for a drugs-and-sex orgy. Next morning the house is strewn with corpses and the meth dealer is castrated as well. Dear old mother proves to be the butcher, and as the caretaker diligently removes the carnage, she devises the means to castrate him, too.

Mother, Jugs and Speed (1976) features Harvey Keitel as a pill-popping ambulance driver. The film's other two stars are Bill Cosby and Raquel Welch. Guess who plays Jugs? *Outland* (1981) has Sean Connery playing an outer-space cop fighting pushers of an amphetamine derivative that drives users mad.

Visions of drug-oriented future societies have been explored in sci-fi novels for nearly a century, but sci-fi films have only examined this area in the last few decades. Foremost among these is George Lucas' *THX-1138* (1971) in which people are controlled with mandatory drug use, constantly reminded by the disembodied stentorian voice of authority coming over the loudspeakers ("If you feel you are not properly sedated, call 344210—failure to do so may result in prosecution for criminal drug evasion"). When one of the couples stop taking their sedatives, emotions, sex and love emerge, but the lowered drug levels are detected and the couple is convicted of drug evasion and sex perversion.

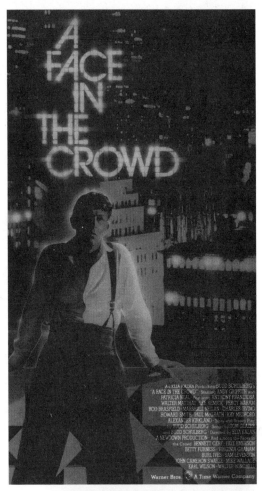

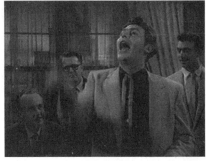

Andy Griffith impresses pharmaceutical chiefs and ad men with his enthusiasm for their caffeine loaded Vitajex tablet.

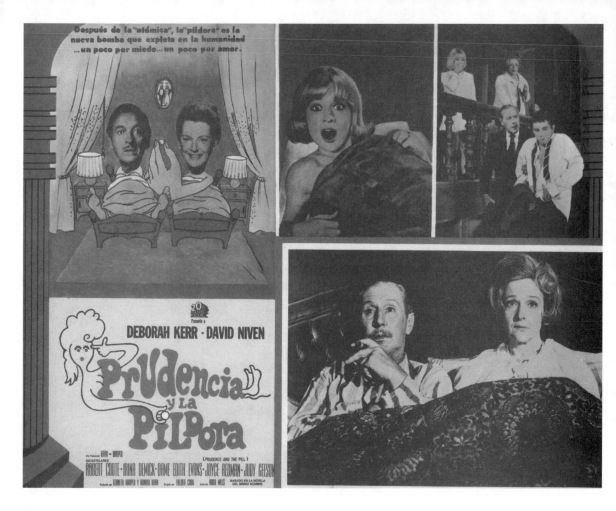

Mexican lobby card for Fielder Cook's *Prudence and The Pill.*

The movie version of Ray Bradbury's novel *Fahrenheit 451* (1966) also shows the citizens preoccupied with drug taking and Julie Christie overdoses on "blues" at the beginning. *Rollerball* (1975) likewise depicts a totalitarian society that keeps order with drugs. The owner of a rollerball team gives his assistant a pill for pleasant dreams and everyone carries his box of little white pills. In Woody Allen's *Sleeper* (1973) people get high by holding a little silver ball, and in Kubrick's *2001: A Space Odyssey* (1968) it is the computer HAL who suggests that troubled astronaut Dave take a stress pill.

In view of their extreme popularity, tranquilizers have for some unexplained reasons appeared in only a few films. Perhaps tranquilized people are cinematically dull people. Richard Widmark mixes tranquilizers and alcohol and wakes up the next day with his memory gone in *The Tunnel of Love* (1958), and Glenn Ford fortifies himself with tranquilizers before murdering a blackmailer in *The Gazebo* (1959). The British *Dr. Crippen* (1963) kills his wife with an overdose of tranquilizers, and Faye Dunaway plays a neurotic model who keeps it together with alcohol and tranquilizers in *Puzzle of a Downfall Child* (1970). *Doctors' Wives* (1971) use tranquilizers and other pills to ease their sorrows, and the judge pops pills to keep cool in *What's Up, Doc?* (1972).

Vincent Price is the head of a ring that uses drugs to pacify young ladies for white-slavery purposes in the European film *House of 1,000 Dolls* (1967), and women are kept drugged in a bizarre brothel where old men pay only to look and touch in the Japanese production, *The House of the Sleeping Virgins* (1968). An international dope ring kidnaps stewardesses and drugs them in the pornie *Fly Now, Pay Later* (1969). The ring smuggles a drug called "khelp" into New York and one of the women is driven insane with an overdose.

Steroid use is presaged in the Italian film *Hercules Pills* (*Le pillole di Ercole,* 1960), which features pills invented by a Chinese scientist that transform men into mountains of muscle. Even Walt Disney's heroes get off on drugs. A football team is given a little extra zip in *The Monkey's Uncle* (1965), and Soupy Sales gets so invigorated that he flies in *Birds Do It* (1966).

Mark of the Vampire (1957) is unique in that pills (rather than munching on jugulars) transmogrify people into night creatures.

Even birth control pills had their fifteen minutes of fame on the silver screen. *Prudence and the Pill* (1968) and *The Girl, the Body, and the Pill* (1967) make cinematic mincemeat out of womankind's new freedom. (*The Girl* was directed by none other than horrormeister Hershell Gordon Lewis!)

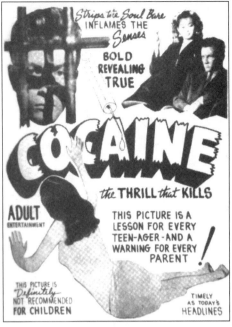

Fractured Flickers Abuse Drugs

Although countless films mention uppers and downers, some drug abuse films actually focus their full attention on these pills as well. *Focus on Downers* (1971), for example, shows that addiction, overdose and death from can result from sudden withdrawal from barbiturates. This film strongly emphasizes death in its dramatized vignettes as do two early 70s Sid Davis films, *Blood Reds* and *The Pill Poppers*. The latter includes material on uppers, which also speed through *Ups/Downs* (1971), *Drug Abuse; Bennies and Goofballs* (1966), *Let's Talk About Pills* (1972), and *Glass Houses* (1972). These four films tend to overemphasize the "speed kills" theme. The personal testimony of thirteen pill poppers in *Glass Houses* is convincingly sordid.

Amphetamines receive special attention in *Speedscene* (1970), *Focus on Speed and Uppers* (1971), *New Drugs, Same Needle* (1968), and *Sports: The Programmed Gladiators* (1971). *Speedscene* presents interesting commentary by users and doctors, but recites the "speed kills" mantra.

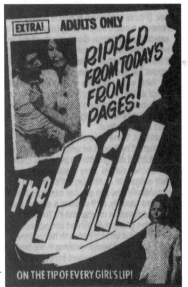

Tranks are singled out for special attention in *The Age of the Tranquilizer,* (1964), and *Mother's Little Helpers* (1968), which originally appeared on television. In case you never were aware that cattle calm their udders with tranks to prevent pre-slaughter hysteria, the 1958 documentary *Tranquilizers, a New Idea in Animal Feeds* provides mankind with a new idea of ways to champion vegetarianism.

Cowboy in a Cage

The pill world grieved at the January 3, 1992 arrest of James Fogle, whose novel, *Drugstore Cowboy,* inspired the beautiful epic movie that defines pill experience.

Fogle was busted in a South Tacoma motel room with some $38,000.00 in pharmaceuticals apparently taken in a series of crash & dash robberies of drugstores. Acting on a tip that a guy named Jim was fiddling with drugs in his room, cops burst in and caught Fogle, wife, Janet, and her 26-year-old son, Tracy Rosi. After gawking at the plethora of pills for a while, the lawmen dragged the family unit down to Pierce County jail. Bond for Fogle was set at a whoppin' $100K and $50K each for his devoted wife and stepson.

The genius author served at least nine prison and jail sentences in his 55 years, logging more than three and a half decades behind bars—often for exactly the type of crime committed by the four youthful protagonists of his benchmark book and movie—the famed crash & dash.

This art form consists of a lightning attack on a pharmacy's shelves and drawers full of luscious pills, while stunned pharmacists and shoppers stand drop-jawed. Such an operation cannot be performed by just any pillhead, as it requires the ability to instantly assess the location and value of hundreds of different pills in just a few moments. Bad judgment cannot only lead to the pokey, but to a haul of useless diuretics, beta blockers and antihistamines.

Judging by what the sheriffs found in Fogle's pad, the old guy hadn't lost his touch. Among the pounds of pills recovered were Demerol, phenobarbitol, codeine, methadone, Ritalin and morphine.

The day he died, Elvis Presley's body contained Valmid, Qaalude, and codeine in therapeutic concentrations and trace levels of chlorpheniramine, Demerol, Valium and morphine (possibly metabolized from the codeine). Also found were Placidyl, pentobarbital, butabarbital, phenobarbital and several unspecified barbiturates. In 1981, Presley's doc, George Nichopoulos, went before the Tennessee Medical Examiner Board because it was found that during the last two and a half years of his life, Presley received more than 19,000 doses of narcotics, stimulants, sedatives, and anti-depressants. Nichopoulos, lost his license in 1995 when the state of Tennessee finally decided he had overprescribed not only to Presley, but Jerry Lee Lewis and other patients as well.

In an attempt to get his curly hair right, Syd Barrett, is said to have slathering it down with a special concoction of hair cream and crushed Mandrax tablets.

Hank Williams was quite fond of sleeping pills and did commercials for drug companies on the radio.

Johnny Cash was arrested for smuggling one thousand Dexedrine tablets from Mexico in October, '65.

The Everly Brothers were prescribed amphetamines in '62.

Janis Joplin took speed and goofballs to help heighten her alcohol-besotted life.

Mick Jagger pounded down Italian amphetamine sulfate/methyl amphetamine hydrochloride tabs in the '60s as he sang "Mother's Little Helper."

Jimi Hendrix died after consuming alcohol and various uppers and downers, as well as 18 times the normal dose of Vesperax, a sleeping pill.

Dorothy Dandridge, the first black woman nominated for the Academy's Best Actress Award, committed suicide by overdosing on a depression pill in 1965.

Actress Carole Landis, star of **One Million B.C.** (1940) and the original "sweater girl" of the silver screen, gulped down a bottle of Seconal tablets in 1948. She was only 29.

Pills of the Stars

Pills have played a juicy role in the lives and deaths of innumerable celebrities. So many "names" have taken so many pills, that only a notable few are listed here.

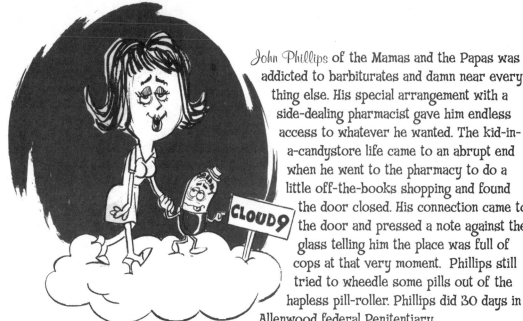

John Phillips of the Mamas and the Papas was addicted to barbiturates and damn near everything else. His special arrangement with a side-dealing pharmacist gave him endless access to whatever he wanted. The kid-in-a-candystore life came to an abrupt end when he went to the pharmacy to do a little off-the-books shopping and found the door closed. His connection came to the door and pressed a note against the glass telling him the place was full of cops at that very moment. Phillips still tried to wheedle some pills out of the hapless pill-roller. Phillips did 30 days in Allenwood federal Penitentiary.

Charles Boyer, considered one of film's most dashing leading men, took the plunge at the age of 78 with the aid of Seconal.

After failing to kill herself after leaping off a bridge in London, model/actress *Gia Scala* resorted to the ever-dependable combo of barbiturates and ethanol in 1972 at the age of 38.

Mario Lanza, the "American Caruso" of the 1950s, supposedly fell victim to alcohol and barbiturates and was reported to have died of a "heart attack" in 1959. Friends believe he was poisoned by the Mafia. Suspiciously, his wife OD'd five months later.

Alan Ladd died in 1964 supposedly as a result of alcohol and sedatives.

In 1968, TV star *Nick Adams* died of a drug overdose, though no syringes, bottles or other drug paraphernalia were found in his home. The coroner claimed booze and an elephant-sized dose of sedatives were found in his body, though no one could explain how he consumed them.

'Lude-head comedian *Freddie Prinze,* star of TV's **Chico and the Man,** had taken half a dozen the day he shot himself to death in 1977 at the tender age of 23. Traces of codeine and morphine were also in his system.

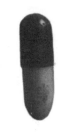

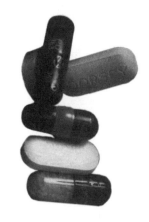

Dan Plato of childhood fame, on the sitcom *Diff'rent Strokes* died May 8, 1999 of suicide by an overdose of Lortab and Soma. In 1992, she was caught and given five years probation for forging a script for Valium.

The constant use of Dexedrine inspired Bill Faires' obsessive work on EC Comics and *Mad* magazine.

The most famous pill suicide might also be the most suspicious. Marilyn Monroe was found dead on the morning of August 5, 1962, lying face down in bed, her hand gripping the telephone, with 47 Nembutal tablets coursing through her system. The first cop on the scene declared that Marilyn had been murdered by someone she "knew and trusted." Conspiracies hold Bobby and/or John F. Kennedy responsible.

The diminutive ex-Cher-svengali-turned-congressman Sonny Bono was said to have died after hitting a tree on a ski slope. Bono's wife claimed he suffered a tremendous pill addiction.

Aimee Semple McPherson, founder of the Foursquare Temple and pioneer of flashy evangelism, overdosed on sleeping pills in 1944 at the age of 53.

"Some fell by laudanum, and some by steel, And death in ambush lay in every pill."
—Sir Samuel Garth (1661–1719), physician, poet

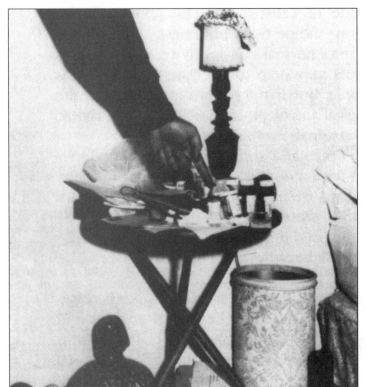

A collection of empty pill bottles on Marilyn Monroe's bedside table. The popular star, who had become increasingly dependent on barbiturates, was found dead of an overdose in August 1962. Most authorities called her death a suicide.

John Bonham overdosed on sleeping pills.

Johnny Rotten and other Sex Pistols got high on amphetamine sulfate, the British legal speed.

Keith Moon died after taking 32 tablets of Herminevrin.

Don Henley of the Eagles was a notable quaalude advocate.

Judy Garland took 40 Ritalin tabs a day in 1968; she was also prescribed Valium and thorazine. she died of a drug overdose on June 15, 1969.

John Belushi regularly consumed as many black beauties and 'ludes as he could fit in his immense stomach.

Nick Drake died of an overdose of anti-depressants.

Andy McCoy (of Hanoi Rocks) was notorious in his native Finland for his stimulating use of stimulants.

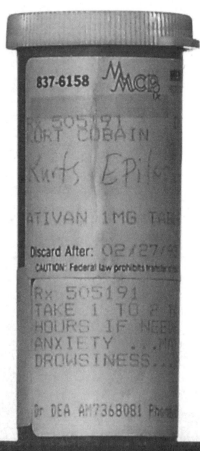
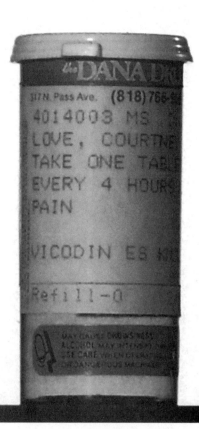

In *The Shah's Last Ride,* William Shawcross recounts how the Shah of Iran took "continual small doses of Valium every day." In 1974, when it was discovered to be afflicted with leukemia, he was able to keep his illness a secret, controlling the disease with chlorambucil pills.

The Shah's sister, Princess Ashraf, took Valium, too, as did their chief bodyguard in exile, Manuel Noriega. An hilarious part of the book comes when Ashraf is so overcome with grief at her situation that she tries to commit suicide with her pills. "Like a robot I went to my room and swallowed a mixture of sleeping pills and Valium," she wrote dramatically, "I lay down as if to go to sleep. But sleep did not come. I stayed wide-awake and I asked myself the question which had been haunting me for months, 'What kind of justice is it . . .' I was like a sleepwalker, drunk with remorse . . . Then I took ten more pills, thinking, This time it will work. But nothing happened and I finally had to accept that when God does not want you, he does not take you."

Speedboat racer George Morales was sentenced to 16 years in the slam for smuggling 'ludes and other drugs into the country for six years. New York Yankees baseball star Joe Pepitone was convicted and sentenced for possessing hundreds of them.

Betty Ford admitted to being hooked on minor tranquilizers for some 14 years, developed dependence due to her arthritis and to help her sleep, after which she entered a treatment program for pills as well as for alcohol. The Betty Ford Center has become the country's most noted addiction complex.

Milton Berle became so attached to tranquilizers he called himself "Miltown Berle."

"And all the sailors who were junkies, they went sailing out to sea, and the white man sold quaaludes to the monkeys, and they all died high up in the trees."

—*Gibby Haynes, 1985*

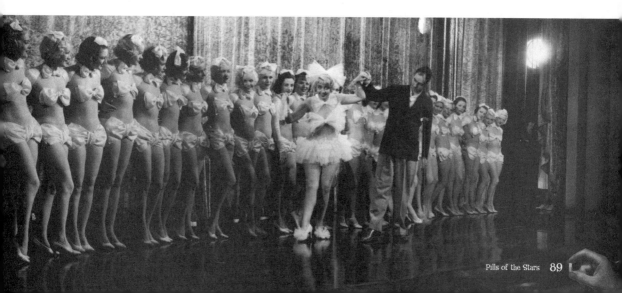

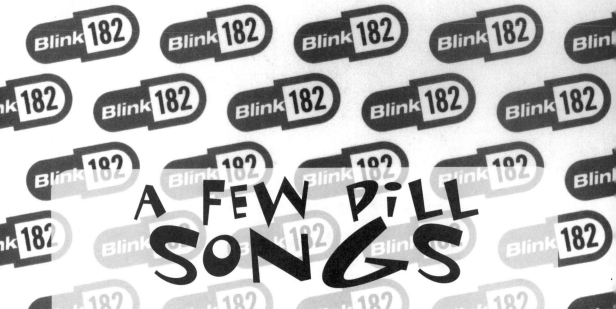

A FEW PILL SONGS

American Music Club I Just Took Sleeping Pills

The Angry Samoans Gimme Sopor "Take a Pill, Take A Pill, Take A Pill, Pill, Pill"

Bay City Rollers Elevator

Beatles Doctor Robert

Bell Noise Chakra "Zoloft, Ritalin—just say all right"

Busta Rhymes Dangerous This song apparently quotes from "Little Blue Pills," the theme song for a public service announcement that ran on New York TV stations during Saturday morning cartoons. The PSA featured a bunch of little blue hand puppets flapping and wiggling against a black background, singing a warning to children about the dangers of eating mom and dad's prescription medicines. Some lyrics: "This is Serious/This Could Make You Delirious/You Should Have A Healthy Fear Of Us/Too Much Of Us Is Dangerous/We're Not Candy/Even Though We Look So Fine And Dandy/When You're Sick/We Come In Handy/But We're Not Candy/Ohhhh Nooooo . . ."

Chin Ho Sleeping Pill Suicide

The Cramps Bop Pills

Dave Dudley Six Days On The Road

Dramarama Anything, Anything "I'll Give You Candy/Give You Diamonds/Give You Pills/Give You Anything You Want/Hundred Dollar Bills"

Dead Kennedys Drug Me

Bo Diddley Pills (Also covered by The New York Dolls and R.E.M.)

Drink Me Little Green Men

Fallen Angels Amphetamine Blue

Family Fodder My Baby Takes Valium

Robbie Fulks She Took A Lot Of Pills and Died

Generation X Valley Of The Dolls

The Godz 714 "Feelin' Fine On My 714"

Green Apple Quick Step Pills

Happy Mondays Pills 'n' Thrills 'n' Bellyaches

Charlie Harper Df 118 (Harper was given them in the hospital after suffering a heart attack.)

The Imposter (aka Elvis Costello) Pills And Soap

The Jam The Bitterest Pill
Jefferson Airplane White Rabbit
The Joneses Ms. 714
L7 Diet Pill
Little Feat Willin' "Weed, Whites and Wine"
Mac Mcnally Little Blue Pill
Marilyn Manson Coma White (aka A Pill To Make You Numb)
Alanis Morrisette Jagged Little Pill
My Own Sweet Pills For Faster Living
Nirvana Lithium
The Other Half Mr. Pharmacist (Also covered by The Fall)
Adam Parfrey The Juggernaut of Entertainment in Contemporary Life
Quicksilver Messenger Service Codeine
The Replacements Valentine
Roger Ruskin Spear Give Me Dr. Rock
Rolling Stones Mother's Little Helper
Street Walkin' Cheetahs Ms. Teen USA
Suede Sleeping Pills
Ray Stevens Jeremiah Peabody's Polyunsaturated Quick-Dissolving, Fast-Acting, Pleasant-Tasting Green and Purple Pills
Squeeze The Dog These Pills
The Tards Just Like You
20/20 Yellow Pill and Nuclear Boy
They Might Be Giants Lie Still Little Bottle
The Who Dr. Jimmy and Mr. Jim
Wings Medicine Jam

Quotes

The desire to take medicine is perhaps the greatest feature which distinguishes man from animals.

—Sir William Osler, *Science and Immortality*, 1904

"Alone, barbiturates can lower the inhibition level of the individual and this explains the popularity of the drugs in teenage and hip circles. Bombed out of their minds, an apartment of people can turn into a modern-day version of the old Roman orgies."

—*The Menace of Pep Pills*

"I gave him the Tylenol to relieve the pain."

—Clive Doyle, one of the few Branch Davidians to survive the fire at Mt. Carmel, Texas describing his reaction to finding a an elderly Davidian shot in the stomach by ATF agents

"Doctors pour in drugs about which they know little to treat diseases of which they know less in human beings of which they know nothing."

—Voltaire, in protest of 18th century medical practices

"Tranquilizer withdrawals can cause: anxiety, stress, de-realization (feelings not in touch with reality), lack of concentration, loss of memory, panic attacks, hyperventilation, insomnia, hyperactivity, depression, over-eating, agoraphobia, suicidal feelings, rage, perception difficulties, hormonal imbalance, muscle pain, numbness, tingling, burning, sore mouth, dental problems, mineral deficiency, hair loss . . ."

—from a self-help book on weaning yourself from prescription drugs

"Is it because as psychotherapists, that is, as people accustomed to using words and verbal insights as a means of inducing improvement in the sick, we have a quasi-religious revulsion against the pill?"

—M. Fleischman, *American Journal of Psychiatry*, 1968, reflecting on the use of psychiatric drugs.

"The FDA, AMA and DEA are in place not to 'save people from themselves' but to provide mob-like professional organizations more money. Individuals should be free to take whatever they want whenever they want. If people want warning stickers attached, fine. But drug laws treat human beings like morons. They're the result of criminal professional organizations and bureaucratic czars and secret government funding."

—anonymous poster to pain-killers email group

"The presence of another drug can keep the body so busy that metabolism of a new drug is delayed. For example, the presence of alcohol keeps the liver so busy that a Seconal or Quaalude will remain in the body two to three times longer than normal."

—*Uppers, Downers and All-Arounders* by Darryl Inaba and William Cohen

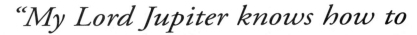

"My Lord Jupiter knows how to

Poppin' Goofballs and Getting All Hopped-Up

The following are slang terms for pills (or drugs that commonly come in pill form) as compiled on a regular basis by the DEA. At times these are inaccurate but cops write 'em like they hear 'em. Many are regional terms (something may mean one thing in L.A. and another in Boston), and some words have multiple meanings.

Amphetamines

A, Aimies, Amp, Bam, Batu, Bennies, Benz, Black And White, Black Beauties, Blackbirds, Black (Or Blue) Mollies, Black Bombers, Blacks, Blanks, Blue Boy, Black Dex, Blue Meth, Bombido, Bombita (injectable desoxyn), Bottles, Brain Ticklers, Brownies, Browns, Bumblebees, Cadillac Express, Ephedrone, Gagers, Gaggers, Goob, Slick Superspeed, Stat, The C, Tweaker Cat, Candy, Cartwheels, Chalk, Chicken Powder, Christmas Trees, Chocolate, Christina, Co-Pilot, Coasts To Coasts, Crank, Crink, Cris, Criss-cross, Cristina, Cristy, Croak, Crosstops, Crossroads, Crystal, Crypto, Dexies, Diet Pills, Disco Pellets, Dominoes, Double Cross, Eye Openers, Fire, Fives, Footballs, Forwards, French Blue, Go Fast, Hanyak, Head Drugs, Hearts, Horseheads, Hot Ice, Ice, In-betweens, Jelly Baby, Jelly Bean, Jugs, Jam, Jam Cecil, L.A., L.A. Ice, Leapers, Lid Poppers, Lightening, Little Bomb, Marathons, Max (Amphetamines Mixed With Ghb), Minibennie, Nugget, Oranges, Peanut Butter, Pellets, Peaches, Pep Pills, Pink Hearts, Pixies, Popcorn Coke, Powder, Purple Hearts, Quartz, Quill, Rhythm, Rippers, Road Dope, Vitamin R (Ritalin), Robin's Eggs, Rosa, Roses, Snap, Snot, Snow Pallets, Snow Seals (When Mixed With Cocaine), Sparkle Plenty, Sparklers, Speed, Splivins, Splash, Star, Super Ice, Sweets, The C, Thrusters, Truck Drivers, Turkey, Turnabout, Tr-6's, Uppers, Uppies, Wake Ups, West Coast (Ritalin), White, Whites, Wonder Star, Yellow Bam.

Opiates

CODEINE: Number 3's, Number 4's, Codes, Schoolboy, Pops
DARVON, DARVOCET: Pink ladies, pumpkin seeds
DILAUDID: Dillies, footballs
FENTANYL: China Girl, China Town, Dance Fever, Friend, Goodfellas, Great Bear, He-Man, Jackpot, King Ivory, Murder 8, Tango & Cash, TNT, Dance Fever, Apache.
METHADONE: Juice, Amidone, Fizzies
PERCODAN: Percs
MORPHINE: Black Pill (Opium Pill), Dreamer, Emsel, First Line, God's Drug, Hong-Yen (Heroin in pill form), Hows, Hocus, Joy Powder, M.S., Miss Emma, Mr. Blue, Morf (or Morph), Unkie, Murphy, M, New Jack Swing (Morphine/Heroin Combo)

sugarcoat a pill. "—Moliere, *Amphitryon*

Depressants and Tranquilizers

Backwards, Bam, Bambs, Bank Bandit Pills, Barb, Barbies, Beans, Blockbusters, Blue, Blue Angels, Blue Birds, Blue Bullets, Blue Devils, Blue Dolls, Blue Heavens, Blue Tips, Bombido, Bombita, Busters, Candy, Chlorals, Christmas Rolls, Christmas Trees, Coral, Dolls, Courage Pills, Dolls, Downer, Downie, Double Trouble, G.B., Gangster Pills, Golf Balls, Goofballs, Goofers, Gorilla Pills, Green Dragons, Green Frog, Idiot Pills, Inbetweens, Jellies, Jelly Bean, Joy Juice, King Kong Pills, Lay Back, Little Bomb, Lib (Librium), M&M, Marshmallow Reds, Mexican Reds, Mickey Finn, Mickey's, Mighty Joe Young, Mother's Little Helper (Valium), Nebbies, Nemmies, Nimbies, Peanut, Peter, Phennies, Phenos, Pink Ladies, Purple Hearts, Rainbows, Reds, Red And Blue, Red Bullets, Red Devil, Seccy, Seggy, Sleeper, Softballs, Stoppers, Strawberries, Stumbler, Tranq, Tooles, Tooties, Tootsies, Tuie, V (Valium), Uncle Miltie, Ups And Downs, Yellow, Yellow Bullets, Yellow Jackets.

ROHYPNOL: Forget Me Drug, Forget Pill, La Rocha, Lunch Money Drug, Mexican Valium, Pingus, R-2, Reynolds, Rib, Roachies, Roapies, Robutal, Roche, Roofies, Ropies, Rophies, Roples, Row-Shay, Ruffies, Ruffles, Wolfies.

QUAALUDES: Lemmon 714's (or just "714s" from the code number imprinted on 300 mg tabs of Quaalude), Ludes, Luds, Disco Biscuit, Billy Boots, Dr. Jekyll and Mr. Hyde, French Quaalude, Heroin for Lovers, Love Drug, Mandrakes, Pillows, Q, Quacks, Quads, Quas, Sopers, Soapers, Sopors, Vitamin Q.

Other Pill Slang:

Kiddie Dope (prescription drugs),
Legal speed (ephedrine),
pseudocaine (phenylpropylnolamine),
mouth worker (one who takes drugs orally).

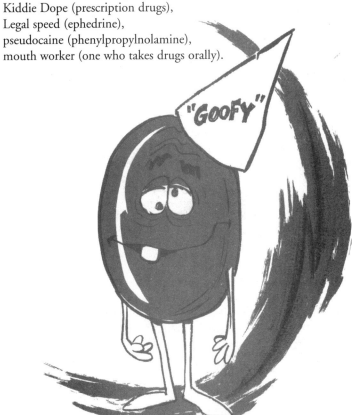

"GOOFY"

1992 Researchers at Merck Sharp & Dohme pharmaceutical house, seeking a powerful blood coagulant, are studying a "provocative and interesting" new substance: vampire-bat saliva. Preliminary research on rabbits showed the saliva to be several times more effective than the next best substance of congealing the bunnies' blood.

1993 Police in Bangkok arrested four male transsexuals and a woman in December and charged them with a crime spree in which the four men, appearing to be female prostitutes, smeared tranquilizer substances on their breasts and enticed their customers to suck them until they passed out, at which point the gang robbed them and fled.

Pill News of the Weird

1994 The Tokyo-based drug firm Dairin announced it would soon market a pre-meal pill to make bowel movements completely odorless. Although the pill was developed principally for the health care market, to improve working conditions for nurses' aides, some commentators in Japan fear that the availability of the pill for consumers will increase Japan's obsession with cleanliness. Psychiatry professor Susumu Oda said that, already, overreaction to unpleasant smells is a cause of unsociable behavior.

1995 The Zhu Ma Dian pharmaceutical company won a lawsuit over a newspaper and a TV station in Liaoning province in China for defamation of the strength of the company's sleeping pills. The newspaper had reported, truthfully, that a couple, distraught over gambling losses, had attempted suicide by swallowing a total of six bottles of the pills, but they wound up only with bad stomach aches. Since the story was reported at the time of the Chinese National Medicines Fair, the company immediately lost about 90 percent of expected sales.

1995 Jay Stanton Liebenow, 37, was arrested in Bethesda, Md., and charged with robbing a CVS pharmacy. According to police, Liebenow successfully robbed the store of drugs, but was caught when he returned a few minutes later because he had forgotten to steal syringes.

1996 Pharmacist Robert Trocki, 59, was arrested and charged with several counts of illegal sale of prescription drugs, including what police said were two instances of giving women birth control pills and pain relievers in exchange for their letting him kiss their feet and sneakers.

1996 The Arkansas State Medical Board ordered Waldo family physician, Jewel Byron Grimmett Jr. to start keeping written records. At a hearing, Grimmett told board members that he has kept all patient histories, including prescription records, only in his head for the 35 years he has been practicing medicine. Grimmett avoided license revocation because he is Waldo's only doctor and he treats about half his patients for free.

1997 *The Sunday Times* of London reported that 300 tons of humanitarian aid from Western countries was sitting in Bosnian warehouses because it is useless. Included were birth control pills with an expiration date of 1986, weight-reduction tablets from Britain, mouthwash from the United States, and chemical waste from Germany. According to the *Times*, some war-zone drivers have been killed transporting these supplies, and, by law, German chemicals cannot be returned, creating a hazardous waste disposal problem for Bosnians.

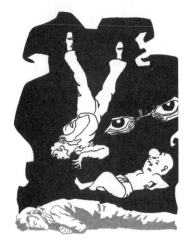

Pills and Suicide

Some pills can kill you. There is an undeniable fascination in that for most people. The idea that something as innocent as swallowing a couple of pills could kill you gives pill-taking an aspect of danger not usually found in such mundane practices. Taking a pill could cause relief, euphoria, nothing at all, a life-changing experience or maybe death. Such a range of outcomes is akin to the thrill of motorcycle-riding or foreign travel.

The centerpiece to Derek Humphrey's bestselling book *Final Exit* was a list of the fatal dosages of 18 different, commonly available pills. Although the rest of the book dealt with such grim topics as suffocating yourself or making a videotaped farewell to keep your surviving and grieving spouse out of prison, the famous chart was most arresting. There it was: How many Darvocets does it takes to kill yourself? Turns out there's quite a lot of pills in a lethal dose. Probably take a bunch of swallows to get 'em all down. Hell, it'd be like eating popcorn or something.

But there is a magic number: 30 of the pills containing 65 mgs propoxyphene each should do the trick. But there are caveats. A footnote points out you'll need to take a sleeping agent (also in overdose quantity) to have the best chance of dying. Oh, and he explicitly advises not to try Darvocet as a way to snuff yourself

That's not much of an endorsement for a drug rated number two on a list of pills most associated with prescription drug-induced deaths. Darvocet *can* kill you—it's just not that reliable. By the way, you've got to take all the pills at one time. The "death dosage" spread throughout a day isn't likely to hurt you.

Instead of encouraging anyone to kill himself, *Final Exit's* list of fatal pills drives home the seriousness of the task. One sleeping pill is not going to do it. Ten won't do it. A whole bottle might not do it. Killing yourself with pills may sound like a good idea, but when it comes down to the nitty gritty—a gun has to be more effective. And if you want to be extra sure—use a shotgun in the tradition of Ernest Hemmingway and Kurt Cobain. Humphrey always recommends a plastic bag over the head to ensure suffocation even when taking a fatal dose of pills.

Humphrey's list, shows that it's so difficult to kill yourself with Valium that attempts to do so make the wannabe corpse look positively stupid. We at *PaGG* take a dim view of this sort of benzodiazepine abuse. Valium and its cousins are valuable members of anyone's medical cabinet and should never be squandered on bogus cries-for-help. Our hint to anyone contemplating such a waste is to substitute a small handful of Allerest—the effect will be roughly similar—and give the benzos to someone who could use them.

"**Some people might wonder why they would turn to their physician when, to put it bluntly, you can just go out and buy a gun and blow your brains out. There's something about pills that feels cleaner and more considerate of the family.**"

—an anonymous doctor quoted in an AP story on suicide

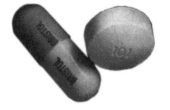

Fatal Doses

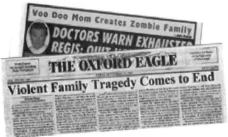

Here is a short list of reported lethal doses of various pills and household substances. Some of them are taken from *Final Exit,* but Pills-a-Go-Go has edited the list.

Amytal (amobarbital)—This short-acting barbiturate isn't as lethal as a barbiturate could be, so you have to swallow at least 90 of the 50 mg pills.

Butabarbital is a little more common but just a little more lethal. Be prepared to swallow at least 100 of the 30 mg doses.

Seconal (secobarbital) was the favorite pill taken by Patty Duke's character in *The Valley of the Dolls,* in which Sharon Tate kills herself with an overdose. But she must have taken a good 50 hits to do it. Less just wouldn't do it. If she were already a user, she'd have needed more.

Primatene Think we're kidding? Phenobarbital is a constituent of the pill, which is available OTC in some states. Since there is only 6 mg of phenobarb in each one, however, it would require something like 700 of these pills to do anyone in. Even then it would have been offset by the gigantic overdose of the stimulant ephedrine. Still, 4.5 grams is enough to kill you, in theory.

Pentobarbital (Nembutol) This one is lethal in doses of around three grams or just 30 of the 100 mg pills. Combining barbiturates will also increase the chances of killing yourself.

Heroin Even experienced junkies sometimes screw their dosage and kill themselves, so opiates can be effective, no doubt. Then again heroin's pretty strong and junkies habitually inject and we're talkin' pills here, so pay attention. You don't have to shoot it. You can swallow it, snort it, smoke it . . . its best feature as a suicide substance is its relative availability. It is sold on the underground market in most cities and towns in the country. There is the problem of standardized dosing and it rarely comes in pill form. To kill yourself with heroin without shooting up you must snort at least five, and more like 10 times, the amount you need to get high. For non-users, such an amount can range from as little as one eighth of a "dime bag" (10 bucks worth) to the whole thing, depending on quality. The only good way to find out how pure the stuff is, is to take it.

Morphine A half-dozen of the 30 mg. pills might kill you. That's 200 mgs and assumes no tolerance at all on the part of the suicide committer. Make sure the tablets are not time-released or you might just go on a pleasant nod. If you're already using morphine, your dose will be considerably higher, depending on the tolerance you have undoubtedly acquired.

Methadone About the same as morphine.

View the evidence and help detectives solve the case.

Evidence:

Contents of Laurie Daniels' carry-on bag, found in the Daniels' shop, behind garage:

- ✔ Handwritten letter from Melanie Daniels to Reggie Simms
- ✔ $72 in currency
- ✔ loose change totalling $3.87
- ✔ bottle of Darvocet (pain pills)
- ✔ bottle of Haldon (sleeping pills)
- ✔ package of Sudafed
- ✔ package of BC Powder
- ✔ pint of gin
- ✔ coffee mug from The Beehive (Pittsburgh, Penn.)
- ✔ rolling papers
- ✔ pack of Camel cigarettes
- ✔ cigarette lighter
- ✔ scrap of paper with number (718-3211)
- ✔ tin of carmex
- ✔ rosary beads
- ✔ two pairs jeans
- ✔ three T-shirts
- ✔ book of stamps
- ✔ half bag of M&Ms
- ✔ (1) sock
- ✔ (1) paperback, "Life After God" by Douglas Coupland
- ✔ walkman cassette player
- ✔ Phür Bürgher cassette
- ✔ (4) unmarked cassettes with music
- ✔ toothbrush/toothpaste
- ✔ hairbrush
- ✔ plastic baby doll (.5″ in length)
- ✔ (3) small crystals
- ✔ (2) unused condoms
- ✔ airline ticket stub/boarding pass

Heaven's Gate RECIPE

It's said (rumored, really) that the Heaven's Gaters decided on phenobarbitol as their Hand of Death in dosages recommended by the do-it-yourself death book, *Final Exit.* It seems they followed his advice to the letter. That there was no one left alive amounts to a good recommendation for Humphrey's book—too bad there's no one from the group available to blurb it.

Of course, the news didn't give us all the details—but there was enough to impart an idea. Typical media style had each member swallowing 50 tablets of phenobarbital as a main course. The dosage of the tablets was not given.

It appears they mixed the unpleasant-tasting pills with applesauce or pudding, as chef Humphrey recommends. And they souped-up the barbiturate overdose with alcohol. Four of them are said to have taken an unspecified amount of hydrocodone.

Presumably they followed the suicide to-do list and laid down on their cots and rested quietly . . . some of them with a plastic bag over their heads as *Final Exit* calls for.

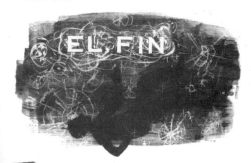

Dilaudid (hydromorphone)—Humphrey says between 100 and 200 mgs is a lethal dose. That means if you got the strongest pill available, you'd need to take 25 of 'em. Got that many in the bottle?

Codeine Here we go, codeine's easy to find and if you've got a prescription for Tylenol 3 you need to eat no fewer than 80 of them to have a crack at dying. (If your prescription even contains 80 hits and if you don't throw up—vomiting is a common side effect of high doses of any opiate.) Then there's tolerance. If you've been taking codeine for very long at all (even a week) you've built up a tolerance and all bets are off with this one. The same goes for all the above opiates.

Valium Humphrey estimates "500 mgs or more" to kill a person. In fact, Valium (diazepam) is not fatal at this dosage. It really isn't fatal in any quantity a person could reasonably be expected to wolf down. In rats, the LD 50 rate (the amount required to kill half the rats) is more than 700 mgs per kilogram of weight. For an adult human, this could easily mean swallowing and fully absorbing a good four or five thousand of the highest strength Valiums made. And then you only got half a chance. Mixed with alcohol and the plastic bag, though . . .

This non-toxicity applies to all the benzodiazepines, whether meant for anxiety or sleep. None of these pills has been shown to kill anyone unless combined with something else (like a gun). These are terrible pills to commit suicide with. Don't use 'em!

Same goes for the benzodiazepines' parent drug, meprobamate. A hundred of the strongest dose (400 mgs) won't kill you. As with so many drugs, tolerance develops pretty quickly for this drug, so if you're on Miltown already, it's an even worse choice.

Even chloral hydrate, the "knock out drop" from a hundred years ago, still marketed today in various forms, doesn't kill a person too easily. One needs a minimum of 50 2 mg doses to approach lethal limits. Other sources have reported a lethal dose to be more than three times this amount.

In the end, a deliberate mixture of pills will do you in most reliably. Mix up, say, fatal doses of morphine and a barbiturate. Then take further precautions not to vomit or otherwise screw up. Taking Compazine or Dramamine can reduce the nausea somewhat. Pills alone, however, are not a sure thing. Sorry.

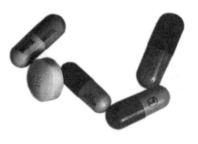

Tranquilizer Chart

The evolution of tranquilizer euphemism in the popular press, 1954–1981.

YEAR	TERMS USED	SOURCE
1954	"Wonder Drugs of 1954"	*Time*
1956	"Happy Pills"	*Changing Times*
	"Aspirin for the Soul"	
1956	"Psychiatric Aspirins"	*Nation*
	"Mental Laxatives"	
1956	"Pacifier for the Frustrated and Frenetic"	*Time*
	"Don't-Give-a-Damn Pills"	
	"Pills for the Mind"	
1956	"Peace of Mind Pills"	*Coronet*
	"Emotional Aspirin"	
1956	"Happy Pills"	*Look*
1956	"Happiness Pills"	*Christian Century*
1957	"Peace of Mind Drugs"	*Today's Health*
1957	"Happiness by Prescription"	*Time*
1959	"Happy Pills"	*Coronet*
1960	"Calming Pills"	*Science NewsLetter*
1960	"Peace of Mind Drugs"	*Time*
1961	"Quiet Pills"	*Today's Health*
1962	"Turkish Bath in a Tablet"	*Reader's Digest*
1963	"Brain Drugs"	*Popular Science Monthly*
1964	"Mind Drugs"	*Science Digest*
1966	"Weak Barbiturates"	*Science News*
	"Weak Alcohol"	
1966	"Mind-Acting Drugs"	*Science News*
1969	"Psychotropes"	*Transaction*
1980	"Bottled Well-Being"	*Time*

from *Small Comfort: A History of the Minor Tranquilizers* by Mickey C. Smith

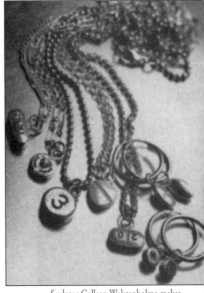

Sculptor Colleen Wolstenholme makes jewelry from antidepressants and tranquilizers.

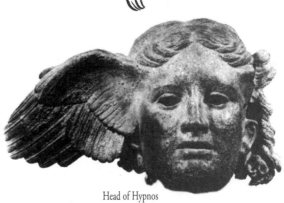

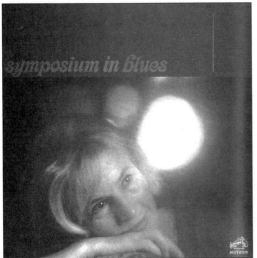

Head of Hypnos

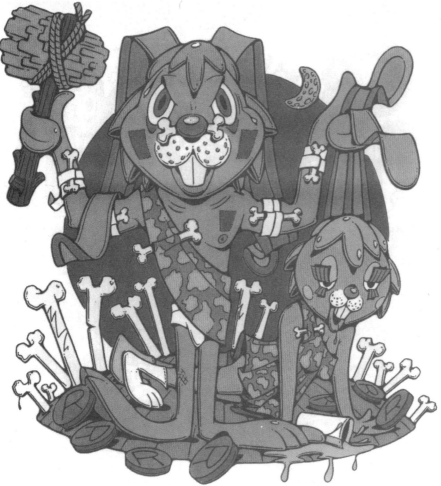

Illustration from Steven Cerio's *ABC Book, A Drug Primer* published by Gates of Heck

Rape Drugs

The concept of a "date rape drug" (sometimes shortened to "rape pill") is not new. Fear of white women being defiled by Chinese who doped their prey with opium was always part of the mythos behind opium prohibition.

Knocking someone out is as old as slipping a "Mickey Finn" into a bar patron's drink to steal his money; a big media fever in the mid-'90s concerned raping a woman after slipping her a "roofie" (Rohypnol). There's nothing new about a "knockout" drop. All that's required is a Central Nervous System (CNS) depressant. Whiskey is plenty sufficient, although the admixture of another CNS depressant would greatly speed the process.

The grandaddy of all knockout drugs is chloral hydrate, which was employed both by swindlers and rapists in the Old West and modern times. A chloral hydrate syrup called Noctec was used by Senator Bob Packwood to help him overpower and feel up female prey. Other substances used as knockout drugs include barbiturates, major and minor tranquilizers, anti-psychotic agents, plant extracts (such as belladonna alkaloids, which induce a "twilight sleep") and, of course, benzodiazepines such as Rohypnol. Don't forget GHB (gamma hydroxybutyrate)!

These drugs are rarely used by themselves —they are either bad-tasting, or too weak without the addition of the very powerful, very available CNS depressant: alcohol. Jeffrey Dahmer used the sleeping pill Halcion (which briefly preceded Rohypnol as the "rape pill") when he fed it to his victims along with lots of beer.

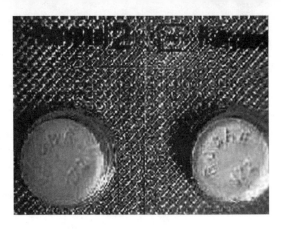

"Rohypnol's real companion value comes in with amphetamines and psychedelics. Say, for instance, you've taken too much speed and you'd like to have a rest, Rohypnol will calm you down quite like nothing you've ever experienced. The result is a warm, fuzzy, very comfortable feeling, free from anxiety, allowing you to drift away in a boat of bizarre and vivid dreams. If you've done an E and are experiencing a drastic or terrifying 'crash', Rohypnol will immediately save you from any emotional trauma, making you feel contented and relaxed, emotionally, mentally and physically." —*Socks,* from Erowid.org website

Most cases of "date rape" involving Rohypnol or GHB have also included alcohol. By itself alcohol has proven powerful enough and easy enough to qualify as a rape drug. In fact, alcohol has been the most popular rape drug throughout history. It still is.

So what the hell are these latest rape drugs? We'll start with the remarkable pill sold around the world for more than 30 years, made by Roche Pharmaceuticals—the same folks who brought you valium and scores of other, similar, drugs.

Rohypnol was invented by the same man who invented Valium and Librium—Leo Sternbach—and has sold in more than 160 countries around the world for more than 25 years. The pill has a record of safety as admirable as Valium or any other benzodiazepine.

Rohypnol is the Roche brand name for flunitrazepam, a benzodiazepine sedative-hypnotic in the same chemical/pharmacological class as Valium, Librium, Xanax, etc. Like others in its family, flunitrazepam works by binding "benzodiazepine receptors," which are part of the larger GABA-A receptor complex. Rohypnol causes marked sedation, muscle-relaxation, relief of anxiety, and sleep. In Europe it is prescribed as a sleeping pill and is used for pre-op sedation. Like all benzos it can relieve psychic tension to the point of mild euphoria. Like all benzos it causes a certain amount of amnesia. Rohypnol causes more amnesia than most, it is also more sedating than most.

Like all benzodiazepines it's incredibly safe even in overdose. But if large doses of flunitrazepam are consumed with large doses of

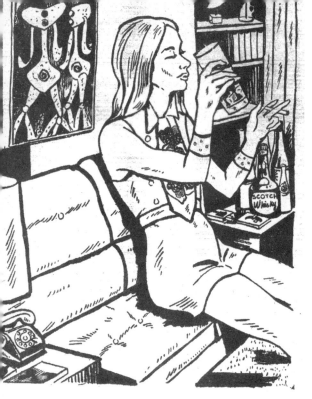

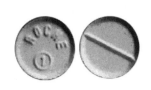

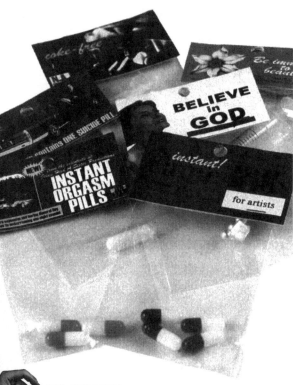

alcohol, the combination is considerably more potent than the pill alone. Such a combo can bring on slowed breathing, general anesthesia, coma, and even death. Rohypnol is the pill Kurt Cobain took with a champagne chaser in a supposed suicide attempt in Italy.

Scare stories about Rohypnol like to remind people that the stuff is ten times stronger than Valium, which, without further explanation, is supposed to give you the idea that it is wildly potent. But like Ativan (lorazepam), Halcion (triazolam), Klonapin (clonazepam), Xanax (alprazolam), and others, the effective dose for flunitrazepam ranges from 0.5 mg to 2 mgs.

These same scare stories repeat the mantra, "never-approved for use in the U.S." The suggestion being that the benevolent FDA has kept us from an overseas danger. But Roche never applied for U.S. approval of Rohypnol. As far as Roche is concerned, there is no reason to go to the trouble and expense of introducing yet another benzo onto a market it already dominates with other products.

Nevertheless, its former "unapproved" status as a schedule IV controlled substance (like Valium) and its import for personal use was permitted until March 6, 1996, when U.S. Customs banned the drug completely, while the DEA prepared to move the pill into Schedule I category. At the same time proposals in Congress tried to criminalize the pill, aping legislation in various states where the pill was already bumped up to Schedule I status. Congress instead enacted the "Drug-Induced Rape Punishment and Prevention Act of 1996," which increased federal penalties for selling and possessing large quantities of flunitrazepam. The Act also calls for the DEA to consider rescheduling flunitrazepam. By now, the rescheduling is a moot issue. The DEA has the authority to reschedule drugs, as does the President. But, what's the point?

GHB is the sodium or potassium salt of gamma-hydroxybutyric acid: sodium or potassium gamma-hydroxybutyrate. Sometimes called sodium oxybate, GHB is used in Europe as a general anaesthetic, and works by binding to its own specific receptor sites on the GABA-B receptor and/or by interfering with dopamine transmission. GHB occurs naturally in the mammalian nervous system as a metabolite of, or precursor to, GABA (gamma-aminobutyric acid).

Compared to most pharmaceuticals it takes fairly large amounts of GHB to get the sedation, and small doses (1–3 g, depending on body weight) produce mild euphoria, heightened sexual interest, disinhibition. Large doses (4 g +) produce heavy sedation, amnesia, general anaesthesia. GHB requires rather large doses to be effective. Because of this, and because GHB has an almost revolting, salty taste, it is difficult to mask the taste of an effective dose of GHB, except with strong alcohol.

Legal status: once available OTC as a nutritional supplement (increases growth hormone production, improves sleep quality), GHB was banned by the F.D.A in 1990. Not a DEA controlled substance, but a scheduled drug in some states (California, Rhode Island, Florida, Texas, others), GHB may be made from readily available precursors—butyrolactone and sodium hydroxide, or ordered from overseas readymade (with questionable legality). Bills have been introduced in Congress which would schedule GHB (either I or III), but no action has been taken as of November 1998.

Any CNS depressant may cause unconsciousness and amnesia (see alcohol). On the other hand, GHB is a more effective general anaesthetic than flunitrazepam. To call either medication a "date rape drug" is, of course, patently unfair. Both have clinical uses, and the vast majority of non-medical use is by willing participants who just want to get stoned.

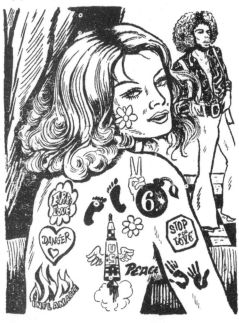

KNOCK-OUT GIRLS

A couple articles appeared in the *FBI Law Enforcement Bulletin* that have to do with pills, and the horrid tortures they inflict on society, and what our fearless men-in-blue can do to stop 'em.

In the *Bulletin's* January, 1993 issue entitled "Knock-out Dates—Flirting with Danger," authors James Schaefer and Murray A. Latzen zero in on what they call "knock-out girls" and the methods they use to render their prey helpless through the use of drugs and then make off with their wallets.

Just picture a well-heeled businessman getting rolled while cheating on his siliconed wife. But as we smile the FBI mag reminds us that 13 people's deaths "have been contributed to" by these chicks—although they don't provide any crucial or critical information.

According to the cop/authors' research, the most favored drugs used by knock-out girls are scopalamine, lorazepam and atropine. As is typical with pill scare stories, they exaggerate the chemicals' effects and fail to take into account the marked effects of large amounts of alcohol—especially when they say these products are typically administered via a cocktail à la Dahmer.

That is when they don't "place a crushed or powdered form of the drug on their lips and then pass it to their victims by a kiss."

Somnolent Culture

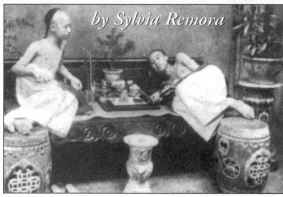

by Sylvia Remora

The world of pills has its own special prejudices that reflect larger truths about Western culture and the society we live in. One of the most blatant and instructive of these prejudices is the widespread fear and contempt that doctors, and patients show toward stimulants.

Except for caffeine and nicotine, most stimulants are reviled and hated. Cocaine has become the target of the war on drugs. Meth labs are treated like nuclear waste dumps and meth chemists are hunted down like diseased animals and thrown into prison for ridiculously long sentences. Doctors who used to make a living prescribing diet pills to bored housewives have gone the way of $15 ounces of marijuana. In contrast, the use of depressants is widely encouraged. The acceptance of alcohol is the most common example of

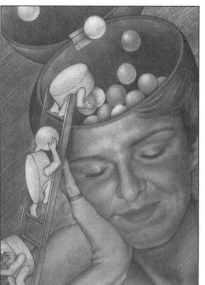

this bias toward drugs that depress body function and mental perception. Doctors frequently prescribe tranquilizers, sedatives and sleeping pills to their troubled patients. Depressants even pop up in our daily conversation; it's common to hear harried co-workers advise each other to "take a Valium" when stress surfaces.

Why do we fear stimulants? Anyone who is normally hyperactive or who indulges in stimulants knows the answer intuitively. People are more comfortable with placid sluggards. To be wide awake is to think, to do, to bounce off the walls and explode in marathon conversations that lead to introspection, prank phone calls, plots and serious societal espionage. To be awake, alert and wired is, in a word, dangerous. The powers that be would rather we all drown our sorrows in booze in front of the television. It keeps us pliant and manageable. It makes us better consumers. Just try to watch TV on speed. By the fifth commercial you'll be ranting against Madison Avenue and you sure as hell won't be ready to go out and buy the crap you see featured in their sluggish, banal advertisements. Living on stimulants makes you realize just how slow everyone else is moving. It's no wonder this shit never changes.

What would happen if all the people who stagger home from their dreary jobs each day stopped dulling their pain with an alcohol or pot-induced stupor each night? What if they popped speed and drank espresso instead? We may never know . . . .

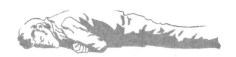

Of all pills, none other elicits such fear and wonder as the amphetamine. Though in recent years amphetamines have come to be re-recognized as a useful drug (what else to use for obesity?), its overall use has dropped by 80–90% since the 1970 Controlled Substances Act put a phobia into doctors who prescribed "pep pills," "bennies" or "goofballs" (speed mixed with barbiturates).

Before the blacklisting, amphetamines were widely and openly recognized as awesome pills. Five to 15 mg of dextroamphetamine banishes fatigue and lifts the spirits of the depressed. Methamphetamine is even stronger and longer-lasting. Amphetamines were also used to treat other mental diseases, including the dreaded Obsessive Compulsive Disorder (which wouldn't find an FDA-approved treatment until 1990 when the anti-depressant Anafranil was introduced). Like characters in a Philip K. Dick novel, we seemed headed for a world where amphetamines would be dispensed from public vending machines.

Alas, it was not to be.

When media demonization failed to persuade the masses into passing up on amphetamines, the force of law was brought down on anything stronger than caffeine. This opened the market for cocaine, and speed was nearly obliterated, even with truck drivers.

Filling the speed void were "amphetamine analogues" . . . supposedly not "real" amphetamines. Like so much else said about pills, this is not the case. Nearly all "analogues" belong to the molecular family of the amphetamine. This family—known as phenethylamines—is quite large. The designer drug Ecstasy (MDMA), ephedrine (Primatene), a top-selling anti-depressant (Wellbutrin), chocolate and even mescaline belong to the phenethylamine familial structure. Hell, only a few strategic atoms differentiate speed from NutraSweet.

Speed is most dangerous to those who want to believe government propaganda, but the slogan "Speed Kills" is statistically unsupported.

The Artist's Friend

Gone With The Wind owes its making to speed. According to film historians, producer David O. Selznick constantly ate benzedrine tablets to fuel consistent 22-hour days. *Dr. Zhivago,* too, was filmed with a cast cruising on speed.

During the filming of *Lawrence of Arabia,* Omar Sharif was such a Dexedrine-head that he was pulled aside and counseled in proper drug use by fellow actor Jack Hawkins. "I was very intense and used to take [speed pills] to make me more excited," explained Sharif.

"And Jack said, 'Dear boy, acting needs sleeping pills.' The secret is to relax; you need energy, but relaxed energy."

Ciao Manhattan staffed its own doctor to administer injections of amphetamines to the cast and crew. High on speed the actors not only performed longer, they exuded a kind of conviviality crucial to the film. The amphets received bad publicity, though, by contributing to the death of Edie Sedgwick, the movie's star.

It's been suggested that Ayn Rand's use of Dexedrine explained why her novels ran over a thousand pages. It's been noted that Rand switched to mescaline, an amphetamine analogue, to help her with some of her books.

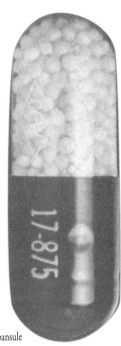

Dexedrine Spansule

APPETITE CONTROL
for compulsive eaters

Adventures in overeating

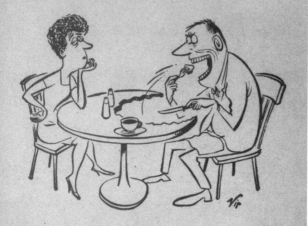

Appetrol®tablets ⊘

meprobamate 400 mg. + dextro-amphetamine sulfate 5 mg.

A Clockwork Orange's Anthony Burgess used speed when writing many of his books, as did Neal Casady and Jack Kerouac and so many other bibliomaniacs. And if these examples aren't enough to convince you that speed and art go hand in hand, consider that Johnny Cash loved Dexedrine so much he landed in jail after being caught smuggling a load into the country from Mexico.

Speed chemists brag how amphetamines fueled Kamikaze pilots and the German army during World War II. In truth, all the armies in the world war were hopped up on speed. American soldiers continued to receive regular rations of Dexedrine in their kits right through the Vietnam War. While Vietnam is generally known to have been rife with drug use, there was lots more speed than heroin or hash, and officially provided, too. To give an idea of the sheer number of dexies downed by GIs in Vietnam, consider this statistic: from 1966 to 1969, American soldiers swallowed more amphetamines than all the American and British soldiers combined for the whole of the Second World War.

In the '50s, speed became almost permanently linked to truck drivers, cramming college students and other examples of stand-up citizens just gettin' the job done. All-American aerospace heroes who broke the sound barrier and risked death in the first manned space flights were bringing speed with them into the Great Void.

As might be expected, it's kept hush-hush that astronauts still take speed with them on their trips into orbit. Every airliner's cockpit is stocked with speed, too, for use by pilots as a safety precaution in case of sudden sleepiness (definitely not an FDA-approved application).

Operation Desert Storm had bomber pilots obliterating Iraqi cities under the influence of speed (hey, doesn't amphetamine use have a mad killer theory?). Luckily, the military was wise enough to dose the pilots with temazepam (Restoril) after returning from bombing Koran-readers into ash.

Perhaps sensing that amphetamines were of great use to the establishment, hippies declared speed an agent of the devil. Allen Ginsberg even issued a warning "ex cathedra" (his words) that "speed kills." This erroneous piece of propaganda has since become axiomatic.

Good morning, Mr. Phelps. Last night, the Stonehurst Chemical Plant was robbed of

Does Speed Really Kill, Allen?

Though it's a widespread belief that amphetamines kill a lot of users, data doesn't bear out the idea at all. In fact, it seems amphetamines are remarkably safe, as was thought from its pharmaceutical beginnings. California criminologist Dr. Roger C. Smith, who headed some drug rehabilitation programs, was responsible for an exhaustive study of amphetamine use. Smith found cases of people mainlining speed in amounts as large as 15,000 mgs in the course of a day, and he discovered that people could easily withstand intravenous injects of 400 and 500 mgs, even if they never took the drug before. The normal dose, orally, is no more than 30 mgs at a time. Five or ten milligrams is more typical.

A study conducted by Drs. Harold and Oriana Kalant of the Addiction Research Foundation in Ontario, Canada and the Department of Pharmacology at the University of Toronto in 1979 found that casual use of amphetamines rarely causes death. All the medical literature until 1963 turned up just nine deaths associated with amphetamine use. By 1979, the entirety of medical literature found 79 cases of death "associated in some way" with amphetamines. Compare this to the hundreds of thousands of alcohol-induced fatalities.

Seven of these amphetamine deaths came from hypertensive crises, i.e., brain hemorrhage. Of these seven deaths, four were found to have happened when speed was mixed with MAOI, a contraindication not known at the time. Three of the speed fatalities were from victims old enough that the hemorrhage was not unusual; and one suffered from cerebral atheroma in the past. Three deaths were from patients younger than 30. Speed may well have killed them. Heart attacks caused by speed killed some people, too, but none of them were clear-cut cases—they were either already sick or took other drugs, such as digitalis, along with amphetamines that could have easily affected the heart.

This is not to promote the idea that no one has ever died on speed. Plenty of people have speed in their system when they croaked. But speed didn't kill them. Apart from several rare, fatal overdoses, speed-users are killed far more often by coronary or vascular diseases caused by mixing speed with other drugs.

In 1967, a Tour de France bicyclist hopped up on speed died of heat asphyxiation as he pumped his bike up a mountain road. Death from speed and hyperthermia is rare, but it's a bad idea to mix speed with prodigious physical exertion at high

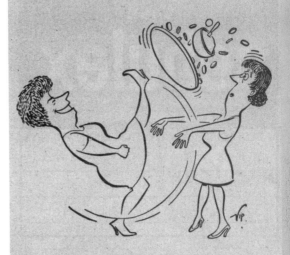
three tons of D-amphetamine sulfate, commonly known as speed.

Speed 107

temperatures. The combo can cause heart failure or burst blood vessels even in seemingly healthy people.

So, once in a blue moon, amphetamines cause death. The rest are killed in accidents. Mundane accidents. Cars are crashed, deadly bacteria is injected into veins, and chronic, high-dose amphetamine use can lead to sustained anorexia and malnutrition. It can even cause tooth decay!

On the other hand, speed has saved more than a few people from death by respiratory depression caused by a heroin overdose. In this way, "speedballs" (heroin and stimulant combos) are almost self-correcting.

Amphetamine-induced Psychosis

The one predictably bad thing speed can do is cause a kind of artificial insanity. Given enough speed in a short enough time, people will begin to exhibit frankly paranoid behavior.

"Amphetamine psychosis" is induced by taking very large amounts of speed for no less than 24 hours. A dose of 10 mgs of amphetamine per hour, every hour, will produce "the CIA is monitoring my thoughts" paranoia in nearly everyone within three days. This sort of paranoia is at least in part truthful. Dr. G. Richard Wendt dosed students with huge combos of Dexedrine and Seconal (goofballs) for the Naval Intelligence/ CIA Operations CHATTER, ARTICHOKE and CASTGATE, to induce hypnotic amnesia. It's possible to bring on psychoses even faster if dosages are doubled or tripled. Strangely enough, this phenomenon doesn't have much to do with sleep deprivation, as had been thought at first. One must discontinue use of the drug to actually stop it.

But a normal dose of dextroamphetamine doesn't exceed more than 30 mgs per day (compared the 2,500+ needed to drive you crazy). Since the induced psychosis is completely reversible upon discontinuation of the drug and letting the subject sleep and recover, large amphetamine usage provides psychiatric researchers good models for paranoia studies.

Depending on your point of view, amphetamines either helped the allies win "The Good War" against the yellow hordes and The Goosesteppers or maybe it helped the Axis to lose their marbles. Either way, speed wins.

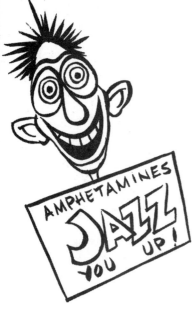

More Evidence of Right-Wing Conspiracy

Now that we know speed is the drug of John Glenn and those magnificent men in their flying machines, it's no shock to discover that none other than arch-conservative William F. Buckley Jr.— CIA man and confidant of the incestuous overlords of the Council of Foreign Relations—takes speed every day and has done so for a good 30 years!

That's right. Buckley's hopped up on Ritalin every single day. It seems Bill owes at least part of his steel-trap mind, rapier wit and maybe some facial tics to a daily dose of methylphenidate hydrochloride. No wonder he came out in favor of the legalization of all drugs and the surrender of the War on Drugs. He was probably terrified.

Terrified by the realization that the DEA controls every aspect of Ritalin, (including its production quotas) and not he nor his doctor nor the chairman of the Republican Party can do a thing about it.

Conventional law enforcement agencies believe that Sam Hibbing, the west's

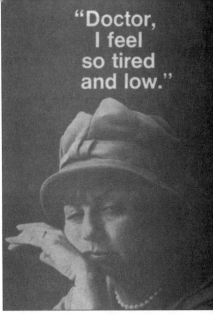

Maybe he was out of town one day, preening for a public banter when he realized he had run out of Ritalin, and tough shit—no doctor was gonna hand him a last-minute Ritalin script. Thanks to the paperwork monstrosities and threats of prosecution, Schedule II drugs are not fillable (or refillable) by phone in any state. Even the precise number of Schedule II pills manufactured each month is a decision made by the DEA only. This idiotic system was responsible for a brief Ritalin shortage in 1994.

The shortage occurred when too many adults were diagnosed with Attention Deficit Disorder and beat the kids to their pills, leaving thousands of terrified mothers to face their monstrous offspring with no help at all. Even if Buckley did get his pills that month, he was, no doubt, held in fearsome thrall by the thought of hyperactive kids going berserk in the streets.

Buckley began to realize that the war on their drugs became a war on his own drugs, too, and he started to denounce naked police power over his private life. Buckley also serves as living proof that daily speed use is not harmful, nor does it lead inexorably to "addiction" and crime.

CIBA's advertisement for William F. Buckley Jr.'s favorite drug.

In a letter to pop-psychologist Peter McWilliams, Buckley answered charges that three straight decades of Ritalin use have transformed him into a "speed freak."

After first explaining that his doctor prescribed Ritalin as a remedy to fainting spells caused by low blood pressure (not an approved use, by the way . . .), Buckley seems a little annoyed at having to defend his usage.

"Big Deal!" he writes, ". . . after 30 years, nobody has detected any change in me, haahahahhhhaaaaaa, eeeeeeee, ooooooooooooooooooo oooooo! Now I'm feeling quite fine, as you can see."

What Is Ritalin?

Ritalin is chemically related to amphetamines but produces less central nervous system arousal than mental stimulation. A cup of coffee raises blood pressure more than Ritalin. Today it's mostly prescribed for hyperactive children, but is also approved for the treatment of narcolepsy. And that's it.

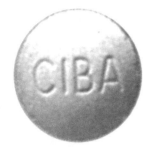

Of course, the approved uses are only a fraction of what Ritalin can do. Before all the FDA noise and regulation in the mid 1960s, CIBA hawked Ritalin to doctors as an anti-depressant. "Buzz" Aldrin, the second man to step on the moon (but the first to pee on it), was given Ritalin for the severe depression he suffered after he got back to earth.

The 1960 *PDR* says Ritalin "restores mental and physical activities to normal or near normal levels . . . induces alertness, a brighter mental outlook and improved psychomotor performance"—a specific recommendation for chronic fatigue and lethargy. It was also suggested for use in helping people recover from general anaesthesia. Useful stuff.

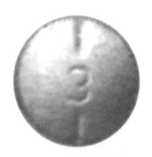

Since then, Ritalin has been advanced in the bad drug hierarchy of Schedule II drugs. Called a "mild stimulant," Ritalin is known to be just as good as Dexedrine. Comparison tests of Ritalin and Dexedrine show Ritalin to be "superior," milligram for milligram, in its ability to excite mental faculties.

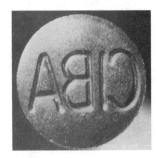

"I'm not about to go out there one-on-one against a guy who is grunting and drooling and coming at me with big, dilated pupils," said one San Diego Charger in the late 1960s, "unless I'm in the same condition." It was reported that his team took more than 10,000 pills, including stimulants, pain killers and downers.

Higher-than-normal rates of violence among returning World War II soldiers in both Japan and Sweden was promptly blamed on speed. In America, police claim speed freaks break out into spontaneous (and murderous) sprees of violence. But, really, there is only one group of violent people whose use of speed can be tied to their violent behavior: football players.

On August 5, 1995, ex-NFL guard Walt Sweeney was awarded more than half a million dollars in back pay plus $4,000 per month for life as a result of disabilities he suffered while a professional football player from 1963 to 1976. Walt's beef wasn't the sprained ankle or broken hand, as you might expect. Walt was pissed because he'd been forced to gobble so much Dexedrine. Walt chowed down on Secanol, steroids, codeine and other pain killers, but his first dose of dex was 100 mgs and it kept going upward from there.

Another Clean-Cut, All-American Speed Freak
Amphetamines and Football

The judge in the case found the NFL liable for injuries because drug-feeding was a matter of NFL policy and considered a "calculated risk." Ending up in the rehab center at age 54, Sweeney says, "I wasn't the Lone Ranger in this." he said "Every team passed out drugs."

Other studies bear him out. Football has become more progressively more violent and drug-driven well into the '70s. Anonymous interviews with 86 players from 15 NFL teams conducted by a team doctor show an interesting distribution of speed according to position.

Linemen consumed far more speed during a game than the quarterback or other players who rely less on brute strength than mental prowess. Statistics also bear out Dexedrine's tendency to provoke awkward behavior in high doses. Nimble gods of the gridiron may have better luck using Ritalin, with its greater effect on mental capacity. Nonetheless, as the charts show, all positions had some use for speed. Tell-all tales since the mid-'70s show that when amphetamines were suppressed, cocaine took its place.

Synthesized by the German scientist L. Edeleano in 1887, and then known as phenylisopropylamine, it was not until 1910 that G. Barger and Sir H. H. Dale investigated the effect of amphetamines on animals. Fear that China could cut off America's supply of natural ephedrine sent scientists looking for alternatives. Amphetamine was hauled out again and proved itself effective, whether inhaled or swallowed. Gordon Alles discovered in 1927 that d-isomer, dextroamphetamine was as much as ten times stronger than its 1-isomer. Alles (1901–1963) apparently did

hidden at a secret location where he plans to package it in pill form and sell some testing on himself with positive results. He's also known for his work on isolating insulin and for his 1939 study on the physiological effects of cannabis, decades before general awareness of medical marijuana.

Meanwhile, over at the drug firm of SmithKline & French, chief chemist F.P. Nabenhauer heard about Alles' experiments and started experimenting with amphetamines with SmithKline's nasal inhaler. It worked like a charm and felt good, too. In 1932, the company bought all patent rights to the stuff from Alles and launched the first speed-driven inhaler that needed no prescription. It probably took less than a few minutes before somebody opened the thing up and sucked out its precious juices. Jack Kerouac broke open inhalers, removed its speed-impregnated folded paper and swished it in his coffee. Nice buzz.

Inhalers provided an easy way to obtain speed while the media fretted about—and thus promoted—new "pep pills." In the mid-'60s, laws were passed to control their use. But as soon as one amphetamine family member was banned, another non-prescription inhaler took its place. This same principle helped increase the popularity of inhalers since competing companies realized SmithKline's patent did not extend to every conceivable variation of the amphetamine theme. More amphetamines were invented and put into more inhalers.

Lawmakers and do-gooders squawked but it was no use. Although SmithKline stopped marketing their inhaler in 1949 (but continues to this day manufacturing speed) they couldn't stop others from making new inhalers. Soon, inhalers were made "abuse proof" by adding nauseating substances like croton oil or pycric acid. This abuse proofing had an unintended effect of creating speed fiends who injected paper strip speed soaked in hot water. It was not until the summer of 1971 that Wyamine inhalers, with their cool dose of 250 mgs of mephentermine, was yanked off the market.

On the other hand, plain old Sudafed (pseudephedrine) was approved for over-the-counter sales in 1976 as well as speedy Afrin (oxymetazoline) nose spray.

Truth be told, there are still amphetamines in nasal inhalers. Vick's (and only Vick's) contains an active ingredient called "desoxyephedrine"—otherwise known as methamphetamine. But it's the L isomer of meth, not the potent dextro isomer. Still, it is possible to extract L-meth and either use it as is, or turn it into a D-L mixture and increase its potency.

Benzedrex inhalers contain 250 mgs. of propylhexadrine—no doubt an amphetamine in the eyes of the law, since there are criminal penalties for its possession!

The quest to stop people from injecting speed has led Abbott, the leading maker of methamphetamine, to formulate the pill Desoxyn so that the active ingredient is intimately bound up with a polymer resin, so that the drug is released into the system more slowly, making it difficult to simply crush up and dissolve. In fact, the damn pills (known as Gradumet tablets) are so hard, it's a job to break them in the first place. Of course, an overnight soaking can do the trick . . .

Benzene ring — Carbon atom — Amino nitrogen atom
"Amine" structure

Serotonin

Epinephrine (adrenalin)

Norepinephrine

An amphetamine compound

it to the underworld at a huge profit. Your mission, should you decide to

Speed 111

METHAMPHETAMINE

S peed use causes not only a reduction in sleep but also in REM and subsequent rebound REM when it wears off.

Because of the government's dogged suppression of legal amphetamines, it has always been profitable to make it at home. Today, most amphetamine is manufactured by illegal "cooks" in clandestine laboratories—many of which are in California. True to the pattern of illegal drug use, one of the strongest versions of amphetamine—methamphetamine—is the one most often made. Although it is sometimes asserted that just about anyone can cook up a batch of meth as long as he has the recipe, this just isn't true. Quite apart from the danger of getting a hellacious prison sentence if you get caught making this stuff. All of the methods used by clandestine chemists to make meth, whether from Phenyl-2-Propanone (P2P) or from ephedrine—the two most common ways—require the product to be reduced or hydrogenated. In simple terms this means using pure hydrogen gas in a sealed container along with heat and pressure. The potential for a violent explosion is very real because of the precise control required and the shitty equipment often used to do it. Add to this the extensive use of flammable solvents like ether and it is no wonder many would-be meth chemists are discovered when they are blown up in their own labs. Most cops would prefer not to wait until a meth chemist begins making his brew—or even waiting until he has assembled all the ingredients—before busting him. Walking into a place full of acetone, ether, open flame and perhaps a couple of idiots is just too dangerous.

Police have shown a real preference for simply selling a person chemical precursors to speed, then busting him for conspiracy to make and sell speed.

Another thing the DEA has done to clamp down on meth manufacture is to assert control over anything that could be made into speed of any kind. Beginning a few years ago, the DEA has gradually outlawed the mail-order business of ephedrine tablets and forced makers to add unnecessary chemicals to the pills to prevent their use in speed making.

These laws are, of course, doomed to failure. There is no ingredient that cannot be thwarted given enough time.

"I tell ya its a full time job trying to stay a step ahead of them," says one underground chemist. "Lately they've been putting a binder in there that is soluble in cold water but insoluble when heated. So you notice you lose all the pills when you do the first extraction and then later it all turns into this gelatinous goo.

"Oh, it's terrible."

AMPHETAMINE

PHENYLPROPANOLAMINE

EPHEDRINE

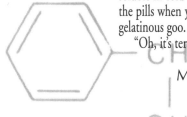

METHAMPHETAMINE $CH_2CHNHCH_3$ with CH_3

AMPHETAMINE $CH-CH-NH$ with H, CH_3, H

PHENYLPROPANOLAMINE $CH-CH-NH$ with OH, CH_3, H

EPHEDRINE $CH-CH-NH$ with OH, CH_3, CH_3

accept it, is to find and recover the speed before Hibbing can distribute it,

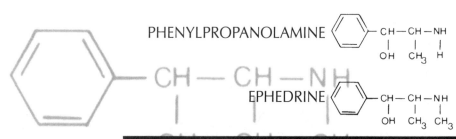

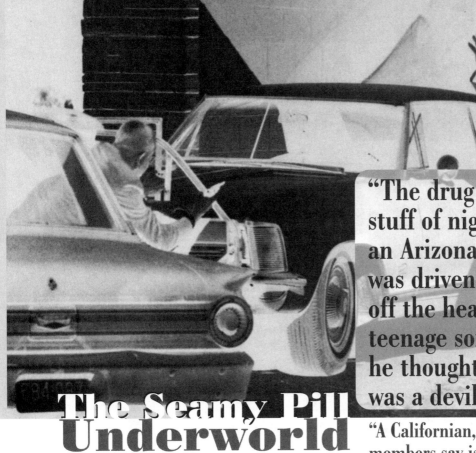

The Seamy Pill Underworld

"**The drug is the stuff of nightmares, an Arizona father was driven to hack off the head of his teenage son because he thought the boy was a devil.**

Tom's voice suddenly came in all too clear, for he was saying: "It's not easy to get really young girls with such big boobies. But that girl with the two guys, she's only sixteen."

"The one with the dark glasses?" Wally asked. "How did you get her to—"

"Like I told you, a coupla drinks with a coupla pills, and for a coupla hunnerd dollars, you're in business!"

"It's the pills that make 'em do it, huh? I mean they did look like straight girls."

"Oh, these are straight girls from, you know, college and secretaries and like that. That one you said—with the dark glasses—she's a college girl. We gave her the pills in a drink and she went crazy. She wanted to take on every man in the bar!"—from BLACK MARKET MEDICINE

It is hard to find a better example of someone more infused with the belief that pills can do anything than Margaret Kreig, authoress of *Black Market Medicine* (1967). Not only is she convinced of the power of pills, she believes in their immaculate holiness—consecrated by pharmaceutical firms, pharmacists and doctors. In the book, the admiring

"A Californian, whose family members say is a loving son, stabbed his 76-year-old father repeatedly, thinking aliens had invaded his body."

"A drug-crazed thief committed point-blank shotgun murders of two teenage companions he mistakenly thought had cheated him, according to Alameda county authorities in California. He denies the killing but said: 'I can tell you that that drug makes me the evilest person in the world.'

"The drug is methamphetamine."

—from the Australian newspaper, *The Dominion*

and to put Hibbing out of business for good. This tape will self-destruct in

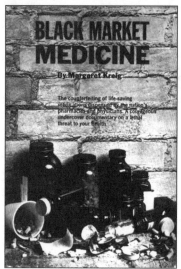

Kreig accompanies fearless FDA agents as they hunt pill counterfeiters and their unlicensed products. For her, even lowly FDA functionaries examining stolen and counterfeit pharmaceuticals become heroic experts in what she calls "Pillistics."

The FDA returns the admiration in a foreword to the book describing what a trooper she was, huddling with them outside seedy warehouses waiting to bust hoods making mislabeled diuretics. She risked her life to bring us the story, they say. It is a courageous undercover documentary.

Although the book was published in 1967, the "action" probably takes place a few years before that. Of course, no place names, times, or other such information is revealed to protect the innocent and ongoing investigations.

This untimeliness is all the better—we are spared any of the normal anti-drug propaganda, which focuses on the abuse potential of drugs rather than the heinous crimes of copyright infringements and lowered profit margins.

In the book, complete with plates showing "peddlers" being arrested by FDA agents springing from dark, bulbous cars, characters named "Big Mex" and "Abe" show remarkable indifference to which drugs they sell.

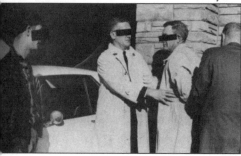

Their conversations—transcribed from wiretaps and bugs—turn easily from discussions of the best markets for geriatric vitamins, to amphetamines, to quinine, to spray-dried lactose to use as a filler. In fact, spray-dried lactose is one of the most sought-after items.

One pill counterfeiter gushes about his favorite inert ingredient:

"It is wonderful stuff," he says, "direct compressible, you don't need any ovens or granulation, all you do is mix your active ingredients with it and it's ready to go."

What's interesting about the dialogue is that it hardly proves these gangsters to be big dangers to society. Other than bad grammar and a lack of respect for the government, these guys are wheeler-dealers who like to please their customers. They talk about taking samples of drugs from the middle of a barrel to minimize getting tricked, and sympathize with "the guy who got stuck on the kilo of expensive hormone—was it cortisone? Turned out to be talcum powder. Wasn't a damn thing they could do about it."

They discuss ways of procuring pill-making equipment and seem to do the work themselves, spending entire nights making pills—making pills until their arms hurt.

Yet it is rare that even Kreig accuses them of manufacturing substandard pills. Just counterfeit in the sense that they were not really made by the proper company.

Still, she blames a lot of society's evils on pills, even including a death house confession by child killer Carl Austin Hall, reminiscent of Bundy's last blatherings about how porno made him do it. The killer, in addition to drinking a fifth of hard liquor a day, ate Benzedrine tablets he bought from a pharmacy with a doctor's prescription. For Kreig, he was the "classic precursor of the contemporary berserk pep-pill addict."

five seconds. Good luck, Jim.—from Mission: Impossible, episode #147, **Speed**

VIAGRA
and the
Boner Test

The normally tightassed twerps at the FDA that are better known for denying drug approval than anything else, waved Viagra through its certification process at a speed that rivaled the agency's approval of NutraSweet. That's a pretty big deal for an agency that has officially denied that prune juice is a laxative and outlawed any advertising that would say such a thing.

The only way the FDA will allow a company to make a claim about a particular pill is if it laid down approximately $20 million and spent years producing literally truckloads of documentation to prove it.

So, discovering their anti-impotence pill was just the beginning for Pfizer, the company that makes Viagra. Before they could sell the pill to help guys get boners, they had to scientifically answer a question that's never been properly answered: namely, what is a boner anyway?

How hard is hard enough? What's the difference between a satisfactory erection and an unsatisfactory one? And how the hell do you prove it?

In other words, if a guy gets an erection in the middle of the night while he's asleep, did he have a boner or not? Could he have used it to fuck, or did it only last for a few seconds, then deflate?

Previous boner tests were fairly crude, most of them being variations on the "Postage stamp test," where a guy was supposed to put stamps on his dick before he went to sleep. If they had fallen off by the time he woke up—the test surmised—then he had an erection. Of course this test reveals more about the glue on the stamps than anything else, and says nothing about *why* or *how* a boner happens.

So, to show how well their pill worked, Pfizer had to investigate the poorly-understood biochemistry and neurobiology of erections. To that end, Pfizer ditched the stamps and millions were poured into development of an extensive self-inventory survey. Called the "International Index of Erectile Function" (or IIEF), Pfizer researchers used the test to measure what had yet to be measured and might have been essentially unmeasurable: sexual performance, sexual desire, along with any changes in them and a way of understanding those changes.

They didn't have much to work with, either.

Like yawning, boners are thought to come from parts of the brain known as the limbic system and the hypothalmus. The limbic system is a nebulous term describing parts of the brain where the conscious and unconscious blur and emotion links up with action. In dogs, these same parts of the brain control barking. Erections and what causes them are a frustrating mystery, seeming to come in three flavors: reflexogenic, psychogenic, and nocturnal.

The first kind are a reaction to direct and physical stimulation—a hand job, say. Even people with broken spinal cords can sometimes get this sort of hard-on, and it is this mechanism that Viagra exploits.

The next kind are brought on by stimulation of the brain. For your average 14-year-old, is might be no more than a glance at a department-store mannequin in the lingerie section. Or it could be the sight of Mary Lou's lovely round ass. Just thinking about her ass can trigger a psychogenic boner.

Nocturnal erections accompany the REM stage of sleep, which is associated with dreaming. Any kind of dream, too. Not just sexual dreams. This is the type of erection men frequently wake up with. It doesn't necessarily have anything to do with sex or sexual stimulation.

And that's about it. Pfizer's tests couldn't elaborate any further. They didn't have to: they figured out the mechanism that causes an erection and how to manipulate it by taking a pill.

The Pharmacological Bullseye

Pfizer's brass ring of pharmaceuticals works by modulating a neurotransmitter called nitric oxide (NO). Although NO was known to be linked to erections, its precise role was unknown. As it turns out, NO is the principle neurotransmitter in the penis that sets off and maintains erections. Nitric oxide carries the

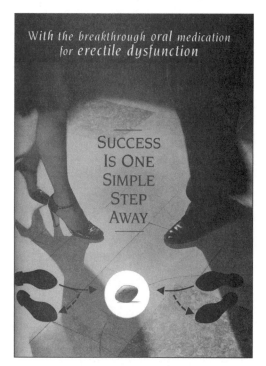

With the breakthrough oral medication for *erectile dysfunction*

SUCCESS
IS ONE
SIMPLE
STEP
AWAY

message "I am horny" to the dick, telling it to do its thing and it is produced on the spot, as a result of sexual stimulation. Nitric oxide is crucial to the chemistry of erections, but it isn't the whole story.

Viagra's action affects just one part of a chain of events leading from sexual stimulation to an erection that is at once Rube Goldbergish and elegant. Simply put, sildenafil increases the amount of that elusive neurotransmitter nitric oxide (NO) produced in response to sexual arousal. Nitric oxide's message is brought to an enzyme that produces smooth muscle relaxation in the corpus cavernosum (the dick) allowing blood to rush in and fill 'er up. It's really what does not happen that is the beauty of sildenafil.

When a guy sees that sweet round ass shimmying down the street, nitric oxide is produced right away. Sildenafil works in the background to block the action of a different enzyme whose job it is to degrade the first "boner-enzyme." As long as Viagra stays in the system (about four hours), this boner-killing enzyme (called phosphodiesterase type 5, or PDE5) is prevented from stopping the boner-inducing enzyme (aka cyclic guanosine monophosphate or cGMP) from doing its work—relaxing the necessary muscles to permit a boner.

Even though a lot of drugs affect enzymes— the chances of finding a specific drug to do a specific thing to any given enzyme are far worse than winning the lottery . . . more like every lottery in the country. On the same day.

Enzymes are produced because of the presence of genes, which makes work in this area a wilderness. For now, it's enough to list all the genes in, say, corn, let alone in humans, where it is impossible to identify and fine tune all the enzymes and neurotransmitters involved in the millions of chemical square-dances taking place in people's bodies.

Like a lot of other milestone drugs (penicillin, heroin, etc.), Viagra was discovered by accident. Pfizer's chemists were originally looking for a medicine to treat angina, a painful effect of heart disease. Instead, they blundered into one of pharmacy's holy grails.

Just say NO to enzymes . . .

Nitric oxide doesn't just appear out of nowhere. It, too, is produced through enzymatic actions from an amino acid (L-Argenine), which the body normally obtains by breaking down proteins, or by building them from other molecules . . . all by the use of enzymes. So far there are three entire classes of enzymes known to make NO and God knows how many there really are.

And, of course the enzyme Viagra knocks out so neatly is one of at least a half dozen such enzymes, (PDE5 is called "5" as opposed to 1,

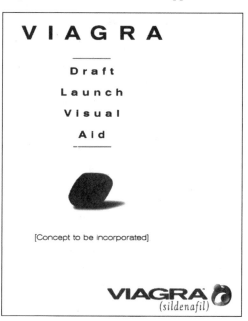

Early design for Roche Viagra ad.

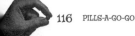

2, 3, 4, or 6). And it's a good thing sildenafil is 4,000 times more powerful at blocking the action of PDE5 rather than, say, PDE3, because PDE3 does its thing in the heart, not the penis. Instead of facilitating erections, Viagra might have caused instant heart failure.

You don't have to be a scientist to fiddle around with enzymes either. Viagra enthusiasts have been looking for ways to enhance the action of their expensive pills by utilizing the reactions between enzymes and other drugs or nutrients.

For instance, that amino acid precursor of nitric oxide, L-Argenine, is available in health food stores and it does increase the potential production of NO. L-Argenine has been added to livestock feed for years—after it was noticed it led to an increase in breeding behavior! Humans who take L-Argenine supplements are only ensuring an ample supply of NO for themselves.

At the other end of the operation, Viagra is broken down in the body like everything else—with enzymes. And that's a good thing, because sildenafil itself doesn't do the job. You're probably not surprised to know that the pill needs to be worked on by enzymes before it will work. Specifically, Viagra is broken down by a "family" of enzymes produced by a gene known as Cytochrome P450. P450 enzymes are responsible for metabolizing a whole bunch of drugs—probably most of them. It is a metabolite of Viagra, produced in the liver, that does most of the work

That's where Viagra hackers have been experimenting by taking substances known to inhibit Viagra's further breakdown and make it last longer. And there are a lot of common substances that can do this. Even drugs like the OTC ulcer medication Tagamet (cimetidine) can exert powerful influences over drug metabolism, usually increasing the time they stay at peak levels in the blood. Tagamet, for instance, can cut alcohol metabolism in half, making a person twice as drunk as normal . . . or allowing someone to consume half their normal ration of booze to get just as drunk as they normally do. So if Tagamet helps one get drunk, can it help one stay horny?

BEFORE VIAGRA
Better Sex Through Pills

Viagra is said to have brought on a sense of misery to trophy wives, formerly guaranteed an easy life dealing with the erectionally deficient. At first considered miraculous, and recently played up in the media for bringing on strokes and heart attacks, Viagra accomplishes what hundreds of years of pill research had promised: the wondrous erection.

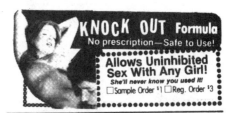

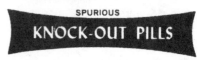

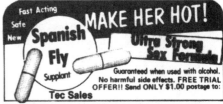

The chemical quest to produce a guaranteed boner produced a spectacular display when Dr. Giles S. Brindley wowed his urologic colleagues at a 1983 Las Vegas convention. He injected papaverine (a constituent of opium) into the base of his penis just before stepping up to the podium to deliver his findings on the substance. As he spoke, his cock grew and stiffened to a point he felt confident enough to impress the audience by opening up his pants to display his erect manhood. Just to prove it wasn't a trick, he wandered among the assembled penis doctors, inviting them to gaze at and even feel his magnificent, purple-headed boner.

Presumably this should have been the beginning of the end for "Spanish Fly," rhino horn, bear gall-bladders and other spurious "aphrodisiacs." It was not.

Not only is using a syringe on your dick painful and unsexy, there is a big difference between a boner and good sex. Boners are mysterious, they pop up at puzzling, unsexual times, and nobody's quite sure why, or even how they ever happen to begin with!

Aphrodisiacs are all about boners—but not necessarily good sex. "Spanish Fly" and other mythical pills promise instant horniness where it otherwise would not happen. In women, aphrodisiacs should quickly transform otherwise prudish women into insatiable sluts. In men, they promise a return to teenage horniness and to give you a big old boner, the biggest, hardest boner you've ever seen. A boner you could use to punch open a paint can.

Until the appearance of Viagra, toiling scientists had not discovered anything besides a healthy dose of puberty that induced willy-nilly boners and bottomless libidos. It was not till 1991 that Eli Lilly (inventors of Prozac) officially gave up their search for a real-life aphrodisiac.

Back in the '60s and early '70s, there was a prescription pill called "Afrodex"—a quasi-alchemical pill that contained yohimbine hydrochloride, nux vomica, a bit of testosterone and other ingredients. It may also have contained amphetamine (the capsule mimicked the look of a "black beauty"). In 1973, it was yanked from the market by cruel and puritanical FDA functionaries.

Afrodex was the first "pro-sexual drug"— a term coined to replace "aphrodisiac" and describe a panoply of pills that truly enhanced sex, and even produced some impressive boners. Here's the scoop:

The FDA is the last place you want to go to get good information on drugs. A purely political organization, the FDA are the guys who force drug companies to swear on the *PDR* that steroids will not enhance athletic ability, that amphetamines will not help in weight loss,

and that Retin-A won't remove wrinkles. If any company dares say these things they will pay dearly. MDMA (the love drug Ecstasy) was legal, prescribed as a psychiatric drug and proving very successful in treating "marital problems" when the FDA summarily banned it.

To get real information on drugs, go to the people who take them, or take them yourself. Or you might ask me. In my role as editor of *Pills-a-Go-Go* and author of books and articles about drugs, I road-tested a number of prosexual substances. I should also add I am a 41-year-old male who enjoys a piece of ass as much as the next man. I like sex and I can't imagine such a thing as bad pussy. The idea that sex could be even better is a concept I would have injected myself with papaverine to explore.

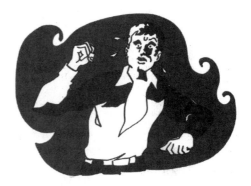

Speed and Sex

Amphetamine use nearly always results in improved mood and lots of energy—two things essential for good sex. It also increases libido and stamina. Amphetamines are also perhaps the FDA's most hated pill and consequently, they are hard to get.

Luckily, there are sideways approaches to achieving the same effects as speed. The best way is to use precursor amino acids such as Phenylalanine and L-Glutamine. These nutrients (available over-the-counter) create the neurotransmitters amphetamines use up. By taking a lot of them you can "fill your tank" and fairly duplicate the effects of speed or cocaine.

Amphetamine use carries its own dangers, all of which stem from prodigious and outlandish overuse of the drug. There are no problems associated with the use of amino acid precursors.

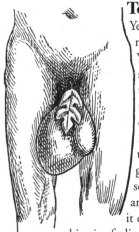

Testosterone

Yep. Testosterone makes you horny. You can feel that sometimes within the first hour of taking it. For me, even a single 10 or 20 mg dose had two effects. First, it gave me a general sense of well-being and vigor. Later on it enhanced my subjective feelings of sex. I became aroused faster and by less stimulation. Each sensation was heightened and my orgasms were almost explosive. This effect wears off after a few hours, then seems to "rebound" days later when another surge in libido occurs. My friends report the same experiences but have gone farther, taking testosterone over longer periods of time. For them, the rebound is even stronger.

Use too much testosterone over too long a period and your balls will just shut down, shrink and wither away. And that's the least of it. Excessive testosterone use can also be rough on your liver, cause serious premature arthritis and cause fast and furious hair growth. It can also make you obnoxiously aggressive and get you screamed at for indiscriminate leering.

On the plus side, most of these ill-effects can be reversed by stopping testosterone, although you will go through a period of marked non-horniness and your excess hair will clog the shower drain.

To use testosterone sensibly, it's a good idea to limit courses to only a few days at a time ("cycling" as weightlifters call it). Liver and other organ damage can be avoided by taking a buccal or sublingual pill designed to dissolve in the mouth and enter the bloodstream from there. There is also a new gel-form of testosterone the user applies to the skin and absorbs it from there.

Wellbutrin

This big red pill is prescribed for depression and is quite effective at relieving it. As a pro-sexual drug, this one's mainly for girls but I took it anyway. If I felt much pro-sexual effect it was too subtle for me. Girls are different, though, so I fed some to my sister who now speaks of the antidepressant pill with a dreamy look in her eyes. "I fantasized a lot on Wellbutrin," she tells me although I am sworn to secrecy about these fantasies (dogs, if you must know). She also described her orgasms as "crashing" and lasting two or three times longer than usual. When masturbating or fucking she said she felt overwhelmed by the sensations and orgasms came upon her in an "untrained" way. They snuck up on her and hit her like a freight train.

A psychiatrist in Richmond, California told me while he was running trials of the drug in 1988 he noticed an unusually strong libido increase among women taking the pill. He said the effect was pronounced enough he had problems with some of the women sneaking away from the ward to get laid.

As with all such drugs, most effects (pro-sexual and otherwise) do not show up for at least a few days, if not weeks. So there's no point in spiking your date's drink with it.

Other anti-depressants are said to cause negative sexual effects, but this is subjective. Prozac, for instance, is associated with a lowering of libido and difficulty in achieving orgasm in both men and women. Yet this may be exactly the kind of effect a "premature ejaculator" would like. In any case, the mood-elevating properties of such drugs go a long way toward removing frustration and other psychological barriers to good sex.

Some antipsychotic medications (notably Mellaril) can also induce a "reverse ejaculation" so that sperm is ejected into the bladder instead of the outside world. It can also favorably influence erections but not reliably enough to recommend as a pro-sexual drug.

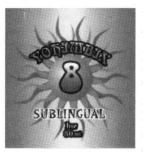

Yohimbe

This is a most promising pill. Its efficacy has even won grudging recognition by the FDA, which admits it "may have activity as an aphrodisiac"— a claim they haven't let anyone use since back when they were kicking Afrodex off the shelves.

In most people it has uniform and positive effects. While yohimbe is non-toxic even at extraordinary doses, a single 500 mg yohimbe pill produced an unpleasant reaction that did zip for my sex life. These effects (pounding heart, watering eyes, raised blood pressure, sweating, etc.) could be mitigated by taking a smaller dose and gradually building up. In any case, they are not dangerous.

A pal of mine follows a twice-a-year regimen of yohimbe and cannot say enough good about it. At an annual San Francisco orgy he attended this year he was something of a conversation piece as he came time and again, sometimes not even losing his erection between bouts. No one would believe he was 44. The way he described it, people gathered around him to practically adore his throbbing member while he laughed. Laughed and jizzed.

His method is to take one 500 mg hit of yohimbe a day for a week, then two the next week, three the next or two. All the time he drinks a cup of yohimbe tea each day. By the end of the 3–4 week period, he reports "obvious and marked" increase in hardness and size of his erections. He also wakes up with the rock-hard and unwieldy boners of his teenage years. Yohimbe, he says, also allows him to remain at a near-orgasmic state for hours.

The pro-sexual effects of his yohimbe treatment last for a "good four or five months" even after he totally discontinues taking the stuff.

And yohimbe is easy to get. So far, the FDA hasn't taken it away and you can get it without a prescription from health food stores around the country. Oh, and if some FDA dude tells you the only valid form of yohimbe is the prescription kind (yohimbine hcl) tell him about the study done by the U.S. Food and Dairy Labs that assayed ten mail-order brands of yohimbe and found all of them to contain plenty of naturally-occurring yohimbine hcl, more than you get in the prescription variety and at a cheaper price, thank you.

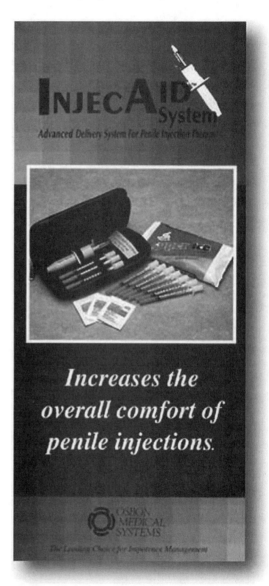

Increases the overall comfort of penile injections.

Papaverine

Ah, Dr. Gile's miracle shot! Like another alkaloid extracted from opium (apomorphine) it really does produce hour-long boners whether you like it or not. Israeli scientists are reportedly working on a cream form of papaverine that eliminates the need for needles and the tissue-damage they can cause.

Before you resort to papaverine, know that the stuff tends to lose its effects over the years. It can also "backfire" on the user by inducing priapism—an unending boner that eventually becomes very painful. Guys who can't get it down after a papaverine shot end up in the emergency room where they may face surgery to release the pent-up blood in the penis. Such surgery can also sever nerves vital to any more erections—thus making them dependent on papaverine shots for life. If you ever do play around with papaverine and have to go to the hospital, try a shot of epinephrine before going under the knife.

It is perhaps not so strange that these opium alkaloids have such pronounced sexual effects. Opium, too, can enhance sexual encounters, even stimulating powerful feelings of love and affection. Although the party line on opium is that it ruins sex, this is not true. Hollywood scallywag and sex-devotee Errol Flynn used it to make love "in ways and manners that I would never believe myself capable of."

The body's internal opiates—endorphins, and hormones from acetycholine to estrogen are closely related, most of these chemicals being produced from the same amino acids, yet working at seemingly disparate sites in the body.

Other Stuff

L-Argenine, another amino acid, has long been used to promote breeding in animals from cows to chickens. Argenine is essential in the production of nitric oxide, a neurotransmitter that has been absolutely linked to erectile function. Gingko biloba, an herb, has also shown pro-sexual properties. Both of these are available without a prescription.

Nearly any drug that elevates mood and promotes health can be a pro-sexual drug. Hell, chocolate, with its myriad congeners known as phenylethylamines, is thought to stimulate the brain in a way that make us feel "in love." These same chemicals bear a striking resemblance to amphetamines, norepinephrine . . . and the outlawed MDMA.

Niacin (vitamin B-3), produces a pronounced "flushing" as it causes blood vessels to dilate, also makes the skin more sensitive to the touch. This flushing is caused by the same his-

tamine release seen (particularly in women) during sexual arousal. "No-flush" niacin tablets have recently joined the market.

There is the chemical, oxytocin available in pill form, released by women in massive amounts during both birth and orgasm. What sort of effect would this have on sexual experience? So far there has been no research into this. Maybe you'd like to give it a try.

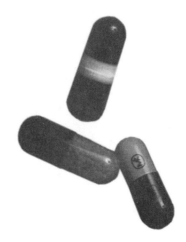

Pill Road Tests

Despite the puritanism of medical science and government goon squads, pills intended to kill pain often create pleasure. What sort of pleasure? You can be sure the secret use of pills wouldn't be described by the *PDR* or any tepid, generic pill book. Before *PaGG*, the relationship of pills to unintended benefit were the mainstay of rumor and urban legend.

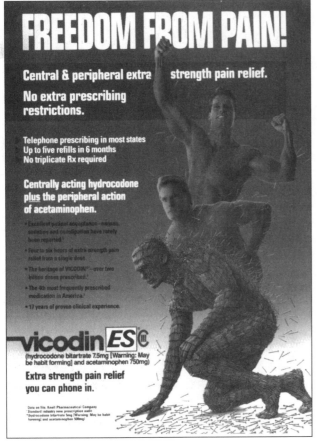

FREEDOM FROM PAIN!

Central & peripheral extra strength pain relief.

No extra prescribing restrictions.

Telephone prescribing in most states
Up to five refills in 6 months
No triplicate Rx required

Centrally acting hydrocodone plus the peripheral action of acetaminophen.

- Excellent patient acceptance—nausea, sedation and constipation have rarely been reported.
- Four to six hours of extra strength pain relief from a single dose.
- The heritage of VICODIN—over two billion doses prescribed.
- The 4th most frequently prescribed medication in America.
- 17 years of proven clinical experience.

vicodin ES ℂ
(hydrocodone bitartrate 7.5mg [Warning: May be habit forming] and acetaminophen 750mg)

Extra strength pain relief you can phone in.

Data on file. Knoll Pharmaceutical Company
Standard industry new prescription audit
[hydrocodone bitartrate 5mg [Warning: May be habit forming] and acetaminophen 500mg]

Pill reviews are perhaps the most important part of *Pills-a-Go-Go*, since they reveal the suppressed and reclaim the forbidden. Pills occupy a legal Purgatory between Heaven and Hell. They don't possess their political or underground advocates, like marijuana, cocaine, and even heroin. Nevertheless, millions of people use pharmaceutical drugs in ways frowned upon by the priests and bully-boys of pilldom.

In *PaGG* reviews, a migraine pill is honestly judged for its capacity to cure a hangover. Or an over-the-counter cough syrup is praised for its ability to turn an experimental user into a reptile. The reviews herein are not—and would never be—sanctioned by the FDA. They're written by non-insiders who consume pills in a quantity, and for reasons, contradicting their ostensible purpose. These wide-ranging informational reports and reviews come from a spectrum of pharmacists, MDs, self-described researchers, and regular Joes who post their discoveries rapturously on the net.

By simply giving honest descriptions, reviews can demystify and deholyize what a pill can and can't do. For example, Tagamet (the first H2 antagonist and now over-the-counter) really is useful against heartburn. It didn't get this FDA-sanctioned claim until 1995, almost 20 years after it was allowed on the prescription market (and was for a while, the biggest selling prescription drug of all time), but nevertheless its anti-heartburn claim was always true. Tagamet also affects alcohol absorption so that blood levels of booze rise twice as fast . . . and stay there. Take a Tagamet before you go drinking and you only need to drink half as much to get drunk. Be aware that your normal ration of beer will get you twice as drunk. Tagamet will also prevent the alcohol from giving you heartburn, especially the next morning. And Tagamet can cause men to grow breasts and develop other feminine characteristics. In fact, the pill is currently used to treat women with simple hirsutism (hairy chicks). That's not an FDA-sanctioned claim, but transsexuals take note!

The Beauty of Hydrocodone

by Pollyanne Hornbeck

I don't know if it's just me and my body chemistry. (I guess that has a lot to do with it), but hydrocodone, or its brand name—the magical and glamorous Vicodin—just seems to fix all my problems. Of course, there is that crankiness and short temper part that comes into play, and the constipation. But if I had an unlimited supply, didn't have to consider my liver or kidneys, and didn't have to worry about hitting a ceiling (which turns into a floor), my life would be so greatly enhanced.

So there's quite a few ifs, ands and buts, but riddle me this, Joker: Why is it so great? Whis it that if I'm tired, it perks me up? If I'm bored, it makes the dullest things tolerable? If I'm sick, it makes me feel better? If I'm in pain, it makes the pain go away? May people say it conks them right out, gives them a tummyache. I'm not one of those people. But it does make me itch, and sometimes I relish it to an embarrassing degree. I know only a handful of other people who feel as I do about hydrocodone. But me and those other people have a similar love affair going on.

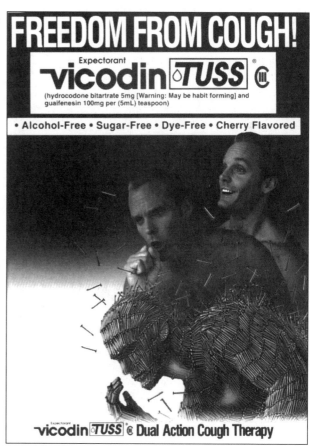

One problem is building up a tolerance and hitting that damned ceiling. Oh, how I long for the days when I could take one and a half 7.5 ES (7.5 mg of hydrocodone in a 750 mg acetaphetamin base) and get a nice buzz going. I guess it's been too short of a time that I've been clean and too long of a time since I've been gobbling them up.

I had a friend that used to love 'em, too. I haven't talked to her in years and I hear that she's clean now. Her name is Courtney Love. She said they made her feel like vacuuming. See, someone besides me felt the beauty of these lovely creatures, making dull work tolerable and even fun. I remember after she went off to Utah to have her first nose job, she came back with quite a supply. And they were pretty generous with refills. She said Utah was where all the porn stars went to get their plastic surgery done. It was cheap and good. Kinda strange, I thought—Utah? But what would I know—look at my nose.

We were living at my friend Lynell dad's house in the Hollywood Hills. Courtney and I had pretty lax schedules and I usually had some money. So she would call up and get a refill. We would split the script. Courtney would weasel some money from a disapproving, scowling-faced Eric Erlandson, and pay me back half. We'd sit on the balcony, eat Vics and drink coffee. Of course, those days didn't last forever. We started gobbling them up too quickly and getting greedy, and even the quack doctors in Utah wouldn't keep up with our requests.

My Hollywood Hills room faced a tiny, twisty street. At two or three o'clock in the morning, I came home blasted from a club, and was hitting the hay when this guy starts honking outside my window. I go out to confront the noisy bastard, who says he's looking for Courtney. I tell him to march down the dark stone steps to her apartment and knock on her fucking door, and not honk outside my window. Then it occurs to me who he is.

I knew that Courtney had her eye on Kurt Cobain. So I pipe up in my drunken annoyance, "Hey, aren't you that guy in that band that sounds like the Pixies?" He mumbles something. An old boyfriend of mine was convinced that Kurt wrote that Polly song about me—with my bad back and the cockatoos flying back and forth in the stairwell between the house and Courtney's room.

Soon I move to Seattle and start up with a whole new group of candy, stealing Percocets from then-boyfriend Greg, who had his tonsils taken out at the age of thirty. Quite painful, they say. I filled his script while he was in the recovery room and immediately ate six before I drove him home. I try to pawn off Tylenol to him to save more Percos for myself. I know Percs are supposed to be stronger than Vicodin—they are Schedule II and triplicates, and Vics are only Schedule III, but they never floated my boat in the same way. Not tingly, orgasmic warmth, only fuzzy and noddy.

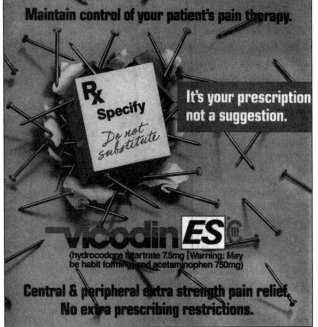

I remember asking a dentist once for some codeine after a root canal, so I could get some sleep. He told me that the Vicodin he prescribed would knock me out. I had to explain to him that it didn't, and it hyped me out, and made me feel like doing all this stuff, and right now I just want to go to sleep and let the pain ebb away in an unconscious state. He was adamant on his point, and continued to disagree with me. I finally got him to write another prescription, but he still didn't believe me and said that he had never heard of anything so preposterous in his life. Well, I know I'm not the only one.

What Elavil Lurks in the Hearts of Men?
by Millicent Grimm

Being a bonafide pillhead, I take opportunity of every situation that arises in my favor. My mom, who, happily for me, is anti-pill, had surgery and a full script of Darvocet laying around. The thought of this tantalized and tingled my mind so much I almost looked forward to visiting her. I'd pop a couple as soon as I got there, since I had to go take a pee after that long drive, and in about 20 minutes I could almost entirely put up with her whining and oppressive negative vibe. After a few visits like this I realized she wasn't taking any of the pills— but I had swallowed the source down to about six hits. So I thought better to take the bottle and let her think she had lost them or thrown them away, than suspiciously leave a lonely hit in the bottle.

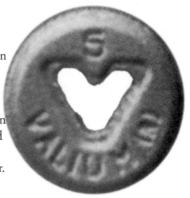

Over a frightfully bad Mother's Day dinner at my boyfriend's gramma's (she can't cook worth a shit) I peeked around in the back bathroom cabinet and found a bunch of pre-1984 Valiums. Back then they didn't have the V cut out of them and they were just little round scored yellow five-milligram tablets. But they were still potent. I also scammed something else . . . maybe some codeines, I don't remember.

I went back to my mom's apartment, but realized I had to start being sneakier. I knew there was nothing left in the medicine cabinet, so I had to get into her bedroom nightstand. I knew I couldn't expect any covering from my boyfriend who is Mr. Anti-Drug, so when I detected a window of safety I went for it. I grabbed lots of little 0.5 Ativans and she had a couple bottles of Elavil. Little tabs and big ones. The bottle of big tabs was nearly full so I grabbed a small handful of the big red 100 mg ones. I figure if little ones are good, big ones must be better, right?

I'll freely take stuff that I recognize or that someone I trust says to go for. But when I got home that night I didn't feel like doing any research and thought I'd just take one since it was getting on in the evening.

I slept hard that night, but in the morning I couldn't really wake up. It was like I was trying to shake off this dense fog surrounding me and was feeling stupid. For the most part of the next three days I was like a zombie. I had no ambition. I felt like one of the stiffs walking around Jack Nicholson in *One Flew Over the Cuckoo's Nest*. I constantly zoned out and fell asleep. I couldn't keep my attention on anything. I wandered around aimlessly, not because I wanted to but because it just seemed that stumbling around was part of my new programming installed by whatever alien being had captured possession of my body and mind.

At the time it seemed like I had really fucked up and maybe was stuck in this state forever. It wasn't interesting or fun like a good acid trip can sometimes be. It was more like a nightmare I couldn't wake up from.

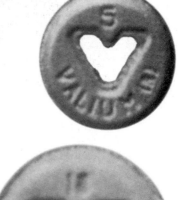

Of course, all this time I couldn't fess up to the B.F. what was up, so I just played that I was straight and started calling around to figure out what the hell I took. Ends up that Elavil can be calming and sleep enhancing in small doses, although the morning fog takes a good while to lift. But the 100 mg dose I popped was pretty massive. It's the kind of medication that you're likely to get if you get taken in and put on suicide watch. Kill the will, calm the culprit.

Elavil is the devil. Look at the last three letters in both words: V-I-L. That's three letters. 3+3=6 and from there it's pretty close to 666!

Guinea-Piggin' for the Last Time

by Itchy DuPont, Pillhead-at-Large

My name's Itchy DuPont and I'm a carpet cleaner. At first glance, carpet cleaning seems like a pretty boring job. Well, guess what? It sure the hell is!

We clean the carpets of the wealthy. Every rug, every room. About two years ago our crew (with the exception of our straight-as-an-arrow boss, John) found a way to make our days a little more enjoyable on the job.

Raid the medicine cabinet!

I'm pretty familiar with most pharmaceuticals, mainly from reading the *PDR* like a kid engrossed in a comic book or an adult reading a great novel. The knowledge gleaned from it pays off almost daily. We'll find something on the job and know what it is, how much to take, and what to expect.

Well, let me tell you a little tale about taking something that I wasn't so sure about on what turned out to be the longest work-day I've ever had.

We arrived at the customer's house—myself, my right-hand man and fellow self-confessed pillhead, Gacy, along with our boss, John.

As John and Gacy brought in the supplies, I locked myself in the bathroom and slowly opened the medicine cabinet. Jackpot. I knew instantly when I saw numerous script bottles with the "drowsy guy" red stickers. That's usually a good sign (not always, but most of the time).

A couple of the bottles were crazy pills, amitryptyline and the like, but two of the bottles read, "take 1 tablet as needed for nerves."

Hmmm, sounded pretty good to me, so I dumped a bunch into my hand. Boy, these things are small, I thought. They were called Lorazepam 2 mg. I had never heard of this particular pill, but I put my *PDR*-education to work and reasoned in a split-second: Nerves, Lorazepam, Diazepam (more commonly known as Valium).

When emotional tension mounts

Valium (diazepam) helps control psychic tension in mild to severe nonpsychotic conditions. Its profile of clinical use extends from pure psychic tension states—where an unremitting build-up of everyday emotional stresses results in disabling tension—to mixed emotional states, where psychic tension intermingles with restlessness, depressive symptoms, vague somatic symptoms or other emotional complaints. Response to Valium (diazepam), many investigators report, may often be achieved without compromising the patient's mental faculties or physical performance.

An indication of the wide usefulness of Valium (diazepam) is illustrated in this partial analysis of reports from over 900 investigators:
From the clinical record of Valium (diazepam)

Diagnosis	Total No. of patients treated	Excellent to good results	Per cent improved
Tension/anxiety associated with			
Psychoneurotic reactions	4593	3773	82%
Depressive symptoms	1327	964	73%
Psychophysiologic disturbances	2950	2410	82%

Cool. Valium was always fun on the job and I knew Gacy would love this good discovery—being a major mother's little helper worshipper.

I figured that these little pills were probably only as strong as about a two mg Valium; possibly a 5 mg (yellow) Valium. But just in case they were as potent as a 10 mg (blue) I would stick to taking only three at first, so I took three. About five minutes later I caught up with Gacy and gave him three, too. He took them . . .

Boy, did we just seriously fuck up, boys and girls. What I didn't know was that this tiny pill packed a mighty punch. Lorazepam (Ativan) comes in three different dosages: .5, 1.0 and 2.0 mg. We just took 6 mgs of a seriously strong tranquilizer. That's like taking 12 of the half-mg pills. It was 9:30 am. and we had a five bedroom house worth of carpet to clean. Our boss was in the next room. It was the start of a crazy, whacked-out, blur of a day.

Twenty minutes later, I was feeling pretty good, pretty mellow, kinda like Jello. But I was scared. I was feeling too good for only twenty minutes. I told Gacy that I thought we had taken too much. Five minutes later Gacy was speaking Chinese. Not really, but he might as well have been. I could comprehend nothing. I was a goober. Spit was flowing freely from my mouth down my chin.

Knowing my job was on the line if John or the customer saw me like this, I played Hide From The Boss—Hide From Everybody, for that matter. Gacy followed me. I can really only remember bits and pieces but I do remember Gacy shaking me awake a few times and I remember doing the same to him. I remember watching him unplug the cleaner and keep going . . . right down to the floor, breaking the fall with his head.

Eventually, it had to happen. We ended up in the same room with John. Gacy was a freak. I tried to act as straight as possible, talking to John, but behind his back, Gacy was sleeping, sitting up on a dining room chair. John turned around and yelled. Nothing. He yelled again. Nothing. Finally, after a vigorous shaking, Gacy woke up. "Wow, man, I fell asleep," he said, forcing out every word.

As fucked-up as I was, I could tell John was pissed. We finally finished up (I have no idea or recollection how) and had about an hour's drive back to the office. Me and Gacy slept sitting up the entire way back, never waking up once.

The next day Gacy forgot to pick me up for work and I had a hell of a time getting up when John finally pounded on my door. Since then, he has made a couple of references to the "bad dope we did that day," but we claimed we were just out late the night before. I think he's just letting us know he's not stupid and don't let it happen again.

There's a lesson in all this, boys and girls. Know what you're taking and leave the unknown up to the guinea pigs. Until next time, remember this little ditty:

Pills are neato
Pills are fun
There's a pill
for everyone!

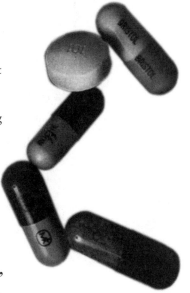

Ephedrine Hydrochloride, *"Your Late Night Friend"*

It's been around in pill form since at least 1923 (in this country anyway) but the chemical has been in use for many hundreds—if not thousands—of years by people all over the world to relieve symptoms of asthma, congestion, and other respiratory complaints. Since it was isolated from the herba ephedra plant, the stuff has proven itself useful in controlling menstrual cramps, raising both blood pressure and

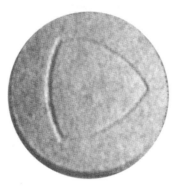

blood sugar, as a cocaine adulterant, a treatment for narcolepsy and even as a remedy to control bedwetting!

But its most dastardly use so far has been as a precursor chemical in the manufacture of illegal methamphetamine, mainly in California. That's one of the reasons an emergency rider attached to a recent bill in the California legislature has made possession of any amount of the stuff illegal.

Luckily, it still remains quite available for the rest of us, and to Californians who order from out of state. By the way, if all else fails, go collect some of the plant (very common in the Southwest, where it is known as Mormon tea) and boil it. The plant contains about 1% ephedrine.

Ephedrine is normally sold as a hydrochloride salt, as it's more stable this way. It is also sold as a sulfate for the same reasons. You can find it at gas stations and convenience stores across the land, where truckers use it to help keep awake. It is the main ingredient in asthma products, but is also sold as an aid to weight loss, because it is "thermogenic"—that is, it speeds the metabolism of the body. A member of the gigantic family of sympathomimetic drugs, it is related to amphetamines as well as other ingredients in OTC cold meds (i.e., Sudafed). Its direct cousins include weight-loss pills Benzphetamine (Didrex), phentermine (Fastin, etc.). It's also related to the stuff found in the notorious Somalian "khat" plant.

Like all those other drugs, ephedrine exerts influence on the central nervous system, but is nowhere near as potent a CNS stimulant as amphetamine, even though they are closely related.

Dosage is something around 25-50 mg a few times per day and any larger doses should be considered with caution. Nevertheless, some OTC "pharmaconauts" have taken doses ten times higher than this and noticed a definite speed-like effect—complete with the unpleasant features of coming down. Also, the drug tends to quickly induce a pronounced shakiness. Definitely not a smooth ride. Frequent or heavy users may find they feel drained. One weightlifter who used the pill to increase his stamina reported that he took ephedrine until he began to suffer from chronic headaches. That was his signal to lay off the pills for awhile and within a short time he was able to resume munching "cross tops." But recall that at real high doses, ephedrine can cause dangerous hypertension.

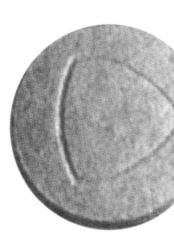

Indeed, studies show that there is some tolerance to the drug, but that this is rapidly lost with only a few days abstinence.

Ephedrine is thought to be synergistic with plain old caffeine and its absorption is increased with antacids. Because ephedrine works partly by stimulating the release of catacholamines in nerve endings, it seems entirely reasonable that the concurrent use of catacholamine precursor amino acids such as tyrosine would potentiate its effect and/or lessen the harsh come-down when the drug wears off.

Ephedrine, Part II

The OTC pill, ephedrine HCl, is headed to be outlawed because it is also such a good precursor in the manufacture of methamphetamine.

Of course, it's not the only precursor, and getting rid of all the ephedrine in the ephedrine world will not stop people from making speed. It's also ironic that amphetamines were first discovered in attempts to synthesize ephedrine in order to avert a shortage of this valuable medicine.

Ephedrine and pseudephedrine (yep, the active ingredient in Sudafed) are really the same thing—just stereoisomers of the very same molecule. That means if you make yourself a cup of Mormon tea (Breathe Easy R), you're getting about half ephedrine and half pseudephedrine. Therefore, it is theoretically possible to use pseudephedrine for anything you use ephedrine for . . . stuffy noses, illegal drugs . . . whatever. The reality of the matter is that changing a molecule like this can be pretty difficult.

One thing we've found is that smoking ephedrine through a base seems to increase the "speedlike" effects of it. Whether this is because smoking is quicker or more efficient way of ingesting the chemical or whether it's because of something else is unclear. However, a look at the figures here shows a striking similarity between ephedrine, amphetamine and cathinone—the supposed active ingredient found in the Khat plant chewed by Somalis, and the street drug methcathinone (or "cat") recently placed on the DEA's shitlist as a dread worse than crack.

Vick's nasal inhalers contain levo-methamphetamine, the mirror image of dextromethamphetamine. And the way the body itself treats these thing is revealing as well. Most of them get metabolized into each other in the body, as it is, so chewing khat leaves may not be much different than taking a few Sudafeds.

Could it be that heating ephedrine and mixing it with a base frees enough hydrogen atoms to form a crude version of cathinone or maybe a substance we can't identify? Would breathing the fumes of Sudafeds cooked in a crack pipe do the same thing?

One reader suggested:

"The best way (to sweeten the smoke) would be to just freebase it. Dissolve it in water, basify with ammonia or about anything and extract from the water with methyl chloride leaving behind any reaction residue or layer. Do a couple of extractions and evaporate off the methyl chloride."

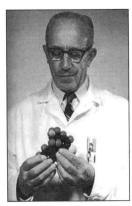

Dr. Leo Sternbach

King Valium and the Benzodiazepines

Valium had a hammerlock on the number one position among the top-selling prescription drugs for nearly all of the 1970s. Introduced in 1963, it replaced Librium (invented by the same scientist, Dr. Leo Sternbach of Hoffman-La Roche) and revolutionized the so-called "minor tranquilizers" that appeared in the 1950s with the invention of Miltown (meprobamate). Valium, like Librium, Serax, and a slew of other hypnotics and tranquilizers is a premiere member of a class of widely-used drugs called benzodiazepines.

Unlike meprobamate, Valium created far less tolerance and, despite its demonizing in the popular media, is not very "addicting" at all. It's true some people become dependent on benzodiazepines, but this is usually the result of a serious chemical imbalance the drug addresses. While a person suffering from a slight case of anxiety may only need, say, .25 mgs of Xanax to obtain relief, someone who is rendered dys-

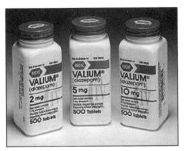

functional by panic attacks seems to be able to soak up four, five, and six mgs a day without being overly sedated. Despite a 24-times greater intake, such people still appear to be pretty nervous!

Unlike meprobamate, a fatal overdose of Valium is not a very plausible way to die. It's been said that the only way to die from too much Valium is to get run over by a truck full of it. State department dweeb Robert McFarlane proved this during his days as an Iran-Contra spy, when he tried to kill himself by trying taking all the Valium he had . . . then getting a good night's sleep.

Research into benzodiazepines has yielded numerous compounds of varying lengths of duration, making them a versatile drug. For instance Halcion (triazolam), like Xanax, is a very short-acting but powerful "benzo" that makes it ideal as a sleeping pill. It has a fast onset of action and a half-life of just four hours. That means taking a Halcion before a long plane flight not only fights jet lag, it allows the user to wake up refreshed, without a sedated, groggy feeling, a sleeping pill "hangover."

Unfortunately, some states, notably New York, have decided that "too many" prescriptions for benzodiazepines were being written for the "wrong reasons." Thus came the introduction of triplicate prescription requirements that effectively deter doctors from prescribing these drugs. Of course, the basic need for such a drug is not eliminated, so doctors have little choice but to either risk prosecution for the nebulous charge of practicing illegal medicine or allowing a patient to suffer. He could also fall back on the older, more addictive and dangerous drugs like Miltown. Records show, when benzodiazepines are strictly controlled, the use of barbiturates and other sedative drugs goes up.

This restriction of benzodiazepines like Valium is disastrous for patients who use them for controlling muscle spasms and convulsions. Instead, doctors are forced to use less-controlled, but mind-numbing anti-psychotics and antihistamines to do a poor imitation of the same job.

To take up the slack caused by government restriction, Valium is a popular item to smuggled into the United States from foreign countries, most notably Mexico, where access to the drug is not nearly so restricted. Quality control in Mexico is not as good as in the U.S., and many of the pills are not up to full strength. Thailand and India are well-known for their counterfeiting of Valium, and pills from these countries are often not even half the potency of the real thing. Adding to a Valium-lover's frustration is the proliferation of generic forms of Valium which can vary quite a lot in their availability. Taste-tests run by your faithful author and others have proven to our satisfaction that only brand name Valium can be counted on to deliver as advertised, though some knock-offs do come close.

This discrepancy is borne out by extensive tests by Valium's makers, which compared their drug to generic competitors using electroencephalographs (EEGs) to monitor the drug's effect on no fewer than 22 brain-wave variables and found generics seriously lacking. The FDA, in contrast, monitored only four EEG variables and, worse yet, allowed a "leeway" of 20 minutes between swallowing the pill and onset of action. To anyone with anxiety, this is far too long and encourages overdoses.

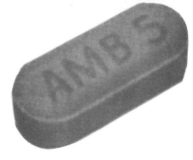

Exactly what causes these differences between generics and brand names is uncertain, although it may be due to different binders and other "inert" ingredients used in non-Roche formulations. Nevertheless, the differences in effects are clear.

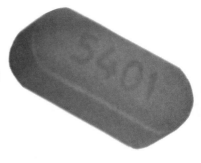

Incidently, is is NOT a good idea to mix benzodiazepines with alcohol. Few drugs react well with alcohol since booze has a strong tendency to alter absorption rates as well as an ability to potentiate any sort of "downer." In the case of Valium and other benzodiazepines this may be because alcohol also binds to GABA (gamma-aminobutyric acid) receptors in the brain. In fact GABA, still available in health food stores, has also demonstrated anti-anxiety and anti-convulsant effects. Next time you get a hankering for vitamin V, I suggest you make a run to your vitamin dealer. In fact, make the run now and stock up before it gets outlawed like so many nutritional supplements have been.

Ultram and Ambien

There are a couple of new pills on the market—both products of legislation-driven research. One interesting example is 1995's introduction of a non-opioid, non-NSAID painkiller called Ultram (tramadol), made by McNeil and Ortho Pharmaceuticals. This is the latest fruit of the so-far fruitless search for a decent painkiller that's not an opiate, which is to say non-addictive.

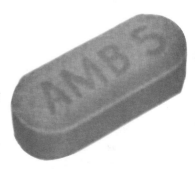

The nature of addiction is debatable to begin with (I mean, if you like something you're gonna do it some more, right?), but the most salient point here is the restrictions put on opioid pain-killers. Most of them are Schedule II and put any physician at risk of being investigated if he or she prescribes them. Below that, in Schedule III, is hydrocodone (Vicodin et al), but lately that drug's been coming under fire and politicians want to bump it up to Schedule II. That leaves only small doses of codeine and good old propoxyphene. But even with these drugs patients get scornful looks from pharmacists and more than one doctor is serving time for prescribing Darvocet to an undercover cop with an agenda.

And then these damn NSAIDs (non-steroidal anti-inflammatories). Not only do they burn holes in the stomach lining, they don't work too damn well. Of all of them, aspirin is still the best.

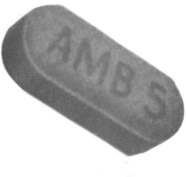

Now there's Ultram and so far it looks pretty good. *PaGG* has road-tested this pill a bit and found it works pretty well on the kinds of pain that usually responds well only to opiates. It stopped normal headaches and relieved chronic neck pain in someone with degenerative disk disease. But it didn't get anyone high unless they took no less than 300 mgs (three times the maximum dosage) and more reliably at 400 mgs.

It should be said at the outset that, although Ultram is supposedly non-opioid, it does bind weakly to the mu receptor (where morphine has a lot of action), so there is recreational possibility. But I didn't feel anything remarkable when I quadrupled the maximum recommended dose. I suspect it could be fun in higher quantities, but my supply ran out. One doctor said he had patients already becoming protective of their Ultram stashes, but this may be simply because it works.

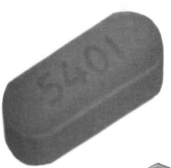

Ultram also has cool-o features mimicking some of the effects of both tricyclic antidepressants and SSRIs by inhibiting re-uptake of both norepinephrine and serotonin. So it may be that people taking Ultram could also be spared some of the psychic misery that pain can cause.

Its main side effects appear to be dizziness, nausea, and constipation—like an opiate. On the other hand it didn't cause much itching, sweating, dry mouth, or vomiting—unlike an opiate. Three stars.

Ambien is the first and so far only non-benzodiazepine minor tranquilizer (from this decade, that is. Meprobamate, etc. is still around). It appears that the main point of this pill is to skirt the repressive "trip script" laws now in force in so many states that virtually prohibit doctors from prescribing any benzodiazepine, Valium or otherwise. These laws require doctors to treat benzos like morphine, and their prescribing "habits" are watched carefully. Patients are also monitored to make sure they don't get "too many" of the pills.

Ambien is technically not a benzodiazepine, but it acts just like one. It fits into benzodiazepine receptors, it fits into GABA receptors. It is also antagonized by Romazicam—a benzo antagonist. *PaGG* has gotten reports that big doses of Ambien (marketed as a sleeping pill) feel something like Quaaludes but our own experience doesn't bear that out. For me, Ambien has proved to be an excellent sleeping aid. It works quickly, reliably, and there is zero grogginess in the morning.

Fen/Phen

When *PaGG* first reviewed it, fen/phen was a Holy Pill. Recommended by *Reader's Digest* and advocated by Oprah Winfrey, the diet pill combo was instantly demonized thanks to a single Mayo Clinic study which concluded fen/phen grew holes in the hearts of some of its takers. In a frenzy of Pill Whore hysteria, fen/phen no longer saved people from morbid obesity, it destroyed heart valves. In September, 1997, the FDA pressured Wyeth-Ayerst Laboratories and Interneuron Pharmaceuticals to stop selling the dexfenluramine (and with it, its parent drug racemic fenfluramine which had been available for decades) half of the magical fen/phen combo. Lawyers across the nation started to chase pill-popping fatties, rubbing their hands in gleeful anticipation of a civil suit downpour. The daddy of fen/phen treatment, Maryland's Dr. Pietr Hitzig, blamed any mishaps on misprescribed dosages by "countless fad diet clinics across the nation." Hitzig's website proudly posted a November, 1998 article about a Mount Sinai Medical Center study that concluded, "Dieters on fen/phen were no more likely to have faulty heart valves than dieters who had never touched the stuff." But the study is too little, too late. It's nearly impossible to save a demonized pill from genocidal inquisition. Fen/Phen remains unavailable. Here's the *PaGG*'zine review:

Illustration from Steven Cerio's *ABC Book, A Drug Primer* published by Gates of Heck

If *Reader's Digest* recommends it, it's got to be wholesome! So here's to the new speed! The May 1995 issue, the magazine extolls the virtues of mixing the drugs fenfluramine and phentermine to obtain very good results in weight loss. The article cites studies at the University of Rochester, which had gone on for three and a half years, showing that people taking the pills lose an average of three times more weight than the control group that didn't get any pills. Not only that, but they kept the weight off—and there hasn't been any evidence of tolerance or other negative effects even in those people who took the pills for years. The *Digest* says, "This much is clear—when you stop taking it [the pills], you gain back the weight. That's why some physicians advise dieters to take the drug for life."

For life, they say.

Fenfluramine, an amphetamine analogue that doesn't stimulate like an amphetamine, seems to increase serotonin levels a lot like Prozac does. Phentermine, another speed analogue that does stimulate quite nicely, cranks up the brain's dopamine supply. For the *Reader's Digest* this is necessary mainly to counteract fenfluramine's "tendency to slow people down." But it is also key in losing weight.

Marinol, The World's Stupidest Pill

As cool as pills are, there are some without much value. Sometimes a pill is such a mistake it's an insult to the rest of the pill world. The worst such pill has got to be Marinol.

Marinol, the synthetic THC pill made by Unimed Pharmaceuticals and distributed by Roxanne Laboratories to stop severe, persistent nausea and vomiting—is unquestionably the stupidest pill in the world. Marinol is supposed to be marijuana in pill form. If that were only true. If such a thing existed, *PaGG* would be very impressed. But such a thing doesn't exist.

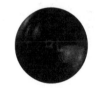

Marijuana can dramatically reduce severe nausea and loss of appetite suffered by cancer patients undergoing chemotherapy. Such a drug is essential to keep a patient in treatment to save his life. Chemotherapy is not only painful and debilitating, it makes people vomit until they are exhausted from dry heaves. Nothing stays down. Some people would literally prefer to die than endure the treatment. Patients who need every bit of strength they can get in a fight for their lives really appreciate a joint. Dope releases them from the hell of persistent nausea and pain and lets them eat. With marijuana they can keep weight on or even gain some while cancer and chemotherapy wage a literal life and death war within the person's body.

But in California, even when medical marijuana is voted into legality, the state shuts down the skunk stores. No one is allowed to have the drug. And cops have shown they are willing to enforce this law even against emaciated, half-dead people in wheelchairs.

A few people fought court battles to win government permission to smoke government-grown weed in government-rolled joints. For awhile it looked like the $2 a joint federal government pot would become part of the pharmacopia. In 1992 the DEA declared any and all marijuana use illegal, even medical use. Besides, they say, there's a pill to take instead.

Marinol is the trade name for Dronabinol, which, chemically, looks exactly like one form of THC that is found in marijuana. Marijuana contains at least 11 different THC molecules and scores of other "cannabinoids," but dronabinol is the "active ingredient" says the government.

If that were true, taking Marinol would feel like smoking marijuana . . . and it doesn't. It's also interesting that the original contender for title of "marijuana pill" mimicked a different THC molecule altogether. They said that particular chemical "the active ingredient." Then some test-dogs started to die off and the pill had to be shit-canned.

Aside from the dubious idea of giving an anti-emetic pill to people who retch everything they swallow, Marinol doesn't cut the pill mustard in other ways. Its effects take hours to kick in, and sometimes don't kick in at all. When Marinol does hit, however, it frequently knocks the patient into an unpleasant stupor, causes hallucinations, paranoid reactions, and depression. Patient after half-dead patient prefers smoking grass.

Marinol is expensive, too. Treatment with it costs between $150 to $180 a month. Marinol's hard to make. Terpene olivitol made in Germany has to be shipped to Southern California, where it is tediously separated by silica gel column chromatography and a tiny amount of nearly "pure" (99%) product is retrieved. Then another lab takes the stuff and makes it into pills (gel caps, really), which it ships off to Ohio for redistribution. All along the way the pills are as closely watched as plutonium. Government guards who keep track of each of these stupid pills every inch of the way generate lots of paperwork, wasting who knows how much money and human effort.

If you're looking for marijuana, just grow the plant and consume it however you want.

Donnagel PG, Requiem for a Faithful Mistress
by Dorian

January 1, 1993, "The Day 'Donna' Died." The "Donna" here is my former beloved mistress: Donnagel PG. She was taken off the market officially at the stroke of midnight on New Year's Eve, 1992. That's what the pharmacist said with a look of satisfaction on his face and a note of triumph in his voice. He felt victorious over us druggies who prefer opiates more than the more respectable, albeit more dangerous, alcohol and tobacco. Its withdrawal from the marketplace had nothing to do with its glorious 24 milligrams per ounce of pure powdered opium. The offending ingredients were the belladonna alkaloids: atropine sulfate, scopolamine hydrobromide, and hyoscyamine sulfate.

Someone, somewhere decided atropine should no longer be available OTC. Now Donnagel exists in a revamped formula that includes neither opium nor belladonna. And why not? Belladonna is a dangerous hallucinogen that causes death when taken in massive doses and at effective doses, it incites vivid sensations of flight. I once added up the amount of these ingredients and discovered it would take more than 40 bottles of Donnagel to equal one effective dose of belladonna. These sinister substances put a nice edge on the Donnagel high and brought "flying dreams" filled with beauty and horror when I chose to sleep. Some may be put off by this sort of

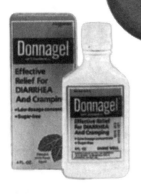

thing, but I'm always up for a great nightmare.

To obtain Donnagel PG you had to ask for it at the pharmacy and sign a Narcotic Exempt Register. This was your word that you had not purchased a narcotic exempt product in the last however many hours. (In Alabama it was 72 hours, in Tennessee and Georgia it was 48.) Much to my dismay, I learned on a trip to New York City, that Donnagel

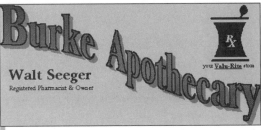

PG was not sold without a prescription there and I practically sent a Manhattan pharmacist scrambling for the phone to bring the law down upon me simply for asking about it. I'm not sure about the rest of the country, but it was available throughout the South without a script. Back then it was a sure-fire way to win a bet: "I bet you I can walk into this Wal-Mart and purchase, sans script, PURE POWDERED OPIUM." Easy money. Usually enough to buy a bottle. Donnagel was "Paregoric equivalent"—a modern-day laudanum, if you will, used to soothe stomach cramps and stop diarrhea. It came in six oz. bottles and featured an acrid flavor that tasted somewhat like banana kisses. From a pharmacy counter I swiped an AH Robins pharmaceutical company promotional fountain pen which featured a rendering of a Curious George-like cartoon monkey, proclaiming, "for that great taste . . . it's the bananas!" I've had friends who gagged at the taste but over a short period of weekend use I developed a connoisseur's palate for Donnagel PG and enjoyed savoring its flavor.

Best, and most important of all, were the effects. About five minutes after drinking an entire bottle, I experienced a rush that was not unlike a mainline heroin rush, albeit on a much, *much* smaller scale. Sort of like Cliff Notes. This was followed by about eight to twelve hours of pleasant euphoria undetectable to those unaware of the wonders of opiates. And no harsh "come-down" either, I always felt invigorated the morning after and seemed to be able to get by with only three or four hours of sleep. Oh, did I ever fall for the siren song of sister opium! The song went something like, "I am Opium! Come with me and sleep in a ditch along the side of the road! Enjoy!"

Yes, I was in love! "Donna" had sisters and cousins, invariably cheaper (about $4 compared to Donna's $7–$11 per bottle) but somewhat homely with ugly names such as Parapectilin and Nastytastin (or something like that). The experience of downing these miserable generic substitutes simulated drinking industrial strength floor cleaner the consistency of egg whites. I almost retch at the recollection!

As with most relationships, there was a downside to Donnagel PG. The side effects included intense dry-mouth and dilation of the pupils, making bright light painful and sunglasses necessary for night time driving. But these were but a small price to pay for the wonderful times I shared with Donna. Grab some Ray-Bans and a Thirstbuster . . . end of problem!

When I found out about Donnagel PG's demise, I was shattered and heartbroken. It was a lonely and bittersweet task, visiting all the pharmacies I could in those waning days, stocking up. Alas, I have one bottle remaining, but haven't been able to bring myself to polish it off. Call me romantic.

Haldol

Haldol (haloperidol) is an anti-psychotic or "major tranquilizer." Other popular anti-psychotics include Thorazine, Mellaril, and Prolixin. Anti-psychotics are used for the treatment of schizophrenia and for the pacification of the unruly, the unseemly, and the hallucinating. Haldol has been used fairly widely in the past, especially in Soviet psychiatric facilities. It may or may not be in common use currently, as dictated by the fads and fashions in the world of medicine.

How anti-psychotics work is not completely understood, but they are known to reduce levels of dopamine, a neurotransmitter linked to movement. Parkinson's Disease is marked by a severe drop in dopamine levels. The symptoms are muscular rigidity and shaking tremors.

The preferred method of administration is orally by tablet, or by liquid if the patient is a crafty devil known to spit out his meds. One person I knew, a recluse who had not left his home for nearly a year except to buy groceries, became uncharacteristically rowdy, claiming that God had talked to him a couple of times. He also trashed his parents' house. He was promptly removed to a local psych ward and was medicated. He was smart enough to hide his pills under his tongue, but not smart enough to settle down and act doped-up. "Pulling an old McMurphy, I am!" he bragged to me when I came to visit. Sure enough, next time I was there he was much calmer and told me of the special orange juice they made him drink in front of them.

Anti-psychotics are favored by the staff of inpatient facilities because of their strong sedative effect. Before, their charges were swearing and growling, playing in their own shit, and masturbating at dinner; now they sure are quiet. A cure would be cool, but peace will do in a pinch. So long as there's always somebody screaming and thrashing around, nobody will ever get a smoke break.

An advertisement in medical journals showed an angry young Hispanic in denim and bandannas snarling at the camera. The copy warned, "He's psychotic, he's violent, and he's threatening your staff." The solution? "Haldol: From Crisis to Control."

There have been reports of "snowing" or spiking the drinking water with anti-psychotics, especially in large, public psychiatric hospitals. While this does produce an atmosphere of tranquility, it is not without risk. The path to synthetic serenity is riddled with uncomfortable and dangerous side effects. Consider a brief excerpt from one warning sheet (or product circular, also known as a package insert): "mask-like faces, drooling, tremors, pill rolling motion, cogwheel rigidity, and shuffling gait." The same sheet also warns doctors that their patients are more likely than usual to drown in their own vomit.

The grand prize side-effect is the drug-induced spaz attack known as tardive dyskinesia (TD). The patient is transformed into a grimacing Energizer Bunny, forever puttering around, puffing his cheeks,

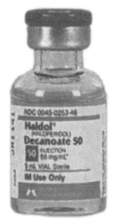

poking his tongue out, twitching his arms. If the patient is kept on these meds for too long, the condition is permanent. This makes ingestion of Haldol or other anti-psychotics a game of psychopharmacological Russian Roulette: if you take the drug, your symptoms will abate for now, but you might be stuck with a permanent case of TD. The odds worsen in direct proportion to the amount ingested.

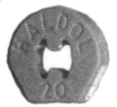

And once you have TD, you might as well stay in the asylum. You would be hard-pressed to distinguish between a raving nut and a perfectly sane person who's been taking his meds too long. Are they shaking their arms and blinking at you to signal that they also know what's being done to get rid of the extra colors, or is it just that they can't keep still no matter how hard they try?

In all likelihood, though, it usually takes years of daily dosing for this to happen. But this is not an uncommon occurrence. If you are committed involuntarily, your case is brought up for review once every six months. (This is rapidly changing: some HMOs and Medicare review patient charts daily and kick them out after a certain time has elapsed, regardless of success or outcome.) A multi-year stay in a state facility is quite possible, if you don't have any friends or family on the outside or if the doctors don't like you. One good way to get the doctors to hate you is to complain about or spit out your pills. Who but a paranoid would claim that the doctors are intentionally hurting them by giving them bad medicine?

Even outpatients aren't safe. A popular tactic for farming madmen out into the community is to make their continued liberty contingent on random urine testing. This is to be sure that they're taking their medications as directed. More difficult customers have slow-release chunks of their assigned anti-psychotic implanted surgically, Norplant-style. No rest for the wacky.

My experience with Haldol is pretty benign, all things considered. I found myself feeling restless after having been admitted to a psychiatric hospital. I got up from my bed and started pacing the halls, bothering no one, just tracing a measured perimeter around the ward.

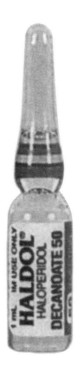

I was challenged shortly after I had begun and asked how I was doing. "I feel restless," I replied. An attendant moved to the hall and watched me but did not interrupt. In about five minutes a nurse asked me to come to the medication window, normally closed at this hour, but this time opened just for me. Ah, personal customer service.

They gave me a wax paper cup of a Kaopectate-looking liquid and told me to drink. I did and felt tired soon after. I went back to bed. The next day I awoke with difficulty and felt groggy. At morning meds, I found something new in my little cup: two small purple tablets with an "H" cut out of the middle—four milligrams of factory-fresh Haldol. Knowing resistance was useless, I ate the new pills. I was quickly transformed into a slow-moving, slow-thinking, slow-talking wretch. I was unable to participate in any of the planned activities. I did not attend the classes they offered. I just lolled around in bed and got up only for meals.

The next morning they gave me two more of the purple pills, and I didn't bother trying to stay awake. I awoke about an hour before the midday meal to hear my juvenile delinquent roommate yelling and singing, leaping from his bed to my bed and back again. The weird thing was, I felt compelled to look at the little bastard. Tried though I might, I could not help turning my head to the left, where he was now jumping on the windowsill. I could not look away. In the stupor, I felt horrified and bad, not knowing of this weakness on my part. I struggled with my neck, but it was hopeless. Then I had an idea: Perhaps it's not that I have to look at him, but that I have to look to the left. By flipping over onto my stomach, I proved myself right . . . or, correct.

An orderly came in and informed me that it was time for arts and crafts. I got up obediently, having been assured that they would tie me up if I caused trouble, and walked down the hall to the activities room, sidestepping to the left as I went.

After arriving, one of the attendants asked me if I could stop looking left. Through my fog I said no, I couldn't. He went away and shortly came back with a nurse. They told me to come back to my room. I did so. They had me take off my shirt and sit facing away from them. I felt a needle prick my back. They had given me an injection of Cogentin, a muscle relaxant.

I had been experiencing an extrapyramidal symptom (EPS), a common Haldol side-effect. The muscles in my back had tightened up involuntarily. If left untreated for too long, the effect can proceed to the throat, causing the muscles there to contract, leading to death by asphyxiation. Luckily for me, my side effect started while I was awake.

Considering both the subjective unpleasantness of not being able to think and a life-and lawsuit-threatening cramp, the doctors decided to see how I coped without the meds. I recovered fully in a couple of days and resolved to be a good quiet inmate after that.

Sailing the Fentanyl Seas
by Will Beifuss

I wanted to try Fentanyl ever since I first heard about it a few years ago. I have tried all of the other pain-killers over the years (my favorite still remains oxycodone) but Fentanyl always managed to elude me. It is the most potent narcotic analgesic available, manufactured by Janssen Pharmaceutica and is available as a liquid for injection under the name Sublimaze, or as a patch that you stick on your skin under the name Duragesic.

I had the opportunity recently to try the patch (or "transdermal system" as they call it) and let me tell you, folks, this is strong stuff. Fentanyl is measured in micrograms, (that's millionths of gram) with 100 mcg equal to 10 mg of Morphine or 15 mg of oxycodone (Percodan) or 75 mg of meperedine (Demerol). The patch I tried delivered 75 mcg/hour of Fentanyl, and lasts for 3 days if left on continuously. In a 24-hour period, it delivers the equivalent pain relief of approximately 250 mg morphine. Now I have never done that much morphine in one day, but I figured if the patch was designed to deliver that amount, then I would give it a try. I did reconsider for just a moment when I read the warning, "Duragesic should ONLY be used in patients who are already on and are tolerant to opioid therapy." But I quickly dismissed this ominous warning as not pertaining to someone like me who has a long history of pharmaceutical use.

My first day on the patch, I put it on as soon as I woke up at 7 am. I resolved to pack as many hours of analgesia into my day as possible. I got ready for work, ever alert for the first signs of the drug's effects. In 45 minutes, the first subtle waves of warmth spread throughout my body. When I arrived at work at 8:30 am., I was getting quite stoned, it had been one-and-a-half hours since I applied the patch, and the effects were equal to about two Percodans. By 9:30 am., I was getting a little concerned—the high was increasing dramatically and an unavoidable somnolence was taking hold of me. By 10:30 am., the high had lost some of its euphoria and become sinisterly heavy and stuporous. My co-workers were giving me suspicious glances as my movements became exaggerated and simple tasks like hanging up the phone became a real challenge. My desk, with its usual office accoutrements, became an obstacle course that required a dexterity I was rapidly losing. By 11:00 am., it felt like I had four Percodans coursing through my bloodstream. Visions of an unwelcome coma coming to claim me became evident and I'd decided I'd better attempt the unsteady expedition to the bathroom to remove the now job-threatening patch. Just then, my supervisor burst in, telling me I was late for the department meeting going on down the hall. I looked in the direction of his voice but found it difficult to focus on his face. I told him I needed to go to the bathroom first and he replied that was out of the question. The president of the company was in attendance at this meeting, and arriving any later would qualify as a serious faux-pas. I lurched to my feet, my head felt like it was full of wet cement, and my body anesthetized. I steadied myself along the desks toward the door, and my supervisor, noticing the difficulty I was having with even this simple task of walking, asked me what the hell was wrong.

I told him I suffered from occasional bouts of vertigo and was having an episode. He seemed to buy my story, although my senses were drowning in a thick sea of Fentanyl intoxication and I could not tell what anyone else was really doing, let alone thinking. He helped me down the corridor to the meeting room and as he opened the door, the room fell silent and all eyes were upon us. I used my supervisor's body as a shield against their prying stares and poured myself into a seat in the back row.

The speaker resumed his presentation but his words were not making sense to me as I drifted in and out of consciousness. The Fentanyl stupor was increasing, I broke out into a cold sweat and was swaying back and forth in my seat. I turned to the person sitting next to me, and failing miserably to make eye contact, muttered something about having bad allergies that day. At this point, I don't remember any more and the rest of the story was related to me by my supervisor, who I fortunately have (or at least had) a good rapport with. Apparently, about 20 minutes after pathetically trying to blame high pollen counts for my condition, I nodded out. When I started to fall out of my chair, I caught myself at the last second and got to my feet. I stood there, eyes closed, vacillating back and forth on rubber legs I could not feel, and then bolted out the door. I was found one hour later passed out on the toilet, with my shirt off and the Fentanyl patch, which I had managed to peel off, stuck in my hair.

A word to the wise—Fentanyl is as potent as anything gets. If you

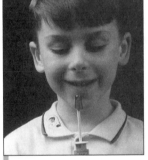

Just approved: The Fentanyl Lollipop, the way Mary Poppins creates junkies of children

acquire some, approach it with the respect and caution this indomitable drug deserves. But don't let my story dissuade you from trying it! Simply remove the patch in two hours until you are ready to set sail again, and then reapply it.

Immodium AD, Over-the-Counter Methadone

There is evidence to believe the OTC anti-diarrhea medication Imodium AD (loperamide hcl) would halt withdrawal symptoms in opiate-dependent humans. We knew it helped morphine-dependent monkeys. We now know that it does the same for human beings addicted not only to plain old opium, but to heroin as well.

None of our information comes from FDA-monitored tests, so don't ask *PaGG* for specifics on numbers and control groups, and, God forbid, the names of any or all informants, as they remain unknown to us, thanks to a no ID double-blind.

Before we begin we'd like to amend something else we reported—namely, that junkies were using Xanax (alprazolam) to improve their heroin highs. Lately the mass media has decided devil drug junkies really use Klonopin —another benzodiazepine like Xanax. This leads us to believe that air-headed reporters haven't considered that the use of any drug in this class (of which Valium is the Undisputed Leader) would be a nice addition to effects achieved by taking heroin.

According to Alexander Shulgin's *Controlled Substances*, loperamide was placed into Schedule V on June 17, 1977, then removed from all scheduling controls on November 3, 1982. Just what prompted this unscheduling is unclear, except that as recently as 1987, it appears most drug textbooks failed to recognize the potential opiate action of loperamide, if not the obvious structural similarities between it and other opiates.

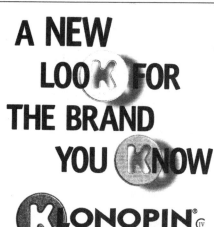

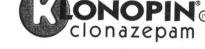

A NEW LOOK FOR THE BRAND YOU KNOW

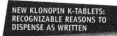

KLONOPIN® (IV)
clonazepam

NEW DISTINCTIVE K-PERFORATED KLONOPIN TABLETS
* Easy to recognize, which may reduce patient medication errors
* The same medication and strengths as before
* Scored 0.5 mg tablets break cleanly in half for divided doses

MANUFACTURED TO MEET THE HIGHEST STANDARDS
* Surpasses USP requirements

NEW KLONOPIN K-TABLETS: RECOGNIZABLE REASONS TO DISPENSE AS WRITTEN

KLONOPIN 2 mg   KLONOPIN 1 mg

KLONOPIN 0.5 mg

As with any benzodiazepine, caution patients about driving, operating machinery and the simultaneous ingestion of alcohol or other CNS depressant drugs. Advise patients to consult a physician before increasing the dose or discontinuing KLONOPIN. Side effects reported with KLONOPIN are those generally associated with benzodiazepines such as drowsiness and impaired coordination.

Please see adjacent page for complete product information.
Copyright © 1996 by Roche Laboratories Inc.
All rights reserved.

Roche Laboratories
A Member of the Roche Group

Shulgin makes a structural comparison of loperamide with methadone and, indeed, there are some striking similarities. But loperamide also exhibits structural similarities to Fentanyl.

In any case, the stuff is obviously an opioid exempt from all scheduling controls—even the minimal ones originally imposed. This is possibly due to a lack of evidence that even high doses of Immodium can get someone high. High dose and long-term consumption of the stuff (as long as two years in some cases), fail the Naloxone Challenge Test, in which a powerful opiate antagonist brings on severe cramps and liquid pinwheel barf sessions if you happen to be addicted or stoned on opiates.

There's not much evidence of tolerance to the stuff, a very un-opiate-like quality that ought to looked into. If it is discovered why loperamide exhibits characteristics of more powerful and abused opiate drugs, yet doesn't require ever-increasing quantities to enjoy its effects, we may be on our way to the holy grail of opiates—the non-addicting high!

So loperamide doesn't get you high very well (although some have reported to *PaGG* a definite feeling of calm and well-being after a normal dose of the stuff.) But it can keep you from jonesing too hard if you're trying to kick Percodans, morphine, heroin, or something. So it's at least partially cross-tolerated.

The Big Immodium Test

Recently, three heroin junkies about to enter withdrawal agreed to try a dose two to three times normal of Imodium AD to see if it would be of any help in kicking their hardcore addictions. They took the drug just as the first symptoms of withdrawal set in—in other words, when it was time for their next "fix." None of the junkies had been tapering or reducing their doses before the test, so all of them were vulnerable to full-on withdrawal.

Happily, all three junkies reported significant relief from the onset of withdrawal symptoms. Loperamide seemed to markedly or even completely eliminate the stereotypical joint and muscle aches, as well as sweating and the restless feeling. One of the kickers felt well enough to go to a job interview and even got the job! On the downside, all three junkies reported nausea—probably caused by consuming a large amount of anise-flavored liquid Immodium. It was decided to use liquid rather than tablets because the liquid form achieves peak plasma levels about twice as fast as the pills. It was agreed that a faster onset would increase the chances of test compliance among these dregs of humanity.

In future tests it would be interesting to see whether loperamide in pill form would eliminate the nausea. We also understand loperamide is also available in cherry-flavored syrup, which might provoke less nausea among those who simply hate the taste of licorice. Interestingly, Janssen Pharmaceuticals, which invented and makes loperamide, also has a patent on another compound called Lofentenil Oxalate—a narcotic analgesic not currently in use. Similarities between the drugs suggest that a few slight differences in the basic molecule could bring about some heavy-duty changes in the effects. This seems even more likely given that Janssen Pharmaceuticals also produces the very powerful opiate fentanyl citrate, known by its trade name of Sublimaz.

Was loperamide discovered by the giant and ingenious pharmaceutical concern as part of its general research on opiates? Could loperamide be transformed into one of its cousins or even another chemical entirely? *PaGG* does not have the resources to adequately research these possibilities other than to speculate on freebasing (oxidizing) the hcl form and see if it doesn't get stronger or yield a smokeable form of loperamide.

Hey, it works with other stuff . . .

The advantages of using loperamide instead of methadone to withdraw from opiate addiction are many. Even name-brand Imodium AD is cheaper than government-issued methadone, and you don't need government permission to take it. You don't have to get up at the crack of dawn to stand in line with a bunch of strangers to get your

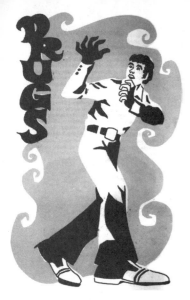

CREATiON of the Drug Fiend

"Suppose it were announced that there were more than a million lepers among our people. Think what a shock that announcement would produce! Yet drug addiction is far more curable than leprosy, far more tragic to its victims, and is spreading like a

dose and you can kick as quickly or slowly as you want since *you* control the dosage.

Some junkies have been known to complain that methadone clinics seem to try to keep them on state-provided dope longer than they would like.

As always, *PaGG* strongly urges any and all readers to consult with their physicians before embarking on any sort of drug therapy, even one using OTC medications. It only makes sense.

Magical Midrin
by Sylvia Remora

If you suffer from migraine headaches, you already may have tried Midrin, an attractive bright red pill with a hot pink band made by Carnrick Laboratories, Inc. Carnrick touts its crimson capsule as "The Headache Capsule" and that's what Midrin does best. It combines acetominophen, isometheptene Mucate (a vasoconstrictor), with a mild sedative into a pleasing little cocktail that chases away those horrid throbbing headaches that can poison an entire day or two.

But Mid is also the perfect party pill. I take two whenever I head out for a beer with the boys. Why? Well, since I'm susceptible to migraines—which are caused in part by dilated blood vessels in the brain—even a small amount of alcohol can give me a whopper of a headache. Alcohol expands those tender brain vessels even more. In fact, two Mids and a latte are a great way to start the day, headache or not!

Midrin is great for hangovers, too. Its sedative (not found in any other pill) effects won't make you drowsy, so close work or heavy machinery is no problem while you're under Mid's influence.

In short, Midrin is a little-known workhorse of a pill that deserves a wider following that it has. Ask your doctor for some today!

L-Glutamine
by Adam Gorightly

Back in ish#11 of *PaGG*, the amino acid L-Glutamine was given mention as an energy booster and fatigue fighter at dosages of around 500 to 1,000 milligrams. I have for many years now been experimenting with cognitive enhancers, the likes of DMAE, Ginkgo Biloba, Choline Chloride and others. L-Glutamine I've found—and concur with the *PaGG* gang—packs a definite punch of energy as well as helping to increase concentration and alertness, more so than I've encountered with other smart drugs and nutrients, and just short of tried and true energy supplements such as amphetamines in the form of cross-tops and black beauties, which I took in younger hop-head years before becoming a responsible member of society.

Anyway, I use the stuff such: 500 mg before lunch, which helps me get a jump on my most lackadaisical/drowsy part of the day, when ofttimes I fall into a "food coma" and feel the need for a nap coming on. L-Glut helps immensely in getting over this low energy part of the day. And even though I may take a 15 minute. nap, under L-Glut it seems like I wake up afterwards more bright eyed and bushy-tailed than in my pre-L-Glutamine incarnation. Lastly, I'll sometimes have a late afternoon early evening blast 500 mg dose just to intensify my evenings at home, whether fueling creative literary efforts, or just simply enjoying another hilarious episode of Martin.

[Mr. Gorightly also wrote us about some non-FDA approved tests involving the OTC "motion sickness" pill called Marezine (cyclizine). He says that some of these friends found that Marezine "induced extremely palpable hallucinations right in front of their astounded eyes. One associate . . . gobbled up about thirteen of these pills and visualized a total hallucination in the guise of a friend of his who walked right up to him, said, 'hello,' and then disappeared."]

Poor Man's PCP, DM Cough Syrup

Dextromethorphan Hydrobromide is the "DM" in DM cough syrup, but you can get it in pill form as a constituent of various solid and liquid-filled tablets. It's also one of the most mystifying drugs in the pharmacopia. Even though it is the king of OTC cough

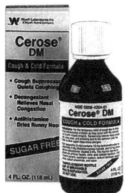

medicines—the drug that replaced codeine as a non-narcotic cough suppressant and is in virtually all OTC cold, flu, and cough remedies, DM is hardly mentioned in most common reference works.

Take a look in the 1993 *PDR*—there's no description of it at all. Rifling the pages of a number of thick, important-looking books here at the *PaGG* research library, we found only sketchy and sometimes contradictory information on DM HBr.

One source called it a "narcotic antagonist" with "very good analgesic" properties. Other descriptions say DM is a cough suppressant only and does not kill pain. It is supposedly non-addicting. It's not supposed to get you high, but legions of high school and college students have a different opinion entirely.

"Full warping of subspace," said one DM experimenter, who took more than the recommended dosage. "Pinhead with expansive arms/legs. Incredible head size. Warping and folding of body. Incredible spatial distortions."

Nearly all experimenters find it enhances or at least changes the way they hear music—especially rhythm. They seem to enjoy the beat of music more and one even expressed a new found enjoyment of the various hisses and pops to be heard between the songs on a tape he was listening to!

For a drug that is related to some powerful anesthetics (like PCP) and is sold all over the place to keep us away from codeine, we find it strikingly stupid that DM is commonly mixed with acetaminophen and guafenisin, which can both destroy your liver. And for a drug that can produce a strange and entertaining experience as well as cause convulsions and possible brain damage all by itself, we think it's high time someone took a gander at the "Robo" experience.

To this end, we begin with an experiment carried out by your faithful author, then we'll look into some of the pharmacological aspects of the stuff before drawing a few conclusions. Here goes:

moral and physical scourge . . . Most of the daylight robberies, daring hold-ups and cruel murders are known to be committed chiefly by drug addicts, who constitute the primary cause of our alarming crime wave. Drug addiction is more communicable and less curable than leprosy. Upon the issue hangs the perpetuation of civilization, the destiny of the world, and the future of the human race."

—Richmond P. Hobson, prohibition crusader and anti-narco propagandist, in a 1928 radio broadcast entitled *The Struggle of Mankind Against Its Deadliest Foe*

The Test

I drank about eight ounces of DM cough syrup. I was feeling kind of achy and wanted to see if it would kill pain. Previous smaller-dose experiments had shown me that the stuff could cause confusion and restlessness, but I couldn't remember how much I'd taken.

Soon enough, pain went away, and I went to bed a couple hours later. It was like midnight. I felt neither awake nor asleep, sort of like a typical narcotic high, but no great shakes. Mildly content, kind of nodding-—just not as pleasant.

At four o'clock in the morning, I woke up suddenly and felt the need to go to Kinko's and shave a week's worth of stubble from my face. These ideas seemed very clear to me.

That seems normal enough, except I HAD A REPTILIAN BRAIN. My whole way of thinking and perceiving changed. It was like I was operating with a medula only.

I had full control over motor functions, but still had the impression that I was ungainly. That's because I felt detached from my body, as if I was inhaling nitrous oxide. I got in the shower and shaved. For all I knew I was hacking my face to pieces—or maybe not. Since I didn't see any blood or feel any pain, I had no worries about it. In fact, "feelings" were so shallow or nonexistent that I probably couldn't have felt anything like anxiety. I lost any sense of time.

I knew I was capable of performing various actions, but could not conceive of any consequences to those actions. Had I looked down and seen another limb, I wouldn't have been surprised at all. I would have just used it. It was very much like being a passenger inside my own body. What was it? It didn't seem too clear.

During this experience I gained the sort of insight associated with acid or dreams. Like in a dream, you aren't surprised by the absurd (an extra limb) and, like an LSD trip, you realize the absurdity of it all. But without hallucinations.

The world became a binary place of dark and light, on/off, safety/danger. When I felt a need, I determined it was hunger and ate almonds until I didn't feel the need any more. Same with water. It was like playing a game. Staying alive, but with no fear at all. I sat down and tried to write down how this felt so I could look at it later. I was very aware that I was stupid. I wrote down the word "Cro-Magnon."

I thought I would have trouble driving, but I had none. I felt "unsafe" confronting the dark street, but then this feeling disappeared when I crawled into the "safe" car. Then I drove to Kinko's, where I parked on a deserted street, and felt quite content waiting for the crossing lights. I knew that it was important to avoid native aggressors like cops, and not provoke them. Luckily there were only a couple of people in the store, and one was a friend. She confirmed what I had seen in the mirror, that my pupils were of different sizes.

I was fucked up.

There was no way I could make any subjective decision or know if I was correctly adhering to social custom. I didn't even know how to modulate my voice. Was this loud? Do I look like a normal human? Outside, my friend shivered, so I asked her if it was cold, because for me there were only two temperatures—tolerable/intolerable (I found that out in the shower). I guess I wasn't cold since I had no urge to change locations.

In no way was this like being drunk, even though I kept thinking I probably looked drunk. But once again, my motor skills were fine.

I understood I was an entity in the big contraption called civilization and certain things were expected of me—but I could not comprehend what the hell they might be.

All the words that came out of my mouth seemed equivalent in meaning. Instead of saying, "reduce it about 90 percent," I could have said, "two eggs and some toast, please," and these two phrases would have been the same. The whole world broke down into elemental parts, each of equal value to the whole, which is to say, of no value at all.

I sat at a table and read a newspaper. It was the most absurd thing I had ever seen. Each story purported to describe a thing or event, or was supposed to convey "news" of a reality of some other location. This seemed stupid. An article on a war in Burma was described as "the war the West forgot." It had an "at-a-glance" chart that said Burma was three times the size of the state of Washington.

This was meaningless, and I knew it. The story did not even begin to describe the tiniest fragment of the reality of that place. From a vague recollection of my pre-reptilian days, I knew of things called "complicated." But the paper's pitiful attempt to categorize individuals as "rebels" or "insurgents," or to describe the reasons for their agony, was literally ridiculous. I laughed outloud.

I found being a reptile kind of pleasant. I was content to sit and monitor my surroundings. I was

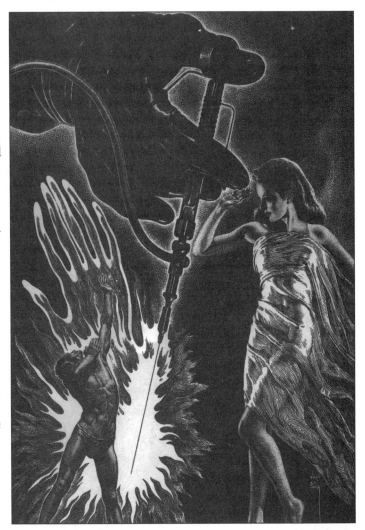

Artwork by Virgil Finlay

alert, but not anxious. If someone had come at me with an axe, I would have acted appropriately. Fight or flight. Every now and then I would do a true "reality check" to make sure I wasn't masturbating or strangling someone due to a vague awareness of non-reptilian expectations. At one point, I ventured across the street to a hamburger place to get something to eat. It was locked up, and yet there were workers inside. This truly confused me, and I considered a way to break in, and make off with food. Luckily, the store opened (now that it was 6 am.) and I entered the front door just like a normal consumer.

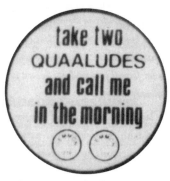

PRESCRIPTION Drug Rap

Prescription

Drugs, they treat

the pain.

If you use too

much, they will

give you no gain.

Con-cen-tra-tion

a thing they can do,

Some help you

think and feel

better too.

"Don't abuse them,"

that's the

prescription.

"Don't abuse them,"

the right decision!

—Another message
from the DEA

It was difficult to remember how to do a money-for-merchandise transaction, and even more difficult to put words into action, but I finally succeeded at the task. I ate bite-by-bite until I was full. If I had become full before finishing the hamburger, I think I would have simply let it fall from my hand.

The life of a reptile may seem boring to us, but boredom has no place in a reptilian brain. If, as a reptile, something started to hurt, I took steps to get away from it. If it felt better over here, that's where I went. Writing this, 24 hours after becoming a reptile, it seems that my neocortex is reconnecting. Soon, I hope to be human again.

As a reptile I still believed in God. I didn't feel like praying (which seemed ludicrous) but there was no diminishing of my belief. Why? is a purely human question. As a reptile, questioning my existence was none of my business. I just didn't care. Become a reptile for a while; it straightens out a thing or two.

The Pharmacology of DM

Here is a description of Dextromethorphan, kindly provided by a colleague in Ohio. In it, he refers to DM as DXM. I put this here so in case you're on cough syrup you can follow the bouncing ball:

"Dextromethorphan acts as a cough suppressant via its agonist (activating) activity at mu-opioid receptors. Unlike codeine, it does not seem to activate other opioid receptors, except for the sigma receptor.

As far as its other effects, DXM is in the same class as ketamine, PCP, MK-801, and several other NMDA open channel blockers/sigma opioid ligans.

The sigma opioid receptor's function is unknown, but it may be implicated in schizophrenia. Sigma opioid agonists produce both the positive and the negative symptoms of schizophrenia, unlike dopaminergics, which produce only the positive symptoms.

The NMDA receptor is a fast ion-channel receptor which is normally activated by the excitory amino acids and possibly potentiated by glycine. There is a second NMDA receptor subtype in the cerebellum (this my account for DXM's perceived effect on motion.) NMDA receptors probably exist in several different subtypes. DXM, ketamine, PCP, and other similar chemicals act as "open channel blockers." Upon the opening of the NMDA channel, the chemicals enter the channel and block ion transfer. DXM is a non-competitive blocker.

In addition to this, there is a second "PCP2" binding site (the PCP1 site is the NMDA open channel block site). This may be a biogenic amine reuptake complex. If so, then this class of chemicals may act as reuptake inhibitors. The role of the PCP2 site is poorly understood.

I don't know offhand the binding of DXM to sigma, PCP1, and PCP2 in comparison to ketamine, MK-801, and PCP. All of these drugs are being studied for their effects in preventing damage to the brain during seizure.

In terms of sources, DXM is available OTC in many countries in tablet form. Robitussin Maximum Strength Cough (not Robitussin DM) contains DXM with nothing else (except a little alcohol). Robitussin DM also contains an expectorant that should not be taken in high doses. A Dose of Robitussin Maximum Strength Cough is two to five full "shots" using the shot glass that comes with the bottle. The usual warnings apply. Additionally, prolonged use of DXM can and has led to psychosis similar to PCP-induced psychosis. Individual differences in NMDA receptors may be at work here, but you're still potentially at risk. I personally wouldn't mix DXM with anything.

Further Ruminations on DM

I must modify my statement about full motor control on DM. For one thing I became very aware of arms and legs. They seemed larger or longer. Although walking was no problem, I felt as if I was loping. Objective observation of people under the influence of DM shows their gestures to be expansive and their strides to be longer than normal. It wouldn't be fair to say that DM has no effect on motor skills. You can easily walk, but I doubt you could play soccer or do ballet.

According to the pharmacological analysis above, DM activates the mu opiate receptor, one of four such receptors identified since the late 1970s, the site where endogenous chemicals called endorphins seem to check pain and elevate mood. The mu receptor is primarily associated with pain relief, while the delta receptor is linked to the euphoric effects caused by either opiates or endorphins. DM is not active at this important site.

The sigma receptor is associated with opiates and endorphins—but not exclusively. As the pharmacological analysis explains, sigma receptors seem linked to schizophrenia. (By the way, when he mentions "positive" aspects of mental illness, he is not speaking qualitatively. Hallucinating, for instance, is a "positive" quality, while becoming silent and withdrawn is considered "negative." In a practical sense, psychiatric medicines such as Thorazine help to curb the "positive" traits, but don't do much about the "negative" ones. Thus, a paranoid schizo dosed with a similar compound may appear more normal, when in actuality he is simply paralyzed. He's still living in his private hell, just unable to react.)

Otherwise DM appears to work in the limbic system, which explains the binary or reptilian experience as this part of the brain is primitive. In essence, the brain (on DM) seems to lose much of its neo-cortex and the user is reduced to a more primitive state. But, not really being a reptile, and not truly disabling the neo-cortex, the user remains human and thus can make some subjective observations—like listening to music in a new way.

The thought that DM could cause psychosis is disturbing. One experimenter who dosed himself on more than half a dozen occasions and took detailed notes, had seizures. After experiencing "full-blown hallucinations," in which he thought he was a flower swaying in the wind, he began convulsing. "I'd all of a sudden get sort of a seizure, and flail around the chair I was sitting in." About 45 minutes of this he fell fast asleep. But he reports waking up "nice and refreshed the next day."

This is something commonly reported: lack of any hangover. Many users said they were energized by the experience. The thought that DM could be neuro-protective is more cheering. It appears that having a stroke or bumping your head while on DM might be like wearing an internal football helmet.

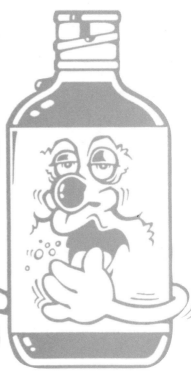

Quaaludes

In 1985 *High Times* featured Quaaludes in their centerfold usually reserved for some voluptuous hunk of pot or hashish. Quaaludes may have been the country's most popular pill, even among hemptsers, who nowadays shun pills. *High Times* also ran a facetious article called "Quaalude Grower's Guide" illustrated with humorously doctored photographs showing earthy 'Lude farmers carefully tending their fields of Quaalude plants. For *High Times* to elevate a pill to plant status is certainly regarded a compliment of the highest order.

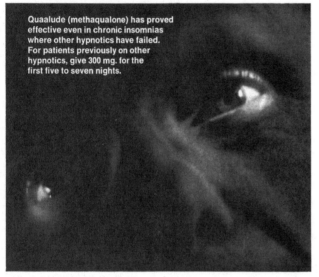

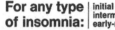

For any type of insomnia: | initial | intermittent | early-morning

Quaalude (methaqualone) has proved effective even in chronic insomnias where other hypnotics have failed. For patients previously on other hypnotics, give 300 mg. for the first five to seven nights.

Prescribing Information:
Usual Adult Dose: For sleep, 150-300 mg. at bedtime. For patients previously on other hypnotics, 300 mg. for five to seven nights. For sedation, 75 mg. after each meal and at bedtime. Not recommended in children under 14. Dosage should be individualized for aged, debilitated or highly agitated patients.
Overdosage: Evacuate gastric contents, maintain adequate ventilation and support blood pressure, if necessary. Hemodialysis may be helpful. Analeptics may increase tonic-clonic spasms.
Contraindications: Quaalude is contraindicated in women who are or may become pregnant.
Warnings: Because drowsiness may occur within 10 to 20 minutes, the patient must be warned against driving a car or operating dangerous machinery while on Quaalude. Pending longer term clinical experience, Quaalude should not be used continuously for periods exceeding three months. Psychological dependence rare. Physical dependence not clearly demonstrated. However, caution needed with addiction-prone patients.
Precautions: Use with caution in patients with anxiety states where impending depression or suicidal tendencies exist, or with impaired hepatic function. Quaalude may potentiate effects of other sedative, analgesic or psychotherapeutic drugs or alcohol.
Adverse Reactions: Mild and transient side effects encountered in less than 5 percent of all patients studied have included headache,

drowsiness, hangover, nausea, fatigue, epigastric discomfort, dizziness, dry mouth, emesis, torpor, restlessness, tachycardia, anorexia, diarrhea, diaphoresis, urticaria, exanthema and transient paresthesia ("pins and needles").
Supplied: Quaalude-150 (150 mg. white, scored tablets)
Quaalude-300 (300 mg. white, scored tablets)
Consult complete literature before prescribing.

New, double-strength
Quaalude®-300
[methaqualone]
prelude to sleep
WILLIAM H. RORER, INC., Fort Washington, Pa. 19034

Originally marketed by Rorer, and introduced in 1965, Quaaludes soon became popular for the pleasant, drunken-like state they produced. Although normally prescribed for sleep, most people preferred to stay awake and enjoy the euphoric serenity the drug gave them.

Of course, soon enough the drug began to get something of a bad reputation. First there was Karen Quinlan who knocked herself into a 10-year coma when she slugged down her Quaaludes with a goodly amount of alcohol. Then there was the case of President Carter's drug advisor Peter Bourne, who was forced to hand in his resignation after it was discovered that he had illegally written a prescription for 'Ludes to his secretary, Ellen Metsky. Afterwards came the Roman Polanski saga, where he drugged a jail-bait Valley girl, and introduced her to a bout of sexual soma in a hillside mansion's jacuzzi.

"There is no question," said a Rorer source, "the press Quaalude received during the Bourne flap added to apprehensions hospitals and private physicians had in prescribing it to patients."

Whether it was because of the drug's seamy reputation or the fact that it made up only two percent of the company's sales, Rorer sold the pill to Lemmon Pharmacal in 1978 for $5 million. But things just got worse for the pill. Several states banned it entirely, placing it in the Schedule I controlled substance category. By November 1983, Lemmon had announced it would cease production of the drug entirely although it planned to keep on distributing the remaining stock until January 31 1984 or until supplies ran out.

Of course, demand for Quaaludes continued. Counterfeit 'Ludes started showing up, mainly from factories in South America. The fake tablets proved to be indistinguishable from the original ones and just as good since they were manufactured from legally made methaqualone from Europe. "Foreign" Quaaludes are known by different brand names, including the famous "Mandrax," aka "mandies."

Sadly, prideless chemists looking for a faster buck started to cut corners. It wasn't long before bootleg 'Ludes began to lose potency and were often adulterated with diazepam or even diphenhydramine or other common antihistamines that can make a person feel drowsy.

Worse, clandestine factories producing methaqualone from inferior, non-pharmaceutical quality precursors and their products were not only sub-strength but often contained poisonous residues and unreacted precursors. Large scale 'Lude manufacturing suffered from another drawback—the sheer amount of the stuff needed to produce its soporific effects. A decent hit of Quaalude contains a minimum of 150 to 300 mg of active ingredient. In comparison to more powerful tranquilizers, such as Valium (for which 10 or 20 mg is sufficient) it meant transporting barrels and barrels of the stuff over international borders, to say nothing of the hassles of storing it. As usual, the illicit drug market favored less bulky and stronger stuff.

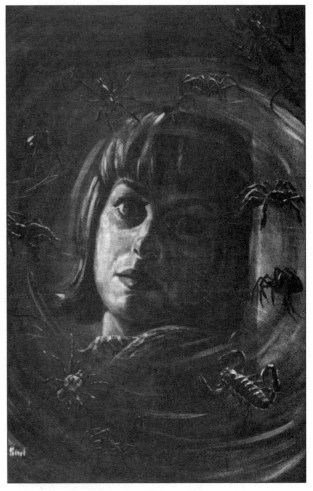

A Desperate Alternative

Back in the 1970s, German scientists playing around with a squiggly little millipede that scurries in the forests of Europe eating wood noticed it secreted a substance that warded off predators whenever the bug was attacked. They called the gunk "glomerin," after the bug's Latin name, Glomeris marginata. As German scientists are wont to do, they meticulously analyzed the stuff and found it to bear an uncanny resemblance to methaqualone.

From there, biologists at Cornell and the University of Missouri ran gladiator contests between the millipede and one of its scariest foes, a starving wolf spider. The result: the majority of millipedes, rolled into a ball and exuding globules of glomerin, fended off the attack. More than a third weren't even bitten. Later, when the researchers force-fed glomerin to the wolf spiders they became disoriented and uncoordinated to the point of being immobilized. When placed on their backs, the spiders couldn't even right themselves and simply lay there for days on end. In the wild, ants would have made short work of them within a couple of hours. Further experiments using higher doses had the predictable result of killing the spiders.

For those who crave 'Ludes, yet are repulsed by sucking on a fearful tree bug, there is an alternative that's perhaps even better than glomerin.

An herb found in parts of India and Bangladesh called "Ash-shoura" contains a compound called Arborine, which bears an even closer resemblance to methaqualone than bug goo. No word yet on how well it works but it seems Ash-shoura is used as medicine in that part of the world.

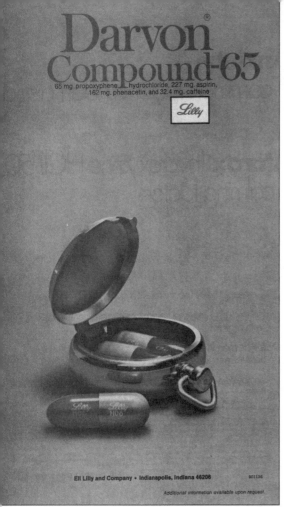

Darvon Compound-65

65 mg. propoxyphene hydrochloride, 227 mg. aspirin, 162 mg. phenacetin, and 32.4 mg. caffeine

Lilly

Eli Lilly and Company • Indianapolis, Indiana 46206

901136

Additional information available upon request.

Darvon

Introduced in 1957, Darvon (propoxyphene) was touted as a "non-narcotic" painkiller that couldn't get you hooked. This was said about it even though it was derived from the methadone, the synthetic opiate that fell into Eli Lilly's hands after WWII. Dr. Irvin C. Kleiderer, the civilian leader of a team of army scientists picking through the remains of the laboratories of I.G. Farben in Eberfeld, Germany found out about the amazing substance (then called "Amidone" or Analgesic #10820). When Kleiderer returned to the States he went to work for Lilly, bringing the formula with him as sort of a war booty. Lilly still makes plenty of methadone but also used it as a model for another analgesic, propoxyphene, first known in pill form as Darvon.

Darvon quickly became the number three selling pill in America. Annual sales were close to $100 million and climbed steadily for years. In 1974 around 1.5 billion of the red and grey capsules were dispensed for pain of nearly any kind. At its sales zenith, it was due for some bad publicity. It was about then that the pill came under vicious attack by the *New York Times* and consumer crusader Dr. Sidney M. Wolfe, who demanded that Darvon be outlawed immediately. The pill, he said, was "less effective in killing pain than aspirin and more lethal than heroin."

Lilly defended itself admirably, and Darvon kept its hold on the number one spot among pain killers. In 1979, the second wave of attacks came, this time from the government. The Secretary of Health Education and Welfare singled out Darvon as a devil drug, personally urging doctors not to prescribe it anymore and patients not to ask for it. His high-handed warning was as effective as talking to a wall. Darvon had become an immediate hit with pill consumers and stayed that way. People loved it!

Instead of dumping Darvon, Lilly was selling Darvon cousins, variations on the propoxyphene theme. There was Darvon mixed with aspirin, there was Darvocet with and without other ingredients and more. Lilly marketed two salts of the same stuff, doled it out in different strengths, put caffeine and acetaminophen into some concoctions. But its most creative strain of Darvon was undoubtedly the now-extinct "Darvo-Tran."

Of course, as it happens with all pills, the higher it rode the harder it fell. When HEW's attempt to harpoon the pill failed, stronger measures were called for.

In 1980, the government ordered Lilly to publish and distribute information on the "dangers" of Darvon to 125,000 doctors nationwide. The plan backfired when sales of Darvon started growing even faster. It seems presenting the facts about Darvon to doctors didn't scare them much at all, and only served to promote the pill. At that point the campaign to kill Darvon was abandoned.

Propoxyphene remains one of Lilly's star pills, though it long ago went off patent. Brand name Darvocet (Propoxyphene napsylate) still captures 20% of the propoxyphene market, and many have come to know and love the red oblong pills as one of their best friends. It still doesn't seem to beat aspirin in objective pain relief, but don't try telling this to people in pain.

Thorazine

No other pill, not even Prozac, has had a greater or more profound and long-lasting effect on the practice of psychiatry than Thorazine. Where Prozac has a fairly subtle effect on a comparatively subtle condition (depression), Thorazine released seriously psychotic patients from the hell of mental hospital confinement.

After Thorazine was introduced in 1954, the doors to insane asylums were thrown open. The population of mental hospitals—once comprising fully half the hospital beds in the country—dwindled and dropped. Today a permanently-committed "insane" person is a rarity.

Although it is sometimes derided as a "chemical straitjacket," Thorazine (and its descendants) remains the only hope for people who have literally lost their minds. The opportunity to subdue a patient and make him receptive to further treatment is crucial; without it the chances for recovery are small. And Thorazine works better than a straitjacket. A straitjacket can only bind an out-of-control mental patient, but a dose of Thorazine calms such a patient enough that he no longer desires to hurt himself, or others. He won't hurl himself into a wall, shit in his pants, or bite off his own tongue. On Thorazine, patients unreachable beyond their own thick cloud of babbling and gesturing became responsive to outside stimuli.

Thorazine also proved itself broadly therapeutic. Very small doses (10–20 mgs) are useful in treating ordinary anxiety. Larger doses (200–600 mgs) silenced the torturous voices of schizophrenia. Still larger doses (1000–2000 mgs) could bring the prototypical "raving maniac" under control.

Invented by French chemists at Rhone Poulenc, SmithKline & French Laboratories obtained the drug in 1952 and, after two

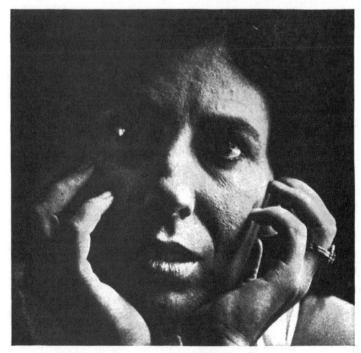

When it's time for Thorazine® brand of chlorpromazine

...can you depend on less?

SmithKline Beecham, the producer of Thorazine, sued a Philadelphia punk rock band who named itself after the famous anti-psychotic pill to change its professional name. The band replied that they already spent $900 on T-shirts and stickers to promote their band and their first album "Coffee, Tea, or Thorazine," but they couldn't buy better promotion than this.

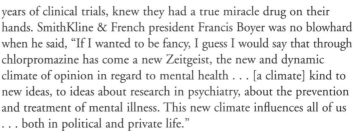

So many bands have named themselves after pills since this suit.

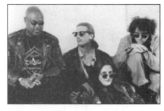

years of clinical trials, knew they had a true miracle drug on their hands. SmithKline & French president Francis Boyer was no blowhard when he said, "If I wanted to be fancy, I guess I would say that through chlorpromazine has come a new Zeitgeist, the new and dynamic climate of opinion in regard to mental health . . . [a climate] kind to new ideas, to ideas about research in psychiatry, about the prevention and treatment of mental illness. This new climate influences all of us . . . both in political and private life."

In addition to its use in treating mental illness, Thorazine was found to stop nausea and vomiting, to treat hiccups—especially the rare and bizarre kind that can go on for years. Thorazine was found to provide supplementary pain relief when used with narcotics, and it was discovered to ease a narcotic addict's discomfort during withdrawal, without the use of additional drugs. These applications may seem insignificant, but the hell of persistent nausea or intractable pain is not insignificant to the person who suffers from them.

Ten years after Thorazine came on the market, so did a slew of related drugs. After further testing, Thorazine was found useful in the treatment of epilepsy and tetanus, and is used with refrigeration as a drastic measure to reduce dangerously high fevers that afflict some cancer patients. Thorazine relieved the physical and mental stress of refrigeration that would have both inhibited the treatment and tortured the patient.

Thorazine is strong—if a normal person were to take even 50 or 100 mgs of thorazine, his mental faculties would definitely slow to a crawl—but that's what's necessary to interrupt the vivid hallucinations and disassociated thoughts of psychosis.

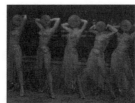

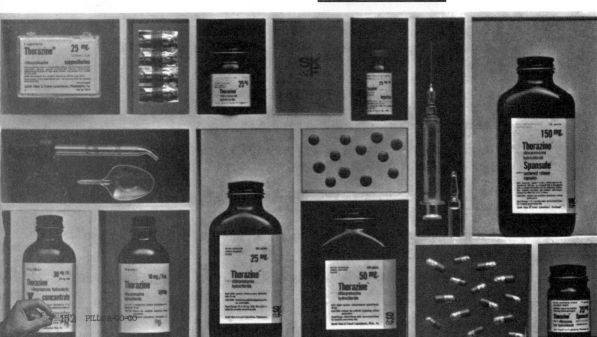

Jet Lag Cure

by Tim Johnson

Having just returned from my 12th business trip to the UK in the past 18 months, I finally came up with a pretty good jet lag protocol (for me at least).

1. Contrary to popular mythology, nap all you want after arrival on the first day. I usually get about two hours of fitful sleep on the first afternoon, local time. If it's still light when you wake up, open the curtains, the light will get you up quickly and help your body clock adjust. I find a walkman with a "sleep inducing" tape, such as WAVEFORM from ABR or the Hemisync tapes of Robert Monroe, a helpful adjunct to this program. I've tried a light and sound machine, but it doesn't seem to have much advantage over the tapes, and gets you stopped by more airport x-ray machines.

2. In the evening of the first day, about one hour before you want to go to sleep, take 3-6 mgs of melatonin, which regulates your body's internal clock; it seems to work best a couple hours after you've eaten or consumed any alcohol. In any case, do NOT have more than two drinks this first evening, as it will interfere with your sleep cycle and may overpotentiate the Dalmane mentioned below. Once mixed with large amounts of alcohol (4-5 pints of British bitter,) I awake with shortness of breath and a pounding heart—not fun! Also, if you're not used to melatonin, it may cause very vivid dreams.

3. Approximately one-half hour before you want to sleep, take 15-30 mgs of Dalmane (flurazepam), a common Rx sleeping pill. If you explain that you're going abroad, most physicians seem willing to prescribe at least small quantities of Dalmane for Jet Lag. I wash it down with a beer, which my MD frowns on, but I weigh more than 200 lbs and the potentiation of the Dalmane by alcohol makes me sleepy very fast. I always fall asleep within an hour.

4. Sometimes, you may awaken after a couple hours, especially if you drank too much the previous evening. This is the worst part of jet lag. If this happens, I suggest immediately taking another 15–30 mgs of Dalmane washed down with beer; however, this is a tough call. It may take a couple hours to fall back to sleep and may leave you quite groggy in the am. Since I generally have to be up and functioning by 8 am. local time the second day, I have a rule of thumb: if I awaken in the middle of the first night, I just listen to a tape in the hope of falling back to sleep. Earlier than 3 am., more Dalmane and beer is indicated. I haven't found melatonin useful for middle-of-the-night episodes, but others may want to give it a try, perhaps in larger quantities.

5. Upon awakening, take some of our "old friend" ephedrine HCl—I use three capsules. That is the equivalent of 20 mg of ephedrine plus 100 mg of tyrosine and some other stuff for burning off fat. Personally, I also take two tablets of the "smart nutrient" Brain Power (500 mg of L-phenylalanine and 1 g of Choline Bitartrate) made by Country Life first thing in the am. A cup or two of coffee a half-hour later completes the wake-up.

Usually, this protocol is sufficient to overcome the eight hour time change between San Francisco and London in one day. If you should start feeling fatigued in the mid-afternoon of day two, I suggest three more Thermoloss caps on an empty stomach, washed down with coffee. Due to this stimulation, you will undoubtedly find yourself very awake late on the second evening.

Prescription drugs pour into U.S.

The top 15 drugs declared over a randomly selected 84-day period:

Valium, anti-anxiety, 928,000 pills.

Rohypnol, the banned "date rape" 338,760 pills.

Tafil, sedative/hypnotic, 284,130 pills.

Tenuate Dospan, stimulant, 111,060 pills.

Asenlix, stimulant, 92,760 pills.

Diminex, stimulant, 79,140 pills.

Neopercodan, narcotic analgesic, 42,550 pills.

Darvon, narcotic analgesic, 37,940 pills.

Qual, sedative/hypnotic, 20,700 pills.

Halcion, sedative/hypnotic, 16,470 pills.

Tylex, narcotic analgesic, 16,230 pills.

Ativan, anti-anxiety, 15,000 pills.

Ritalin, stimulant, 13,380 pills.

Somalgesic, muscle relaxant, 10,890 pills.

Xanax, anti-anxiety, 7,680 pills.

DRUG IDENTIFICATION Bible

edited by Tim Marnell $24.95

This 306 page book, chock-full of information, is undoubtedly the best reference work of its kind. Like any of the better "pill books" it provides full-color pictures of pills. Unlike the rest of them (including the *PDR*) this book has pictures of nearly ALL the pills you'd care about 602 of the estimated 620 pills and capsules controlled by the DEA.

That means this "bible" has sharp pix of bland generic speed tablets alongside fancy-pants brand-name pills anybody can recognize. This is the book to have along while scavenging the

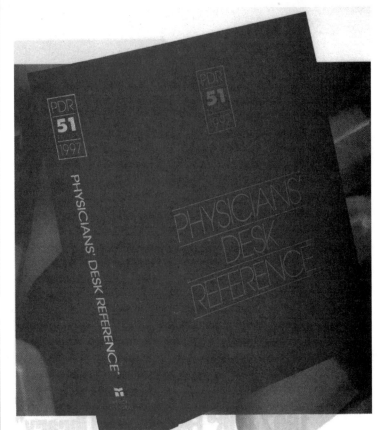

Mighty Morphin' *PDR*

Not matter which category you choose to rate books—weight, number of pages, notoriety . . . the *Physician's Desk Reference* is the mother of all pill books. Alternating cover colors between blue and red each year the *PDR* is widely considered to be THE book for information on prescription and non-prescription drugs. No doctor is without one and no self-respecting pillhead (or even mild-mannered, in-the-closet pill fan) is without at least one. As docs get their free copies each year the old ones get passed down through various folks in the office and osmose into the populace. Lots of people have a 1988 or-so copy and *PDR*s can easily be found in used book stores at various prices, depending mostly on their age.

Old ones are worthwhile to have around to look up drugs taken off the market or to see what they used to say about a pill before the lawsuits came in. Old *PDR*s can be free, too. Just ask your doc if he's got an old one you can have. Or ask your sister's boyfriend, the occupational therapist, to nab you one. Nobody really pays for a *PDR*. *PDR*s are strewn all over the place, being handed out gratis to every single doctor in the country and the chief pharmacist of every U.S. hospital with more than 25 beds. Free copies are also distributed to "other health-care professionals in pharmacies, dentistry, nursing homes, hospitals, and schools of nursing."

You can even buy the damn thing for like 70 bucks.

The oldest *PDR* in the *PaGG* Research Library is from 1960. Back then, the book was only a couple inches thick and was not full of all the cover-your-ass FDA bullshit that makes up most of the book we know today. Back then, there were pills with neato names like "Darvo-Tran" and pills that were prescribed for "harried housewife syndrome." On the other hand it didn't have nearly so many pills and there was no color picture section for EZ identification.

Today's *PDR* is thick and has nearly 3,000 pages and is sometimes said to include every single pill sold in America. Would that this were true. If the *PDR* has any major failing it is this common misbelief. It is true that the enormous tome can stop a .32 caliber hollowpoint, but it doesn't have all the pills you can buy at the store.

It has almost every one and it probably has any pill the doc is likely to give you. But it's not complete. Here's why.

If you haven't figured it out yet, the *PDR* is not so much a book as a big-ass advertising flyer. Drug companies pay *PDR*'s publisher, Medical Economics Company Inc. in Oradell, New Jersey, to have their pills listed and described. That's why the pills are arranged by manufacturer, not alphabetically or by type or something. It's the pill companies who are essentially taking out ad space in a publication with no other copy. Pill companies pay more to get into the color picture section. Pills that aren't big sellers don't rate much space in the *PDR*. Little pharmaceutical companies specializing in vitamins or generic drugs can't afford to get their pills listed although they sometimes can afford a simple list of their products, with no descriptions at all.

So if you don't pony up, you don't get in the book. It doesn't matter if you're the maker of the Fountain of Youth nasal spray, the *PDR* is not a charity operation, it is a serious publishing enterprise.

Something around three quarters of a million *PDR*s are distributed nationwide every year. Its spin-off, the *PDR* for Nonprescription Drugs, prints up and hands out more than 300,000 copies. Even the puny and obscure *PDR* for Opthalmology has a circulation of better than 13,500. And then there are the supplements sent out from time to time to update the damn thing with new drugs, new dosage forms etc.

There is also the *PDR* on CD ROM, which is beginning to make sense because the 1994 *PDR* weighs more than seven pounds—more than a laptop computer. The cool thing about the CD is that you can cross-reference things by side-effects or other parameters that would be nigh impossible to do with the book.

The *PDR*'s popularity with pillheads has prompted the company to put out a "layman's version" without so much technical jargon and sell it to the general public. In its first year on the market, the *PDR Family Guide* sold 250,000 copies.

The propensity of pharmaceutical advertisers invading non-traditional advertising space (like newspapers) is making the book even more popular.

So your friend, the venerable *PDR*, is really just an advanced species of the calendars, penlights, and prescription pads with an advertisement every 20 sheets. It's a promotional device. It's there to influence prescription writing and to keep doctors abreast of what the hell some of their patients are talking about when they come in jabbering about the latest prescription pill ad they saw in *Time* magazine.

Truth be told, the *PDR* doesn't seem to be nearly as fascinating to physicians as it is to the rest of us. Doctors don't spend as much time poring through the *PDR* as some of their patients, who treat it like

shag carpet after a party, or shaking down grandma's medicine cabinet. Calling the pharmacy is always a drag and often they don't have the information anyway.

As if that weren't enough, the book has a list of another 7,000 non-controlled pills, tablets and capsules organized by serial number, letter code, or whatever other identifying hallmarks a pill has. By decoding these digits you can tell what the drug is, its strength and who makes it.

It's sure to impress your friends!

The book also covers "street" drugs like heroin, PCP, etc. Each section has an accurate chemical description (including an outline of synthesis!), history of the drug, its various forms, and, of course, plenty of color photos showing the processing of a drug as it makes its way from field or lab to your open mouth.

No drug is too obscure. For example, there are descriptions and pictures of the manufacture of Royal Nepalese Temple Balls, Thai sticks, and other items seldom seen in the street. This section also surveys a drug's potency and popularity on the street over the years. There is more—such as the Mexican Cannabis Crop Calendar.

Even though the book is packed with info, none of it is filler and none of it is propaganda. *The Drug Identification Bible* is a reference tool only and it does the job superbly.

some Holy Book of Knowledge. In the past, there was a kind of implied agreement among doctors not to let the *PDR* fall into the "wrong hands." The *PDR*, even an old one, was a precious thing to a layman. It was a peek into the alchemist's book of potions and spells—forbidden secrets of pill lore. This *PDR* scarcity is rapidly falling by the wayside and now many patients are able to find a particular pill's entry with the alacrity of an idiot-savant.

Some people seem to have whole sections of the book memorized, even the words they don't understand. Sometimes the knowledge gained from the *PDR* is quite helpful in a quick raid of a stranger's medicine cabinet, while poorly understood information can cause confusion leading to mistakes in self-prescribing with other people's pills.

The *PDR* might be enjoying a wider readership than ever before, but that may not bode well for the publisher. Pillheads love the *PDR* and the doctors know it. Sometimes medical journals publish letters from MDs about how a *PDR* was the root of a patient's problem or advising each other to look with suspicion on patients who refer to one.

The loss of mystique may cause the downfall of the traditional *PDR* as king of the pill books. As it moves from the shelves of the health care elite to the lumpen patients, doctors may start to shun the thing as just another popular pill book like all those glossy paperbacks you see at B. Dalton's. But that may not happen quite yet.

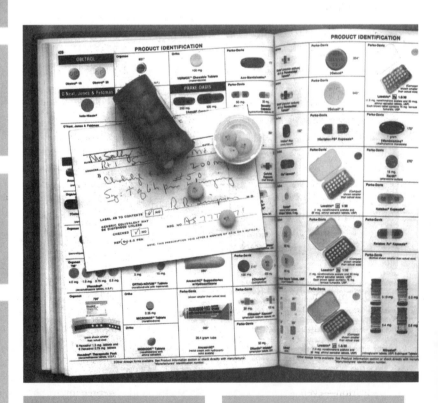

Scheduling Madness

Drugs classified Schedule I and II are considered roughly equal in terms of their dangerousness, except that drugs in Schedule I (LSD, heroin, etc.) are considered bereft of medical benefit and are thus prohibited from use for any reason but forensic labs or experimental purposes licensed by the federal government.

Schedule II drugs (amphetamines, morphine, cocaine, etc.) are considered useful. Because of their supposedly immense danger, Schedule II drugs are limited in their manufacture. Refills are forbidden. Phone-in scripts for these drugs are discouraged but they are possible—if the amount is small, if it is an emergency and even then the physical piece of paper must follow withing 48 hours. Doctors who dare prescribe Schedule II drugs must submit to rigorous accounting procedures to help police agencies track every prescription they write for these drugs.

Schedule II drugs are also limited by the number of doses prescribed at one time. This presents problems for a patient receiving a high dose of a schedule II medicine. This restriction can force a person to fill their prescription every week, because to have enough medicine to last longer than that is illegal. These patients are effectively prevented from going on vacation—even a spontaneous road trip!

And, unlike other medicines, physicians may not prescribe Schedule II meds for any reason except those ailments deemed "legitimate" by the government. It is a crime for a doctor to prescribe

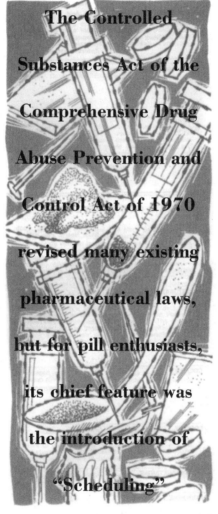

The Controlled Substances Act of the Comprehensive Drug Abuse Prevention and Control Act of 1970 revised many existing pharmaceutical laws, but for pill enthusiasts, its chief feature was the introduction of "Scheduling"

Ritalin to an Alzheimer patient just because it seems to help. Ritalin is not approved for that purpose. State licensing agencies will bar a physician from practicing medicine if they discover he or she has prescribed more of a drug than the law deems acceptable. As you might guess, this decision is made without any regard to the patients being treated—whether they're doing well or badly—the law's the law. It's not medicine.

It is this serious threat that causes doctors to withhold morphine and other opiate painkillers from cancer patients, people with severed spinal cords, and especially those suffering from chronic, debilitating pain. The doctor is simply too frightened to prescribe the drugs.

The lack of sufficient pain treatment is the most obvious and hateful perversion of medicine caused by government's control of medicine.

Schedule III and IV drugs have "currently accepted medical use in treatment in United States." These drugs are deemed to have a lower abuse potential and are less likely to cause the dreaded "addiction." Abuse may lead to "limited physical or psychological dependence" relative to the drugs of the preceding Schedules. Most psychoactive drugs fall into these categories even if they have no abuse potential at all. Prozac, for instance, is a Schedule IV drug even though it doesn't get you high. But some people enjoy relief from depression or rage, so perhaps that may be construed as getting high or "abuse." Patients who decide they prefer living without such burdens might take their medicine every day, which could be called "addiction" or even "abuse."

Then there are Schedule V substances, most of which contain "limited quantities of certain narcotic and stimulant drugs generally for anti-tussive, anti-diarrhea and analgesic purposes. Schedule V substances may be dispensed without a prescription, but only by a pharmacist, who must also maintain a record book of these purchases. Schedule V is set aside for those drugs deemed to have some abuse potential but which fall into a kind of time-honored self-medication tradition. A good example of this is codeine cough syrup. In small amounts, codeine is Schedule V and can be purchased by any adult willing to sign his or her name in a register for inspection by the police. Schedule V drugs may be further restricted (even abolished) by state laws. Some states, like California, have just about eliminated this class of drugs.

The federal government may do the same. Since 1970, the number of medicines available in the Schedule V category has diminished. Paregoric, a diarrhea medication containing morphine, is now banned. So is the venerable cough syrup, Terpin Hydrate. Neither ban was subject to any sort of citizen's consensus. They were simply ordered by the head of the FDA, whose orders are not subject to review except by the President of the United States.

Once a substance is scheduled, its status rarely changes—a petition to do so may be initiated by the DEA, the Department of Health and Human Services, the drug's manufacturer, a medical association, or (theoretically) a single citizen.

When a drug does change schedules, it can go anywhere. For example, in 1973, the DEA bumped phenobarbital, secobarbital and amobarbital from Schedule III to II. (Nevertheless, in some states, phenobarbitol remained an OTC ingredient in Primatene tablets until about 1990.)

Restrictions might also be loosened. In 1976, when the newly-invented anti-dirreaha drug, loperamide (Imodium AD) was introduced, it was initially subject to very tight restrictions. Then it began a slow journey of decontrol as it was first eased from Schedule II into schedule V. Then it entered kind of Schedule V purgatory where the DEA monitored the drug closely for three years. In 1982 loperamide was approved for OTC status.

It is possible for a drug to exist in more than one Schedule at the same time. Codeine pro-vides an example of such a multi-dimensional med. As an ingredient in cough syrups, codeine is in Schedule V. But, if codeine turns up as an ingredient in a pill or if the amount grows relative to the other ingredients in a medicine, it moves up to Schedule III. Pure codeine in any amount is Schedule II. It is very possible for a person to buy a larger amount of codeine without a prescription as a schedule V cough syrup than he would get from a physician in any other schedule.

Codeine is a versatile drug indeed! One good thing about the scheduling scheme for pillheads is the way the government determines "abuse potential." Just how can someone know if a drug is too fun? The answer is to ask someone who has fun with the drug!

The term "potential for abuse" is not clearly defined in the law, so the government relies on signs that people are having too much fun with a particular pill to know when to look into it. Among the tell-tale signs of fun are too many reports of "significant diversion" of a drug from legitimate channels. One sure sign of abuse is the discovery that people are taking the drug "on their own initiative." Once the warning bells have gone off, the FDA assembles a select group of pill-heads to help them understand what the hell is so fun.

In these special post-marketing tests, pillheads and others who take drugs without permission are solicitated to come in and party. After sufficient fun has been had, the pill-poppers are asked to rate the suspect pills as compared to other, similar drugs. Carefully noting dosages and subjective descriptions of a pill's non-FDA approved "fun" effects, the cops decide if they need to further restrict the drug and by how much.

The FDA takes their tests of a pill's fun qualities seriously. To measure the fun-ness of a drug they insist on bonafide recreational users. Investigators looking into the fun potential of a new painkiller seek out regular, even addicted, users of opiates, and will exclude people who use drugs for pain, and not just to have fun. Even if the patient enjoys his medicine, a "legitimate" user presumably doesn't know how to have a good time with his stash.

Because of tests like this you find (in the PDR) that "experienced" users of benzodiazepines pronounced the new "non-benzodiazepine" drug Ambien to be similar in effect to, say, ten milligrams of Valium, when taken in larger than normal doses. But that's purely from a recreational point of view.

A similar investigation into the hedonistic effects of Johnson & Johnson's "non-opiate" painkiller, Ultram (tramadol) was probably already in the works even before the pill was released in Spring, 1995.

Because the chemical structure of Ultram varies slightly from "the morphine rule"—the strict chemical definition of an opioid—the pill's manufacturer, Johnson & Johnson, has been able to claim the pill is non-narcotic and keep it out of any schedule.

This is important for the company's bottom line because doctors become reluctant to prescribe pills once they are scheduled, and that reluctance only increases as a pill is moved up into more restrictive classifications. The doctors' reluctance comes from a (justifiable) fear that it could come back to haunt them later. Even Schedule IV drugs like Valium or Darvocet have been used to prove a doctor's incompetence, deprive him of his license to practice medicine and send him to jail. Once a pill is controlled, it is officially abusable and "addictive." It is also countable, which means the evil can be quantified and a previously invisible crime is plain to see.

Just as Roche lobbied so hard for so long to keep Valium unscheduled, Eli Lilly fought to prevent Darvocet from being stigmatized. Despite their fights, both Darvocet and Valium became Scheduled. Darvocet's active ingredient, propoxyphene, derived from methadone, clearly met the structural requirements of the "morphine rule."

Pill classification is substantially political in nature, as seen by both unclassified and classified pills. While the Schedules' legal definitions have an air of precision and certainty, some meds (like amyl nitrate) have bounced back and forth between controlled and non-controlled and back, when politicians tried to decide if a pill was "abused" or not.

Such confusion is to be expected from politicians who are already trying to practice mass medicine. But Scheduling even gets worse. Here they try to restrict medications they cannot any better than the conditions they are meant to treat. This confusion is compounded when the language of chemistry is forced into the already dense prose of legalese!

Narcocrats base evaluations on a drug's potential for abuse by reports about changes in behavior and mood in would-be bonafide pill-head "abusers!" Drugs are far too subjective to measure in this way. All legalese based on this subjective data is bound to look ridiculous.

No controlled drug was meant to be "abused." Such drugs are the fruit of costly research, made all the more expensive by having to leap through the official FDA obstacle course. If it is lucky, a pill makes it to market a decade after the approval process begins. The last thing any pharmaceutical company needs is to have a new pills damned as "abusable." Unlike Hollywood, which seems to benefit by a small official restriction—say, an R rating, drug companies do not want the government to restrict movement of the pill to customer. That is all that Schedules do.

It's not as if the Schedules make a hell of a lot of sense, either.

Heroin, which was once prescribed, has pharmacological features that make it a valued and useful medicine. Of course, in the U.S. it remains forbidden. Yet a drug such as Soma (carisoprodol) remains unscheduled and uncontrolled, even though it has been known for years and years as a pretty decent party drug.

Rohypnol's abrupt placement into Schedule I was the predictable fate for a pill that has been dubbed "the rape drug" by the national media. The truth about the "roofie" is awfully mundane.

The fact is, Rohypnol has never been approved for use in the United States by the FDA mostly because Roche doesn't seem to have bothered to ladle out the millions to apply for such approval because the minor tranquilizer market already dominated by Librium, Valium and all their chemical cousins.

If any drug is commonly and reliably used to intoxicate a girl so she cannot defend herself against sexual attack, it is grain alcohol. In a few thousand years of formal and informal tests, results show a bottle of vodka to be the "drug of choice" for such predators.

There are also drugs that, besides showing up simultaneously in two or three of the five schedules, manage to find themselves in as restrictive a category as Schedule II (cocaine, morphine, etc.) and are also sold over-the-counter! The finest example of this is back when Americans found speed from nasal inhalers!

This sort of misunderstanding is something like the way heroin escaped regulation, even in the Harrison Act—medical views as interpreted by laymen deemed heroin sufficiently different from morphine, that it wasn't treated as harshly. A 1924 law was required to specifically outlaw heroin.

Schedule II Narcotics

ALFENTA Controlled ingredient: alfentanil hydrocholoride

CODEINE PHOSPHATE INJECTION Controlled ingredient: codeine phosphate

DEMEROL Controlled ingredient: meperidine hydrochloride

DILAUDID Controlled ingredient: hydromorphone hydrocloride

DOLOPHINE Controlled ingredient: methadone hydrochloride

DURAGESIC PATCH Controlled ingredient: fenatyl

HYDROMORPHONE HYDROCHLORIDE Controlled ingredient: hydromorphone hydrocloride

INNOVAR Controlled ingredients fentany citrate. Other ingredient: droperidol

METHADONE HCI DISKETS Controlled ingredient: methadone hydrochloride

MORPHINE SULFATE (INJECTION AND TABLETS) Controlled ingredient: morphine sulfate

MS CONTIN Controlled ingredient: morphine sulfate

ORAMORPH SR Controlled ingredient: morphine sulfate

OXYCODONE & APAP Controlled ingredient: oxycodone hydrochloride. Other ingredient: acetaminophen

PERCODAN Controlled ingredients: oxycodone hydrochloride, oxycodone terephthalate. Other ingredient: aspirin

PERCODAN-DEMI Controlled ingredients: oxycodone hydrochloride, oxycodone terephthalate. Other ingredient: aspirin

PERCOCET Controlled ingredient: oxycodone hydrochloride. Other ingredient: acetaminophen

SUFENTA Controlled ingredient: sufentanil citrate

TYLOX Controlled ingredients: oxycodone hydrochloride, oxycodone terephthalate. Other ingredient: acetaminophen

Schedule III Narcotics

ACETAMINOPHEN WITH CODEINE Controlled ingredient: codeine phosphate. Other ingredient: acetaminophen

ASPIRIN WITH CODEINE Controlled ingredient: codeine phosphate. Other ingredient: aspirin

FIORINAL WITH CODEINE Controlled ingredients: codeine phosphate, butalbital. Other Ingredients: aspirin, caffeine

LORCET Controlled ingredient: hydrocodone bitartrate. Other ingredient: acetaminophen

LORTAB Controlled ingredient: hydrocodone bitartrate. Other ingredient: acetaminophen

LORTAB ASA Controlled ingredient: hydrocodone bitartrate. Other ingredient: aspirin

PHENAPNEN WITH CODEINE Controlled ingredient: codeine phosphate. Other ingredient: acetaminophen

PHENAPHEN-650 WITH CODEINE Controlled ingredient: codeine phosphate. Other ingredient: acetaminophen

SYNALGOS Controlled ingredient: dihydrocodeine. Other ingredients: aspirin, caffeine

TUSSIONEX Controlled ingredient: dihydrocodeine. Other ingredient: phenyltoloxamine

TYLENOL WITH CODEINE Controlled ingredient: codeine phosphate. Other ingredient: acetaminophen

VICODIN Controlled ingredient: hydrocodone bitartrate 5 mg. Other ingredient: acetaminophen 500 mg

VICODIN ES Controlled ingredient: hydrocodone bitartrate 7.5 mg. Other ingredient: acetaminophen 750 mg

Schedule IV Narcotics

DAVOCET-N 100 Controlled ingredient: propoxyphene napsylate. Other ingredient: acetaminophen

DARVON Controlled ingredient: propoxyphene hydrochloride

DARVON COMPOUND-65 Controlled ingredient: propoxyphene hydrochloride. Other ingredients: aspirin, caffeine

DARVON-N Controlled ingredient: propoxyphene napsylate

TALCEN Controlled ingredient: pentazocine hydrochloride. Other ingredient: acetaminophen

TALWIN NX Controlled ingredient: pentazocine hydrochloride. Other ingredient: naloxone hydrochloride

WYGESIC Controlled ingredient: propoxyphene hydrochloride. Other ingredient: acetaminophen

Schedule II Depressants

AMYTAL SODIUM Controlled ingredient: amobarbital sodium

DORIDEN Controlled ingredient: glutethimide

NEMBUTAL SODIUM Controlled ingredient: pentobarbital sodium

TUINAL Controlled ingredients: amobarbital sodium, secobarbital sodium

Schedule IV Depressants

ATIVAN Controlled ingredient: lorazepam

CENTRAX Controlled ingredient: prazepam

CHLORAL HYDRATE Controlled ingredient: chloral hydrate

DALMANE Controlled ingredient: flurazepam hydrochloride

EQUANIL Controlled ingredient: meprobamate

HALCION Controlled ingredient: triazolam

LIBRIUM Controlled ingredient: chlordiazepoxide hydrochloride

MILTOWN Controlled ingredient: meprobamate

PLACIDYL Controlled ingredient: ethchlorvynol

RESTORIL Controlled ingredient: temazepam

SERAX Controlled ingredient: oxazepam

TRANXENE Controlled ingredient: clorazepate dipotassium

VALIUM Controlled ingredient: diazepam

XANAX Controlled ingredient: alprazolam

Schedule II Stimulants

BIPHETAMINE Controlled ingredients: amphetamine, dextroamphetamine

DEXEDRINE Controlled ingredient: dextroamphetamine sulfate

DESOXYN Controlled ingredient: methamphetamine hydrochloride

METHYLPHENIDATE HYDROCHLORIDE Controlled ingredient: methylphenidate hydrochloride

RITALIN Controlled ingredient: methylphenidate hydrochloride

Schedule III Stimulants

DIDREX Controlled ingredient: benzphetamine hydrochloride

PLEGINE Controlled ingredient: phendimetrazine tartrate

Schedule IV Stimulants

ADIPEX-P Controlled ingredient: phentermine hydrochloride

TENUATE Controlled ingredient: diethylpropion hydrochloride

TENUATE DOSPAN Controlled ingredient: diethylpropion hydrochloride

FASTIN Controlled ingredient: phentermine hydrochloride

IONAMIN Controlled ingredient: phentermine hydrochloride

MAZANOR Controlled ingredient: mazindol

SANOREX Controlled ingredient: mazindol

Schedule II Cannabis

MARINOL Controlled ingredient: dronabinol

Schedule III Steroids

ANADROL Controlled ingredient: oxymetholone

ANDROID-25 Controlled ingredient: methytestosterone

EQUIPOSE Controlled ingredient: boldenone undecylenate

DEPO-TESTOSTERONE Controlled ingredients: oxymetholone, testosterone cypionate

DIANABOL Controlled ingredient: methandrostenoleone

FINAJET Controlled ingredient: trenbolone acetate

PARABOLIN Controlled ingredient: trenbolone

SUSTANON Controlled ingredient: testosterone esters

TESTOSTERONE Controlled ingredient: testosterone

WINSTROL Controlled ingredient: stanozolol

BY PRESCRIPTION ONLY

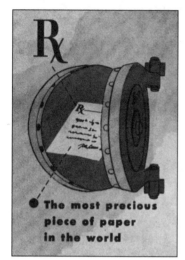

The most precious piece of paper in the world

Before the 1950s, a prescription had neither the legal status nor the legal ramifications it has today. Even after the Harrison Act, a prescription was more or less the same thing it had been for hundreds of years: an order from a physician to a pharmacist to provide his patient with a certain medicine in a certain form along with instructions on how to take it.

Until very recently, pharmacists made most of the medicines they sold. They mixed them from stocks taken from the apothecary's shelves of ingredients, compounded with mortar and pestle and other druggist's supplies that have now nearly disappeared from drugstores—the mortar & pestle has now become a symbol only.

The original use of a prescription and its history is covered later in the book, where the esteemed document is examined, deconstructed and decoded for your reading pleasure. For now it's enough to know it wasn't long ago that a prescription was none of Big Brother's business, a matter solely between patient, doctor and pharmacist. The concept of "refills" did not exist. None of the quirky features now required by the government to monitor and control drug sales were there before. There was certainly nothing like the central computer logging each prescription in a multi-state area or the triplicate hard copies of today.

All "demon drugs" were sold without restriction or supervision by authorities of any kind—certainly not the government and its police agencies. This includes those drugs purchased with a prescription. And yet the nation did not go to hell in a handbasket!

The history of heroin's legal status reveals a clownish parade led by politicians making laws about drugs they do not understand with language they fail to comprehend. As T. Metzger points out in his *Birth of Heroin and the Demonization of the Dope Fiend,* there are two heroins: the chemical compound diacetylmorphine, a rather unremarkable drug used for more than a century for a variety of reasons, and the symbolic heroin, responsible for incalculable depravity and decay.

Heroin was originally marketed by Bayer as a cough medicine. Although the drug was (and still is) used as a substitute for morphine—even in cases of morphine habituation where maintainance—not prison or ostracism—was the preferred treatment. Heroin was never seriously considered non-habit-forming nor a "cure" for morphine addiction. That's another manufactured legend designed to appeal to our egos, so we can pat ourselves on the back and brag about how right we are!

In late 19th century America,

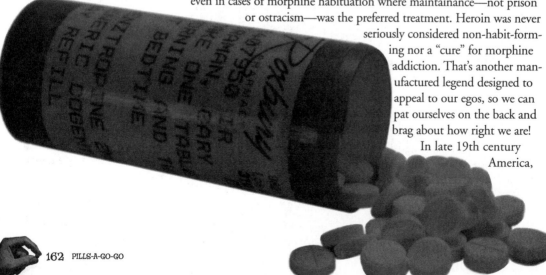

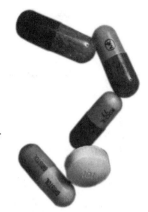

even cocaine was put to more medical uses—treating sinusitis, hay fever, morphine addiction and chronic fatigue.

After their introduction in the 1930s, amphetamines, too, were sold by doctor's prescription and in OTC products, a practice that continued until the Drug Law Avalanche of the 1970s. Instead of being feared as a tool of Satan, amphetamines were praised for their safety record and the long list of medical problems they could treat: petit mal epilepsy and head injury were recognized problems speed could help alleviate, along with Parkinson's, depression, asthma, nasal congestion, barbiturate and opiate poisoning, hyperkinesia in children, narcolepsy and obesity.

Methamphetamine, especially, proved to be a rather successful tool to help patients withdraw from opiate addiction.

Fake prescriptions were first used to obtain state-mandated drugs during the years of alcohol Prohibition. Though the U.S. Pharmacopoeia dropped whisky and brandy from its official list of medicines in 1916, doctors were still able to prescribe them and pharmacies could legally fill these prescriptions during the height of the Prohibition.

Thousands of doctors, pharmacists and drug manufacturers applied for licenses to prescribe and sell liquor—for medicinal purposes, not for fun. By 1928, physicians were making an estimated $40,000,000 annually by writing prescriptions for whisky.

SCRIPT ABBREVIATIONS

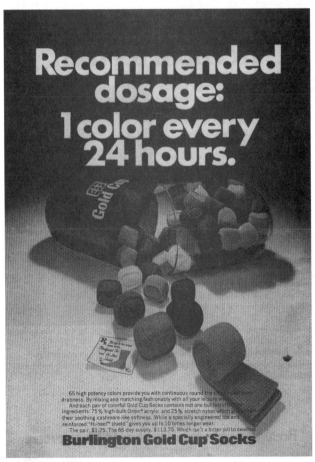

"T"	*Take 1*
"T" "T"	*Take 2*
"T" "T" "T"	*Take 3*
po	*By mouth*
pc	*After meals*
hs	*At bedtime*
bid	*Twice a Day*
tid	*3x a day*
qid	*4x a day*
qh	*Every Hour*
q2h	*Every 2 hours*
q	*Every*
d	*Day*
qd	*Once a day, every day*
c	*With*
et	*And*
mg	*Milligram*
x	*Times*
tabs	*Tablets*
ss	*½ (half)*
prn	*As needed*

HOW TO FORCE A SCRIPT

After visiting the high priests of medical care, our pill-gramage is commemorated by a scrap of paper elevated to near-holy status. Its scrawled and coded instructions are written for a specially-empowered medicine monk (the pharmacist) who is the only person permitted to transform it into a bottle of pills for you ... and you alone.

The secular punishment for writing your own prescription can be harsh—as you might imagine of the punishment for blasphemy and fraud. Those desperados who do try it risk being caught in the steely gaze of the pharmacist, whose uncanny powers alert him to the bogus document with a mere glance. Towering over the rabble crowding at the apothocary's altar, he raises an eyebrow in disgust—then summons the Inquisition.

A lot of people think there's some kind of special ink or invisible marking or some other hi-tech way of making the prescription pad distinct. Except in those few states where a triplicate prescription is required (for certain drugs) or in Indiana, where all scripts must now be written on a supposedly forgery-proof pad, this is not the case at all.

Usually, a prescription is just a piece of paper—not even as elaborate as a check or a supermarket coupon. There is no bar code, magnetic ink, or watermark. Though some doctors might use carbonless pads to keep copies of the prescriptions they write, the vast majority of prescriptions are written on normal white pieces of paper from preprinted pads. You can easily photocopy one and make a decent fake script for yourself. There is no latent "VOID" hiding in a background pattern. There isn't even a background pattern like is commonly found on checks. There is also nothing to show erasures, no sequential numbering, nothing. So the easiest way to make a fake script is to photocopy a real one and use it to make a decent blank for yourself.

Prescription for heroin in 1910.

A prescription will occasionally be printed on colored paper and marked with the message, "This document has a [green] background." Whiting this out will be sufficient to defeat this crafty measure. Or else photocopy your fake script onto appropriately colored paper.

Besides photocopying an existing prescription, you can also create a pad of prescription blanks for an entirely fictitious doctor using a computer and any decent desktop publishing software. If you do this, you should know that each state has a sort of model form which doesn't vary too much, so copy a real prescription and don't vary from the form. Even the little box to be checked when the doc instructs the pharmacist to "dispense as written" has to be one of a few designated sizes, a tip not many people know, including doctors.

R

The little document itself can come in many sizes and shapes, but generally they are a one quarter-page rectangle (4.25″ × 5.5″). And when you cut it, use a paper cutter—not scissors—because bored-to-death, anal-retentive pharmacists will easily spot your uneven edges. If you cannot access a paper-cutter then you might do a good enough job with a ruler (or better yet, a T-square) and a fresh razor blade. Even if you're really careful, there will still be one or two places on the edge that are slightly off. Remedy this by bending/crumpling the paper so the pharmacist won't be able to see it.

It is also a big plus to make the prescription look like it was torn from a pad. You might be able to do this by really making a pad but that may require asking the help at the photocopy place to do this for you and you cannot risk exposing yourself like that. So the next best thing is to touch-up only the thin edge of the top or the side of the "script" with a red felt-tip pen. Then comes a hint of rubber cement to simulate the gummed edge of the pad and your fake script is complete. Now it's time for the more artistic part—writing the fake prescription.

The main thing "protecting" widespread prescription forgery is ignorance about what is on the prescription and an almost superstitious belief that there is something there the pharmacist can pick up on. Hence, the urban legends of invisible marks, etc. There is nothing special about the prescription paper or anything printed on it. All of it is very straightforward, yet pharmacists can spot alterations and forgeries miles away. How do they do it?

The answer lies partly in the subtle things that are written in the prescription by the doctor—not any special message to the pharmacist—but the peculiar way scripts are written: The vestiges of Latin, the probability of a certain doctor prescribing a particular drug, the presence or absence of recognizable patterns every pharmacist internalizes. And of course, the doctor's signature.

Pharmacists do recognize doctors' signatures, and if the signature is wrong an alarm will go off in his head. But that's not usually what tips him off. (However, a good forger will spend lots of time learning to mimic signatures. To really imitate a signature, it must vary slightly each time used. No one signs their name exactly the same way every time.)

The doctor's true signature resides in the way he or she writes the prescription in the first place. For one thing there are those Latin holdovers and their modern equivalents. These days they are mixed-up more often than not. Indeed, a prescription written entirely in Latin or with medical symbols would be highly suspect.

SOME EXAMPLES OF PRESCRIPTIONESE

The first part of the script is called the "superscription" and is the pre-printed RX, which is the shortening of the Latin command "mix thou."

The next part of the script is the "inscription," and today, alas, it is gone. Here's where the doc told the pharmacist which ingredients to use. Today he just names a pill. The next part of the prescription (called the "subscription") is where the doctor used to tell the pharmacist how to dispense what he just made. We normally don't find any of the old stuff except for perhaps "M" meaning misce (mix in Latin).

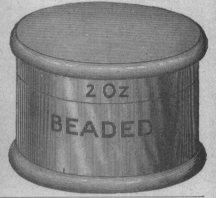
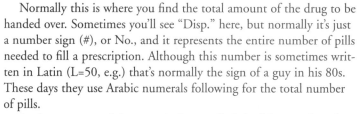
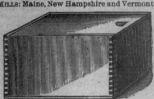

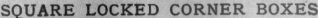
Normally this is where you find the total amount of the drug to be handed over. Sometimes you'll see "Disp." here, but normally it's just a number sign (#), or No., and it represents the entire number of pills needed to fill a prescription. Although this number is sometimes written in Latin (L=50, e.g.) that's normally the sign of a guy in his 80s. These days they use Arabic numerals following for the total number of pills.

At the next part of the prescription—called the "signature"—where dosage is given, doctors almost always write "Sig:" (short for signature). They don't write it out or abbreviate it any further, nor do they write "dosage." They also don't write the word "take" since this is implied already.

Like a check, a prescription is simply a message to an agency to carry out an order. That means the thing could be written on a napkin or even given orally.

There are other things the doc might want to stick on the script, and has the option of using Latin phrases and abbreviations or else English words or abbreviations. For example, he or she can write "before meals" or else "a.c." (Latin.) He or she can write "as needed" or else "p.r.m." (Latin.) In this case, it's up to the doc. However, he or she is likely to add something in English after such directions like "for pain" or "for sleep" or something.

Hence, "Vicodin #30, t.i.d. for pain" means you get 30 hits of Vicodin and you take them three times a day. It can be seen the doc has prescribed a 10 day supply. If you add a "1" in front of the 30 and expect to get 130 tablets (and you might if the pharmacist is an old lady with bad eyesight), you're taking a chance. Some multiple of three is wiser. Ninety sounds better than 130. Same goes for alteration of refills.

A few final words of advice: first, a good script banger should be familiar with prescribing laws. Some drugs cannot be refilled more than a certain number of times depending on the schedule. Some Schedule II drugs are even restricted by the absolute number of pills dispensed per prescription. To learn about this stuff, read the pharmaceutical industry's trade mags. *Drug Topics* is particularly good.

Second, remember that your prescription must fit into the normal patterns of the world of professional medicine—as stupid as that world may be. Besides the large number of internal consistencies within a prescription, the prescription itself should fit into a normal pattern. Prescriptions coming from old doc Whitehead, the pediatrician, are likely to be for medications (and dosages) associated with children. Prescriptions coming from an emergency ward will be for drugs of the type and quantity for a short time. Prescriptions for narcotics come from such likely places as oncologists and dentists. If they come from either one, however, they are very likely to be accompanied by another prescription for a logically related drug, say, something for nausea or an antibiotic to stave off infection. And these drugs, too, will tend to mesh in a coherent fashion and may very well be written on the same piece of paper.

Third, a single piece of paper can have as many as four or five prescriptions on it, though one or two is the norm.

Finally, when you've got everything right and ready, go to a small pharmacy on a Sunday afternoon. Dress like a reasonable person and try to get an old lady to help you. Be nice, give her your script, and if she asks any questions, tell a simple story. If she asks you to come back in much more than 15 minutes, don't.

This is how the majority of script-forgers get caught. While they wait for their prescriptions, the pharmacist calls the cops. Yet a 20 minute wait isn't unreasonable, depending on the amount of traffic in the store. And hanging around the counter is itself suspicious behavior.

THE SECRET CODE NUMBER

Each prescription for a "scheduled drug" must be accompanied by a serial number the DEA has assigned physicians since the Controlled Substances Act of 1970. Drugs are Scheduled One through Five, with

---

The Secret Code Number

AB 375987 $\times 2 = 46$ $46 + 16 = 62$ AB3759872

$= 16$ (check digit is final digit)

AK 479966 $\times 2 = 44$ $44 + 19 = 63$ AK4799663

$= 19$

Tips for Prescribers of Controlled Substances

1. Keep all prescription blanks in a safe place where they can't be stolen easily. Minimize the number of prescription pads in use.

2. Write a prescription order for Schedule II controlled substances in ink or indelible pencil or use a typewriter. The order must be signed by the physician.

3. Write out the actual amount prescribed in addition to giving an Arabic number or Roman numeral—to discourage alterations of the prescription order.

4. Avoid writing a prescription order for a large quantity of controlled substances unless it is absolutely determined that such a quantity is necessary.

5. Maintain only a minimum stock of controlled substances in the medical bag.

6. The medical bag should be taken by the physician while away from the automobile or locked in the trunk.

7. Be cautious when a patient mentions that another physician had been prescribing a controlled substance for him/her. Consult

Schedule I being most restricted of all and Schedule V requiring only a pharmacist's consent. As a practical matter, though, this number is printed or written on every prescription a doctor writes. If you're inventing a fictitious doctor, trying to make up a DEA number off the top of your head really will get you caught—if you don't know the secret code. Here it is:

The numbers always start out with A or B and are then followed by another letter. The first letter is A for physicians who got their numbers before approximately 1980, thereafter they begin with B. This may not be a hard and fast rule, but it seems generally true.

The next letter is the first letter of the doctor's last name! So old Doc Smith's number will begin AS. But the number stays the same no matter what Smith does with his or her name. So if old Doc Smith is a woman who married J. Paul Getty, her number will still remain the same, beginning with AS.

The next numbers are the registration number, with the final digit being the "check digit." A "check digit" is a number that can be used to verify the rest of the number by corresponding to the proper algorithm. Credit cards have check digits at the end and the algorithms are more or less secret. This greatly lessens the chances of someone just making up a number.

In the case of the DEA registration number, the algorithm is as follows: the final digit (that is, the "check digit") will equal the last digit of the sum of a) the addition of the second, forth, and sixth digits times two plus b) the sum of the addition of the first, third and fifth digits. That sounds confusing, but as far as algorithms go, it's kid's stuff.

Warning: There may well be a major exception to this method of producing a DEA registration number. We suggest you check the above method with reliable internet posters.

ALTERING AN ACTUAL SCRIPT

Of course, there's always the crude Beaver Cleaver-type method of altering numbers to get higher numbers, turning a 5 into an 8 for instance.

A much smarter trick to double the amount of any prescription plays upon the pharmacist's mortal fear of making a dispensing error, along with his fawning desire to make sure no one complains to the management or worse . . . the Pharmacy Board.

To do this you have to already have a supply of the same medicine, but in another, smaller dose. Here's how it goes:

Take your prescription for 30 2 mg Klonopins and have it filled. Wander around the store, be somewhat curt with the pharmacist if you feel like it (so he knows you mean business), but politely respond when he calls out your name to pick up your freshly-counted pills. Pay for the bottle, which he has already placed in a paper sack and perhaps even stapled shut with your receipt inside. Listen to his spiel about when to take the thing and act like you're fascinated with the instructions. This is "patient counseling" and its the closest the pharmacist ever gets to fulfilling his role as Trusted Figure in the Community. It may also be required by law.

Then bid him farewell and leave the store.

Once you are in your car or other appropriate place, you remove your bottle, pour out the 2 mg Klonopins and replace them with your stash of 30 1 mg pills.

It's up to you when to return with your embarrassing, job-threatening "mistake." You may not want to do it right away, but an hour later is not really too soon. Of course, if your make your purchase in the morning and return that evening you can be pretty sure your pharmacist has been released for the day and a new one is on duty. This just makes things easier.

When making your complaint, remember to be polite and non-accusatory. Pharmacists are unbelievably sensitive about this and you hold his whole future in his hands. He will be plenty obsequious already. If you treat him like a human being he will be overcome with gratitude and relief. Even if he suspects a scam, he knows there's no way to prove it and if it really was a dispensing error and he argues with you about it, he might well find himself answering to the Pharmacy Board.

He'll fix the mistake. He may give you some coupons for free tampons or product samples of the latest OTC pill. You cannot pull this scam on him again, though, not for awhile anyway.

THE ULTIMATE SCAM

DEA officials are so steamed about a successful drug diversion scam they won't say where or how many times it has been pulled. It sounds like a neat trick. Here's how it works:

Posing as a legitimate businessperson, the perp rents a store, hires a pharmacist, stocks the store with plenty of pills and announces a grand opening. Then, just before the big day, the perp loads all the pills into his van and leaves.

That's that. And the coolest thing is, so much of it, from leasing the store to buying the pills, can be done on credit.

the physician or the hospital records—or else examine the patient thoroughly and decide a controlled drug product should be prescribed.

8. A prescription blank should be used for writing a prescription order—and not for noted or memos. A drug abuser could easily erase the message and use the blank to forge a prescription order.

9. Never sign prescription blanks in advance.

10. Maintain an accurate record of controlled substance products disposed—as required by the Controlled Substances Act and its regulations.

11. Assist the pharmacist when he/she telephones to verify information about a prescription order. A corresponding responsibility rests with the pharmacist who dispenses the prescription order.

12. Phone the nearest DEA field office to obtain or furnish information. The call will be held in the strictest confidence.

Helpful hints from the DEA's 1990 pamphlet, *Physician's Manual: An Informational Outline of the Controlled Substances Act of 1970.*

The Fate of Pills in the Managed Care New World Order

Early in 1994, the first tangible traces of "health care reform" began trickling into most doctors' offices.

Even though there isn't yet a definitive National Health Care Program, complete with computer chips embedded in every citizen's forehead and helicopters spraying Prozac over the inner cities to keep the natives docile—the future is with us now.

It's visible in the pills you get. And don't get.

Insurance companies, HMOs and individual hospitals have lately started issuing "formularies" to doctors around the country that list a compendium of drug therapies either endorsed or at least recognized as beneficial by some organization (governmental or private). Sometimes a formulary issues guidelines as to how each medicine should be used.

Often a formulary is national.

Notable differences in national formularies might be, for instance, that Canada recognizes a therapeutic use in heroin to control severe pain, while the United States formulary does not. In the same vein, the Mexican National Formulary recognizes the use of a native plant called "chicalote" as being an analgesic. There is no chicalote to be found in the U.S. counterpart (although the plant grows in this country).

These differences reflect the prevailing medical opinion of a country, along with certain cultural considerations. Of course, heroin is a strong analgesic. It's just that, in America, it's been so demonized that it is probably impossible to consider it as medicine. Canada takes a lot of its culture from Britain, where heroin was (and still is) a medicine. In the case of chicalote, there is probably no history of its use here or in Canada and so it doesn't even occur to those putting together the formulary to include the plant, however useful it may be.

And I can't think of any formulary that recommends chewing a piece of willow bark to fight off a fever or control pain. Even though willow bark will do both these things, it's considered to be a bit old-fashioned and nowhere near as effective as the aspirin we derive from the bark.

In other words, a formulary is built on the consensus of opinion and experience by medical practitioners. Formularies can therefore reflect biases peculiar to its region or staff. One hospital may prefer the use of Drug A over Drug B because a drug's representative shows up at the hospital with free samples.

At a local hospital level, especially, cost can mean something too. A certain drug company might simply cut a better deal than its rival. As bulk-buyers, hospitals can often get drugs at a discount. Or a drug might have other inherent advantages that aren't strictly medical. Hospitals like to use acetaminophen more than aspirin not because Tylenol is "better" than aspirin—it's just less likely to cause immediate stomach problems exposing the hospital to complaints, grousing, maybe even lawsuits. Tylenol might ultimately damage a patient's liver, but the damage won't show up for a long time.

But usually such things aren't written down

A Mere

and passed around as policy. It isn't good medicine for an accountant to standardize treatments from on high, since the doctor and patient are supposed to be unique entities. Since medicine and the economy are changing all the time, it's not wise to link the two very closely.

Insurance companies didn't used to have such extensive formularies. The practice of medicine was left to degreed practitioners, and insurance companies concerned themselves with how much they would charge and pay out. Perhaps they classified certain treatments as "experimental" or capped the price of treatment at a certain price. Everyone has heard horror stories about people not getting life-saving treatments because an insurer refuses to pay.

You don't hear any stories today about a patient being made to chew on a piece of willow bark because the insurance company has decided that aspirin is too expensive. And no patient has yet been asked to slug down rum and bite a bullet as anesthesia for outpatient surgery. But we're on the way.

Cost-Consciousness Gone Berserk

Some insurance company formularies are only a few pages long and humbly suggest to physicians that they consider using generic instead of brand names whenever possible. Others go so far as to list some of the most commonly prescribed pills and suggest alternatives, such as the cheaper Tagamet for Pepcid. But then some insurers require a patient to suffer a few months of Rolaids before they're even allowed at the Tagamet. Here's where it starts getting ugly.

The most shocking "suggestions" from insurers arrive in thick book form and are blatantly, even unabashedly, based on one thing only: cost. The most egregious formularies seemed to be based on a model produced by Blue Cross/Blue Shield. These formularies make no effort to candycoat their message—use the cheapest possible medicine and stay away from certain pills.

Most formularies come with a prominent

Formulary

warning that its contents are not to be copied or duplicated in any form. In other words, Doc, don't go showing this to your patients or anybody else.

Then the formulary explains in gentler terms that Big Brother will be watching:

"We encourage you to refer to the Formulary before prescribing for your patients," begins one section. "At a later date, you will be provided with a computerized report that will indicate your Formulary compliance, as well as other pertinent prescribing information." The book then advises of Pre-Authorization, "a system to intervene before the prescription is dispensed. It is a form of prospective Drug Utilization Review (DUR) to promote rational drug therapy."

After these warnings, the formulary gets down to business.

Benadryl—The New Miracle Drug!

One need only flip to any part of the formulary to see what is going on. For example, in the section on treatments for Parkinson's dis-

ease we find that the formularies most often recommend the use of Benadryl as a first-line therapy for this degenerative disease of the nerves.

Benadryl? You mean the allergy pill?

That's right. Patients first diagnosed with this condition, which will slowly destroy them, are to be fed these particular antihistamine pills because one of their side effects is to slow down some of the involuntary shaking these patients have.

Only after Benadryl has been proven ineffective (and even the formulary admits no more than one in four patients will show any improvement with this antique medication) the patient gets to come back and try the next pill on the list: Symmetrel.

Symmetrel is much better. Even the formulary says it proves useful in half the patients who try it. True, it does have the drawback that it stops working in almost all patients within 6-12 weeks after starting on it, but by this time the company has been spared the cost of a real drug for months. Hell, the patient may have even died or given up by this time. But, in case this jerk (who by now is literally jerking around) comes whining back to the doc, then he's allowed to have Sinemet.

Sinemet is what he might have gotten in the first place since it usually proves therapeutic for the first few years of this horrible, progressive disease. After a few years, it stops working, too, and only then can the doctor start using the more powerful (and expensive) drugs.

Benadryl is not only a good medicine for people with Parkinson's, according to these formularies. Hell, that allergy pill is also good for anxiety and tension. That's why they recommend patients—so tortured by anxiety they seek a physician—to swallow the same pill that is so useful against Parkinson's.

And it's true that most people are practically knocked out by Benadryl. This antihistamine is well-known for its "sedative" effects—normally considered so disagreeable that a slew of antihistamines have been developed to overcome this drawback. Later, if the patient seems to genuinely need some kind of tranquilizer, the doctor is permitted to prescribe off-patent forms of Valium or Librium. After that, a couple of other anti-histamines (Vistaril, Atarax) may be prescribed along with chloral hydrate.

In case you don't remember what chloral hydrate is, it's the stuff invented about 100 years ago that gave us the term "knock-out drops." Sure, chloral hydrate isn't used much anymore, and it can be fatal, but, c'mon, it's cheap.

In May 1997, the National Alliance for the Mentally Ill took out three full-page ads in California newspapers regarding formulary restriction. The ads read, "Caution, Your HMO May Be Dangerous to Your Health."

It seems a patient with anxiety is going to have to visit the doctor at least three times before he or she will get any of the newer, more specific drugs like Xanax or Buspar. Although formularies deny it, price—not efficacy or potential danger to the patient—is the dominating factor in prescribing medications.

This has good points, too. For instance, morphine will be making a comeback as first-line therapy for severe pain. In one hospital, which may have cut a special deal with a certain drug company, methadone will be considered first in treating severe pain. In another hospital, dexedrine will be preferred over more expensive Ritalin to treat hyperactive kids and even venerable old opium may well be making a comeback as a treatment for diarrhea and pain.

And muscle pain patients will finally be reintroduced to their old favorites: Valium and Soma, long before they'll have to start taking (more expensive) Flexeril and Norgesic. These last two might work well enough, but they do absolutely nothing for your partying needs. (Hint: if you feel anxious or sleepless, tell the doctor you've got a pulled back muscle! That way you can skip the Benadryl and go straight to Valium.)

Of course for depression, nobody's getting Prozac right off the bat since that stuff and its relatives are way too costly. One insurance provider is openly against Prozac and its similarly priced cousins, complaining it's gotten too much good press. The same insurer explicitly tells doctors they may prescribe Prozac for "major depression" only "as second-line therapy when less costly drugs have failed or are contraindicated."

Nope, depressed people who show up at the doctor's office won't be getting Prozac anymore. Now they'll get . . . Benadryl. Just kidding. None of the formularies recommend Benadryl for depression, but they may as well, since Elavil, introduced in the early 1970s, is the first drug of choice to alleviate depression.

The cool thing about Elavil is, if you're thinking about putting a gun to your head and you take an Elavil, you quickly lose the will to blow your head off. You also lose the will to talk to anyone or even feed yourself, but, hell, it's better than being depressed isn't it?

The new rules mean you have to be mighty depressed and above all determined to get the latest in anti-depressants. As seems to be the rule, you'll have to visit the doc three times before you can have a pill proven to relieve depression without turning you into a zombie. Maybe four visits for Prozac, Paxil, or Zoloft.

Three's A Charm

This three-times-before-you-get-relief rule seems based on the HMO style of health care. Yes, HMOs pay for everything in the world, but to get to specialized help, the patient must break through successive walls of RNs, PAs and interns before a real doctor is called on the scene. This may ensure that a doctor's time is taken up only with patients with proven needs, but it can be exhausting (maybe too exhausting) for a sick person.

The other economy measure lurking in the new formularies is the shifting of cost to the patient by using OTC drugs. At the time the formularies began appearing, Naprosyn was suggested by many as an alternative to other, more expensive anti-inflammatories. Now that this pill is going over-the-counter, the cost may shift away from the insurance company to the consumer, who must buy any OTC-available drugs—like Benadryl. Or Tagamet.

Soon, drug research will stop and physicians can start hawking cold pills on the streets, as Benadryl is recognized for the cure-all it must be.

One silver lining to this strategy, of course, is to make self-medication more possible for everyone. Who knows, if things get bad enough economically, we may see the day when OTC heroin will once again compete with willow bark extract as a remedy not only for pain, but Parkinson's, depression, "women's ailments," cancer, polio, gout. . . . ▬

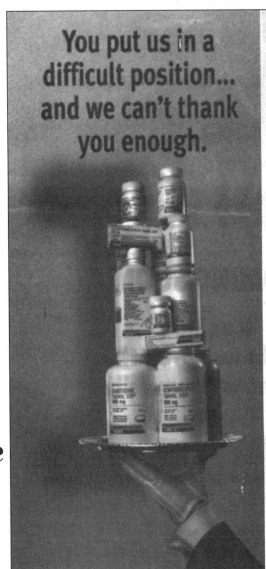

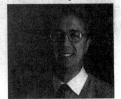
Generic Drugs Just Don't Win . . .

In 1998, prices for brand name prescription drugs rose 4%, while prices for generics dropped 2.7%.

Recently, the *Wall Street Journal* examined why generics have so little success competing with their name-brand counterparts. "Despite the fact that every generic approved by the FDA has been found by the agency to be precisely the same chemical, with the same dosage and equivalent absorption rate, and with the same manufacturing consistency that brand manufacturers must have," brand names still win. Generics just don't have equivalent advertising muscle.

Drugs are assigned brand names and sold on the market when when their founding pharmaceutical companies undergo the extraordinary expensive patent procedures. Unless pharmaceutical companies find ways to satisfy some FDA requirement or another, drug patents usually last a total of 17 years, after which any pharmaceutical firm can produce its generic version called by its chemical name.

Price differences between generic and trade name can range between 50% to over 500% at the retail level.

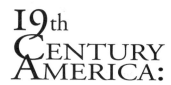

19th CENTURY AMERICA:
a
"Dope Fiend's Paradise"

The United States of America during the nineteenth century could quite properly be described as a "dope fiend's paradise."

Opium was on legal sale conveniently and at low prices throughout the century, morphine came into common use during and after the Civil War, and heroin was marketed toward the end of the century. These opiates and countless pharmaceutical preparations containing them "were as freely accessible as aspirin is today." They flowed mostly through five broad channels of distribution, all of them quite legal:

1. Physicians dispensed opiates directly to patients, or wrote prescriptions for them.
2. Drugstores sold opiates over-the -counter to customers without a prescription.
3. Grocery and general stores as well as pharmacies stocked and sold opiates. An 1883–1885 survey of the state of Iowa, which then had a population of less than 2,000,000, found 3,000 stores in the state where opiates were on sale, and this did not include the physicians who dispensed opiates directly.
4. For users unable or unwilling to patronize a nearby store, opiates could be ordered by mail.
5. Finally, there were countless patent medicines on the market containing opium or morphine. They were sold under such names as Ayer's Cherry Pectoral, Mrs. Winslow's Soothing Syrup, Darby's Carminative, Godfrey's Cordial, McMunn's Elixir of Opium, Dover's Powder, and so on. Some were teething syrups for young children, some were "soothing syrups," some were recommended for diarrhea and dysentery or for "women's trouble." They were widely advertised in newspapers and magazines and on billboards as "pain-killers," "cough mixtures," "women's friends, "consumption cures," and so on. One wholesale drug house, it is said, distributed more than 600 proprietary medicines and other products containing opiates.

Most of the opium consumed in the United States during the nineteenth century was legally imported. Morphine was legally manufactured here from the imported opium. But opium poppies were also legally grown within the United States. One early reference—perhaps the earliest—was in a letter from a Philadelphia physician, Dr. Thomas Bond, who wrote to a Pennsylvania farmer on August 24, 1781: "The opium you sent is pure and of good quality. I hope you will take care of the seed." During the War of 1812, opium was scarce, but "some parties produced it in New Hampshire and sold the product at from $10 to $12 per pound."

In 1871 a Massachusetts official reported:

There are so many channels through which the drug may be brought into the State, that I suppose it would be almost impossible to determine how much foreign opium is used here; but it may easily be shown that the home production increases every year. Opium has been recently made from white poppies, cultivated for the purpose, in Vermont, New Hampshire, and Connecticut, the annual production being estimated by hundreds of pounds, and this has generally been absorbed in the communities where it is made. It has also been brought here from Florida and Louisiana, while comparatively large quantities are regularly sent east from California and Arizona, where its cultivation is becoming an important branch of industry, ten acres of poppies being said to yield, in Arizona, twelve hundred pounds of opium.

Opiate use was frowned upon in some circles as immoral—a vice akin to dancing, smoking, theater-going, gambling, or sexual promiscuity. But while deemed immoral, it is important to note that opiate use in the nineteenth century was not subject to the moral sanctions current today. Employees were not fired for addiction. Wives did not divorce their addicted husbands, or husbands their addicted wives. Children were not taken from their homes and lodged in foster homes or institutions because one or both parents were addicted. Addicts continued to participate fully in the life of the community. Addicted children and young people continued to go to school, Sunday School, and college. Thus, the nineteenth century avoided one of the most disastrous effects of current narcotics laws and attitudes—the rise of a deviant addict subculture, cut off from respectable society and without a "road back" to respectability.

Our nineteenth-century forbears correctly perceived the major objection to the opiates. They are addicting. Though the word "addiction" was seldom used during the nineteenth century, the phenomenon was well understood. The true nature of the narcotic evil becomes visible, the *Catholic World* article pointed out, when someone who has been using an opiate for some time attempts to give up its use. Suddenly his eyes are opened to his folly and he realizes the startling fact that he is in the toils of a serpent as merciless as the boa-constrictor and as relentless as fate. With a firm determination to free himself he discontinues its use. Now his sufferings begin and steadily increase until they become unbearable. The tortures of Dives are his; but unlike that miser, he has only to stretch forth his hand to find oceans with which to satisfy his thirst. That human nature is not often equal to so extraordinary a self-denial affords little cause for astonishment. . . . Again and again he essays release from a bondage so humiliating, but meets with failure only, and at last submits to his fate a con-firmed opium-eater.

Our nineteenth-century forbears also perceived opiate use as a "will-weakening" vice—for surely, they insisted, a man or woman of strong will could stop if he tried hard enough. The fact was generally known that addicts deprived of their opiates (when hospitalized for some illness unrelated to their addiction, for example) would lie or even steal to get their drug, and addicts "cured" of their addiction repeatedly relapsed. Hence there was much talk of the moral degener-ation caused by the opiates.

Nevertheless, there was very little popular support for a law banning these substances. "Powerful organizations for the suppression . . . of alcoholic stimulants exist throughout the land," the 1881 article in the *Catholic World* noted, but there were no similar anti-opiate organiza-tions.

The reason for this lack of demand for opiate prohibition was quite simple: the drugs were not viewed as a menace to society and they were not in fact a menace.

—Edward M. Brecher and the
Editors of Consumer Reports Magazine,
The Consumers Union Report on Licit and Illicit Drugs

Drug Law
A Brief and Sordid History

"Unless we put medical freedom into the Constitution, the time will come when medicine will organize itself into an undercover dictatorship."

—Dr. Benjamin Rush, physician and signer of the Declaration of Independence.

The passage of the Pure Food and Drug Act in 1906, regulating the labeling of medicines to disclose the presence of certain ingredients, was the first breach of the world of medicine by the federal government.

It popped America's drug law cherry, you might say. After this, further regulation seemed nothing more than a slight alteration of the status quo. The 1906 Act heralded the final years of an America that would seem unreal to us today. It is probably just as difficult to grasp the enormity of government control of medicine today in comparison to the utter lack of such restrictions at the time. Americans saw no place for any government claim to any but the most public aspects of their lives.

The world of restrictions on commerce was essentially a vacuum; a void. Unless a business was a blatant and commonly recognized crime it was presumed legal. And no substance on earth required a citizen to provide special credentials or "good reason" to have or buy. Drugs were an item of commerce, without negative or suspicious connotations. Obviously the distinction between "hard" or "soft" drugs would have been lost on Americans at that time.

Let's imagine that the government suddenly claimed dominion over electronics, where one was forced to obtain a degree or pay licensing fees to gain permission to solder or operate a photocopier. What if agencies governing electronics grew so robust a person could face jail for being caught with too many batteries? What if these agencies, recognizing the necessity of batteries for so many evil purposes, strictly limited their production and required that everyone dealing in batteries—from manufacturer to consumer—to record detailed information about them and be required to account for them at any given time? Can you imagine facing a mandatory prison sentence for illegal possession of batteries, or arguing for leniency because they were for personal use and not for resale?

Say the prison sentence was determined by the specific number of batteries possessed? If you can imagine that, then you can easily imagine some milquetoast civil rights group patting itself on the back for its tireless lobbying to base punishment on the number of volts available at the time of apprehension and not just the number of batteries? Finally, they would brag, finally the law is based on rational thinking!

This analogy is no more ludicrous than how Americans at the turn-of-the-century would consider the government's role in controlling the use of drugs, or for that matter, anything.

Alcohol

But, alcohol (obviously a drug, among other things) was once outlawed. For 13 years the possession of alcohol earned Americans prison. At first, the sentence was six months. Successive government crackdowns "got tough"—until booze meant a then-draconian sentence of five years.

Then, Prohibition was abandoned. It ruined enough lives, corrupted enough government entities, and the people finally were able to repeal the awful laws. The tragedy was called a "noble experiment" in the attempt to save face and, weirdly enough, the repeal of Prohibition is often trotted out as an example of how "the system works." As if its destruction was repaired. . . .

The "problem" of habit-forming drugs did not exist before the turn of the century. Terminology had to be invented and defined before "addicts" could be identified and punished. At the time the word "addict" meant something close to "fan." A person might be a novel-reading addict or a snow-skiing addict, but there was no such thing, really, as a drug addict. The idea of government saving people from "bad" medicine, or of ostracizing and punishing users of morphine, just did not compute. This was true as late as 1916 when the Supreme Court failed to comprehend how the nation's first drug control law (the Harrison

Act, which masqueraded as a tax law) could be construed to limit a citizen's access to opium or other "narcotics."

It took a sustained propaganda campaign that took advantage of social upheavals and fears, like evil foe of the First World War and the precedent of alcohol prohibition, to invent and drive home the concept of evil narcotic use.

The creation of the "dope fiend," or "addict" sparked a few squabbles between druggists and physicians. It was considered improper role for government to be in the business of licensing or otherwise certifying what constituted real medicine or even who was a doctor! States that ever passed laws restricting medicine had repealed them within a few years of their passage.

In the years before and after the Harrison Act became law, various factions in the field of medicine coalesced into pressure groups, all vying for the title of legitimate. The American Medical Association (AMA), which was to emerge the victor—and reigning champion— was a only a splinter group at the beginning of the century.

The litmus test for true legitimacy soon came to turn on the medical practitioner's relationship with dope fiends. The more a doctor could be associated with "dope fiends," the easier it was to discredit him, toss him in prison and otherwise shove him out of the way.

In 1901, a prescient American Pharmacy Association formed a Committee on the Acquirement of the Drug Habit which cited, defined and then heartily opposed "drug abuse." To solve this new-found problem, the APA recommended regulating the sale of drugs. Though the APA never directly gained the control it sought, it remained a heavy influence on the drug legislation that would soon come to dominate the medical establishment.

Dr. Rush's fears of a covert medical dictatorship resulting from a lack of Constitutional vigilance were realized when, one year after gaining the hotly-disputed income tax, Congress passed the Harrison Act in 1914, the country's first attempt to restrict drug use on a national level. The federal government relied on its new-found power to tax as the way it could regulate

Important Dates in Pill History

1765 John Morgan founds the first medical school in the U.S. at the College of Pennsylvania.

1775 William Withering introduces digitalis, in the form of foxglove, as a cure for congestive heart disease.

1800 Nitrous Oxide ("laughing gas") is discovered by English scientist Humphry Davy, who proposes its use as an anesthetic. At the time, many of Davy's neighbors considered him a dangerous lunatic and sorcerer and ran him out of town.

1805 German chemist Friedrich Wilhelm Adam Serturner isolates and describes morphine. It is the first alkaloid ever isolated and prompts pharmaceutical scientists to tease out more such alkaloids from plant drugs of every kind. The beginning of the age of the "active ingredient."

1820 Eleven physicians meet in Washington D.C. to establish the U.S. Pharmacopeia, first compendium of standard drugs for the country.

circa 1825 Eli Whitney, inventor of the cotton gin, tortured by enlargement of the prostate is forced to invent the flexible catheter to relieve his bladder and his pain. It is possible the same gizmo was invented by a similarly-plagued Benjamin Franklin in 1784.

1831 Chloroform is discovered by American scientist Samueal Guthrie.

1832 Codeine isolated by French pharmacist Pierre Robiquet.

1847 The American Medical Association is born.

Cocaine is isolated.

1852 The American Pharmaceutical Association is founded; the Association's 1856 Constitution lists one of its goals as "To as much as possible restrict the dispensing and sale of medicines to regularly educated druggists and apothecaries."

1853 Dr. Alexander Wood develops an impractical syringe, without refinements, such as a point made by Frenchman Charles Pravaz.

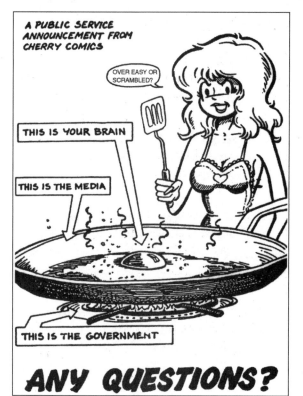

medical products. In this case it was opium, a few opium derivatives and cocaine.

Almost immediately, newly-minted Narcotics cops began tossing Harrison Act violators in prison, and the few federal prisons that existed were soon overcrowded. (Early drafts of the Act restricted sales of caffeine, so maybe we should count ourselves lucky we can still buy a Mountain Dew without facing ten years in the federal slam or a Jolt Cola, which would mandate a life sentence!)

The Harrison Act never intended to restrain itself to tax law, though government officials continued this charade for a number of years as a means to accustom citizens to the rapid expansion of federal police power. The Act was also explained as the means the U.S. government could comply with non-binding treaties drawn up by a few extremely wealthy citizens to control opium production and sales worldwide. The power to conduct these treaties, with all their domestic control and intrigues, rested conveniently with the President.

The Harrison Act's true purpose revealed itself as federal authority over social control. Drug commerce was quickly placed under the beady eyes of the Treasury Department, already home to alcohol prohibition agents.

While alcohol prohibition and its Constitutional Amendment was repealed when the populace, disgusted by a shocking increase in police corruption and organized crime, practically threatened politicians to correct their error. But drug prohibition and control over medicine and countless other industries lives on today. The original idea of the Harrison Act to provide protection against fraud and raise a few dollars for General Welfare has grown into a mega-regulatory civic nightmare, in which citizens who use drugs that were commonly taken and sold over-the-counter in pharmacies, are treated as the most horrible criminals and incarcerated by the millions in a civil war known as the War on Drugs.

To its ever-lasting shame, the American Medical Association backed the Harrison Act, ignoring the protests of doctors outside the Association, along with pharmacists, drug manufacturers and the public. It took the AMA five years to consolidate its power and be granted exclusive rights to define the meaning and practice of medicine.

It probably didn't even take a year before it became apparent the government was not satisfied with simply taxing opium at a measly dollar per year, nor was the Act merely a way of encouraging better record-keeping of possibly dangerous drugs. The Harrison Act went far beyond bookkeeping and barged right into the practice of medicine. Through its front group, the government used its power to decide who was a doctor, and the meaning and practice of medicine. So it goes with pacts with the devil.

Doctors originally joined the AMA to avoid becoming employees of large medical corporations and remain small-time capitalist professionals. To obtain doctors' backing, the AMA Act included explicit wording that MDs believed would leave them free to practice medicine (and distribute it) as they saw fit:

"Nothing," read the Harrison Act ". . . in this section shall apply . . . to the dispensing or distribution of any of the aforesaid drugs to a patient by a physician, dentist, or veterinary surgeon registered under this Act."

Yet this very phrase gave the government the power to distinguish between legitimate medical practice and the seamy selling of drugs to degenerates.

To make sure everyone ponied up the Harrison Act taxes, 162 IRS agents were taken from enforcing income tax and placed in the Treasury Department's Miscellaneous Division in 1915. The ex-tax cops vigorously enforced the Act in ways its backers had apparently never foreseen. The moment the Harrison Act went into effect, people, mostly doctors, were dragged off to prison—at times without any trial! In the spring of 1916 the law was challenged at the highest level: the Supreme Court.

The Supreme Court's first drug case is known as United States v. Jin Fuey Moy. In this case the government argued that giving morphine to a morphine addict was not "legitimate medicine," but rather, a criminal act. Although the Treasury Department had no authority to regulate the practice of medicine, it declared addiction was not a medical condition, but a moral failing. Doing anything to aid and comfort the "dope fiend" (an interchangeable term with "addict") was grounds for criminal prosecution.

The Justices (7-2) overwhelmingly found against the government. In the judges' opinion, the Harrison Act was "a police measure that strained all the powers of the legislature." The judges continued: the Harrison Act took on "the appearance of a taxing measure in order to give it a coating of constitutionality." The Harrison Act was a tax only, said the Court, and could not be construed as a restrictive law on drugs. If that's what the Act was meant for, they wrote, it was unconstitutional.

Government prosecutors tried to claim the Act was required by two international treaties that preceded it: the Shanghai Convention of 1909 and the Hague Opium Convention of 1912, both of which had attempted to control a worldwide opium "epidemic"—especially in China, where U.S. economic interests sought to dislodge the overbearing, opium-mongering British.

Writing for the majority, Oliver Wendell Holmes attacked the law's validity as fulfillment of a treaty. Such an argument was "to say the least, another grave question." The Act was a tax law, not a treaty, and had no link to the conventions, which had nothing to do with U.S. narcotics control in the first place.

1862 President Lincoln appoints a chemist, Charles M. Wetherill, to serve in the new Department of Agriculture. This was the beginning of the Bureau of Chemistry, which becomes the FDA in the Department of Health and Human Services.

1864 German chemist Adolf von Baeyer synthesizes barbituric acid, the parent of all barbiturates. Apocryphal stories say he named his discovery after a saint, a girlfriend, or his wife, all named Barbara.

1865 British physician Josph Baron Lister discovers the use of disinfectants in surgery reduces the death rate from 45% to 15%.

1874 Diacetylmorphine (aka Heroin) is first synthesized by C.R.A. Wright, at St. Mary's hospital in London, England. He feeds some to a few dogs, one of them barfs "a little" and that wraps it up for Wright, who wasn't too impressed with heroin. He doesn't even bother to shelve the stuff.

1876 Lydia Pinkham of Lynn, MA, starts advertising her famous patent medicine aimed at treating "female problems." It is mainly alcohol.

1881 Louis Pasteur develops develops a vaccine that protects sheep and cattle from anthrax.

1884 Cocaine is first used as a local anesthetic.

1885 Louis Pasteur is back again: this time with a vaccine to protect humans from rabies. He uses it to save the life of a boy bitten by a rabid dog.

1890 Surgeon and morphine addict William Halsted introduces the practice of wearing sterilized rubber gloves during surgery.

In Germany, Emil von Behring develops a vaccine against tetanus and diphtheria. Robert Koch discovers tuberculin will cure tuberculosis.

Also in Germany, diacetylmorphine is discovered again by W. Dankwortt, of Bayer Pharmaceuticals. Nobody notices until eight years later when division head Heinrich Dreser plucks it from the shelf and takes credit for the new sensation: Heroin. Dreser had also picked up the aspirin file, but considered the stuff too dangerous to market until a year after putting heroin on the market.

This judicial hard-line vanished suddenly in 1919 when the Supreme Court, presented with two cases nearly identical to Jin Fuey Moy, did an about-face, coming down hard on a doctor who prescribed morphine to a morphine addict and the pharmacist who sold it to him (United States v. Webb et. al).

By allowing the criminal prosecution of both the doctor and the pharmacist who dispensed the drug, the Court had apparently seen the light. Even though the parties concerned were licensed and paid taxes, they still violated the "tax law." Prescribing morphine merely for the comfort of the addict had become, in the words of the court, "so plain a perversion of meaning [of the Act] that no discussion of the subject is required."

So there. No further discussion. The decision was narrow (5–4), but two of the Justices had been replaced. But this alone was not enough to tip the Harrison Act scales in favor of the Government. One of the judges had to change his mind. In this case it was none other than Chief Justice Holmes, whose inexplicable decision to switch sides provided the vote that upheld the Act. The previously fiery defender of individual rights and freedom took a hairpin turn in his legal reasoning, the first in a series of decisions in which he would find exceptions to most of the Constitution he once upheld.

After Holmes' shift, the Supreme Court finally agreed with the cops, and 25,000 doctors were prosecuted for violations of the Harrison Act between 1919 and 1924. What happened in the three years between Jin Fuey Moy and Webb to account for such an abrupt and radical change?

Professor David Musto (author of *The American Disease*) theorized that the change of heart during those three years was due to World War I. In that time "drug addiction" was successfully propagandized as a problem foisted on good clean Americans by heathens from abroad. Indeed, the U.S. press, including the *New York Times*, published shocking reports of supposed German plots to introduce addicting drugs into U.S. Army training centers, and lacing candy with drugs, then handing them out to schoolchildren. These drugs were so fiendish that eating just one piece of the evil candy would transform cherub-faced innocents into raving heroin

maniacs. One of the most fascinating stories in the *New York Times* told of a dastardly German plot to spike toothpaste with addictive drugs and then export the stuff to its enemies, who would become so dope-addled the Hun would have no trouble conquering the nation. That's just how fiendish these foreigners were. Addiction was a matter of national security.

Between 1916 and 1919, years leading up to and during the first World War, the government had taken serious interest in controlling the population, monitoring its thoughts, and guiding its prevailing opinions. It was the dawn of what has been called "The Surveillance State."

For one thing, the Court's two new Justices 1919 were Woodrow Wilson appointees (Brandeis and Clarke). Brandeis, especially, was a great supporter of government supervision over all aspects of life where "the public good" could be invoked. During these years, Wilson personally promoted an updated Sedition law and a vaguely worded Espionage Act. The law introduced the "clear and present danger" argument to free speech. These laws made almost any anti-government speech or action tantamount to treason and deserving of a long prison sentence. In 1917 Wilson established a government Censorship Board to control all publications in the country. It's an historical memory hole that President Wilson was able to suppress many books by a supposedly free press.

Although he won re-election on the slogan, "He kept us out of war!" (even as he invaded Mexico in the famous bombardment of Vera Cruz), Wilson wasted no time in calling for forced conscription into a national army sent to fight in a European war, in which the United States had no direct interest. During the war, Eugene Debs, a socialist union organizer, exhorted young men to disobey the government and refuse to go to war. Arrested under Wilson's Sedition Act, Debs was sentenced to 10 years in prison (an exceptionally harsh sentence in those days). When his case reached the Supreme Court, the government prevailed.

Woodrow Wilson, inventor of the League of Nations—the early version of the United Nations—viewed his primary role as a conductor of foreign policy; unfortunately, Wilson believed there wasn't much in the way of domestic law that didn't come under that heading. Buried within the Versailles Treaty, forced on all the players to end World War I, was a clause binding every signatory to the Opium Convention convened by the United States. Countries that previously refused to join the effort to suppress Asian economy, had just been drafted.

Foreign Policy? National Security? What's That Got To Do With Medicine?

The Harrison Act forced the hand of the U.S. government to bring its policing of international treaties to domestic shores. In the case, drugs, due to treaties signed at the international Anti-Opium Convention. Like most drug laws that followed, the Harrison Act ruled by administrative fiat. And it made such things possible as the Palmer Raids, when government agents hunted down and deported (or imprisoned) "communists" during the "Red Scare" of 1919–1920.

Although alcohol Prohibition was repealed in just over a decade, drug laws have stayed and flourished without Congressional approval, constitutional amendment, or popular referendum.

By linking drug laws (and the practice of medicine) to the executive office, and by using "foreign policy" as an excuse to enforce them, the laws could never be repealed or even challenged, since they were never properly enacted to begin with!

In 1930, the Federal Bureau of Narcotics 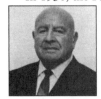 (FBN) was established, with Harry Anslinger, a former prohibitionist, as its head.

As a result of the Harrison Act, so many drug prisoners jammed federal prisons that the government worked overtime to build more. To ease some of the pressure, the government decided drug addiction could be viewed as a disease, making it possible to order enforced detoxification under lock and key. Thousands of drug and alcohol felons began to popular "drug farms" built in 1938 at Fort Worth, Texas, and Lexington, Kentucky. Prisons overflowed into "treatment" farms where the sentence had all the same features of prison! With alcohol prohibition in effect until 1933,

1893 Aspirin is invented by Felix Hoffman as an improvement on an earlier variant of salicylic acid used by Hermann Kolbe.

1887 Amphetamine is first synthesized by German scientist L. Edeleano, who called his invention phenylisopropylamine, then shelved it.

1903 Veronal becomes the first barbiturate marketed in the U.S.

1906 The passage of the Pure Food and Drug Act attacks the pharmaceutical industry by requiring the labels of "narcotics" containing concoctions to disclose its ingredients. A proto-Food and Drug Administration is formed to oversee regulation this regulation and goes hog wild.

1910 Modern chemotherapy is born with the introduction of the arsenic-based drug, Salvarsan (arsphenamine). Known even then as a "magic bullet," it is used to treat syphilis.

Army Medical Corps Major Frank Woodcury introduces the use of iodine tincture as a disinfectant for wounds.

1912 Phenobarbital, one of the derivatives of barbituric acid, goes on sale in the United States under the trade name of Luminal.

Polish-American biochemist Casimir Funk coins the term "vitamin" to describe a class of food substances known to be essential to health.

1923 Albert Calmette and Camille Guerin develop a vaccine for tuberculosis, a French bacteriologist, Gaston Ramon introduces a more effective diphtheria vaccine and, acetylene is first used as an anesthetic. Today the gas is used for welding.

1925 In U.S. v. Linder, the Supreme Court rules drug addiction to be a medical condition for which it is not illegal to prescribe opiates. This decision was ignored by drug cops at the time—and still is.

1927 Gordon Alles works extensively with the nearly forgotten chemical, phenylisoproplyamine, which he calls amphetamine. He discovers the d-isomer, dextroamphetamine, is far stronger than its l-isomer. Fearlessly experimenting on himself and his friends, Alles rapidly proved "dex" unsurpassed in relieving nasal decongestion. Pharmaceutical firm, SmithKline & French buys all the scientist's patents.

there was more than a decade when nearly any drug but tobacco and caffeine could land a citizen in jail or in a treatment camp until he was "cured."

Despite all the new prisons, drug farms and federal agents hired to enforce the "dangerous drugs" or "narcotics" laws, the anti-drug effort was still in low gear compared to what was to come. By World War II, the federal government had given birth to a sizeable police agency for drugs that saw spasms of growth every few years, eventually turning it into a cop enterprise rivaling the FBI.

Picking Up Speed

After WWII, drugs were still associated with evil foreigners, but focus shifted from the German Hun to evil Communists and their plot to take over the world. This scare tactic was no different or unbelievable than stories about German toothpaste laced with narcotics, but it worked just as well. (As late as 1981, New York governor Hugh Carey claimed "The epidemic of gold-chain snatching in the city is the result of a Russian design to wreck America by flooding the nation with deadly heroin.") By the end of WWII, heroin replaced opium on the street, as Italian gangs usurped the mostly Jewish gangs that once held sway.

Anti-drug legislation and rhetoric in the '50s was especially severe: at one point the death penalty was adopted for anyone caught selling heroin to a minor. The Boggs Amendment to the Harrison Act, passed in 1951, upped the penalties for all drug crimes, outlined mandatory minimums, prohibited probation for all but the first violation and instituted a predecessor to today's "three strikes" law, with convictions of 10–20 years for three violations.

The Narcotics Control Act of 1956 enforced mandatory prison terms for offenders, even though the Supreme Court had, three decades earlier, ruled addiction to be a medical condition and not a crime. Those convicted were automatically placed on three years' supervised probation after serving any prison sentence. Any further drug use ("relapse") resulted in more incarceration. Those convicted three times of drug use would also be remanded to a

federal drug farm to serve an indeterminate sentence. In other words, the prisoner would be found guilty of "criminality" (and not of a particular crime) and as a result, land in prison for months or years.

Drug felons were also denied passports, lest they spend all their time traveling the world only to flood the country with drugs. Though passports have never been required to travel to Mexico, one woman titillated senators when she testified for over a year she had smuggled more than $1,000 worth of heroin a week across the border by stuffing the smack in her vagina. Drug use also became sufficient grounds to exclude any would-be immigrants. (These laws were later declared violations of the Eighth Amendment.)

Narcotics officers got permission to carry guns in 1956. For reasons unknown to sentient beings, the two decades following WWII are known as the "classical" era of narcotics control. Drugs, especially heroin, were so fixed with the concept of evil in the public mind that any use was inexcusable. Like Frankenstein's monster, drug abuse was revived when Kennedy took office in 1960. The "Big H" remained the chemical focus of the public and drug experts, but not for long. Heroin remained the worst possible drug, but since the '60s it had a gaggle of other illicit substances with which to share the spotlight.

Prescription Drug Abuse

In the mid-'60s the idea of prescription drug abuse was put in people's heads by hysterical articles in the mass media. Amphetamines, barbiturates and their chemical relatives were singled out, as they became more associated with random hedonism than "legitimate" medicine. Amphetamines were logically popular, due to their ability to suppress the appetite, focus concentration and provide extra energy. (U.S. troops were issued them in WWII for those very reasons.) Barbiturates, doled out by docs since the teens, were big-time psychiatric cures by the mid-'50s, treating anxiety, mania, and alcoholism, along with insomnia.

Both drugs were considered part of medicine until it was realized that millions of these pills were consumed illegitimately each year—scammed or bought on the black market as "uppers" and "downers."

Although one of the biggest speed users around (getting his regular speed injections from the original Doctor Feelgood), Kennedy jumped on the bandwagon to decry indiscriminate use of drugs and appointed an advisory committee to glorify their suppression. Among the recommendations of the committee was that amphetamines be more tightly controlled, and in 1965, the Drug Abuse Control Amendments were enacted to address the abuse of stimulants and depressants—as well as hallucinogens. Dr. Timothy Leary was already dropping acid by 1960, as it and other psychedelics were nearly all discovered or developed by government spy agencies who experimented with them on a large scale at universities.

LSD, along with barbiturates, amphetamines and substances with similar effects were classified as "dangerous drugs" by the 1965 law. Versions of this law had been grinding through congress for years, dying slowly as lobbyists for pharmaceutical companies methodically gutted and stomped them. But this one managed to struggle through. Methamphetamine, which had escaped all drug controls until this time, came within a hair's breadth of being outlawed as politicians misunderstood the pharmaceutical lobby's official line: that they didn't care about methamphetamine. They realized their mistake only after being informed by Abbott Labs that as the nation's only manufacturer of methamphetamine, and purveyor of two very popular methamphetamine products, they certainly did object to outlawing the stuff.

So the law was revised to prohibit only liquid, injectable methamphetamine, which made up only 1% of the methamphetamine market and was therefore tolerable to Abbott.

The next year, the Bureau of Drug Abuse Control (BDAC) was created and staffed with 100 agents, all devoted to policing these "dangerous drugs."

But it was apparent pills would never become the focus of drug control, either by the government or puritanical anti-drug crusaders. How could things approved of by the best members of the community be Bad? Pills were medicine.

1930 The Porter Act creates Federal Bureau of Narcotics, with Harry Anslinger at its head carves its role out of the Treasury's Alcohol Prohibition department.

Ernest H. Volwiler and Donalee L. Tabern synthesize the still-popular barbiturate, Nembutal (pentobarbital).

1932 German scientist Gerhard Domagk invents the first sulfa drug, Prontosil, the first of the so-called "wonder drugs."

In America, SmithKline begins marketing its famous Benzedrine inhaler, with their patented compound, dextroamphetamine. It's a hit.

1936 Volwiler and Talbern are back this year with their latest barbiturate concoction: sodium pentothal. Used to induce a deep sleep it is also dubbed "truth serum," because of the profound state of suggestibility it induces.

Swiss chemists figure out the active part of Prontosil is a metabolite called sulfanilamide. From then on sulfanilamide becomes the basic sulfa drug, spawning sulfapyridine the next year and, in 1939, sulfathiazole.

1938 Congress whips up the Food, Drug, and Cosmetic Act (FDC), putting the finishing touches on the FDA, giving it jurisdiction over food and drugs. The Act requires new drugs to be proven safe before marketing and takes a major step toward total pill regulation by establishing the modest, reasonable concept of "prescription medicine." Prescription status is determined by the drug's manufacturer.

Dr. Albert Hoffman, a chemist at Sandoz laboratories in Basle, Switzerland, synthesizes LSD. The 25th in a series of compounds based on rye ergot, Hoffman puts it on a shelf and gets back to work. Five years later he accidentally ingests some of it, and reports on its effects.

1940 Two scientists at Oxford University get hold of some purified penicillin and show how it can be used as an antibiotic. Although it had been discovered in 1928 by English scientist Alexander Fleming, it had, of course, been shelved.

And there were too many other, scarier things, to worry about: mind-melting psychedelics, marijuana-tokin' war protesters. Even cocaine, which could be found making the party circuit late in the decade.

In 1968, President Johnson consolidated the Federal Bureau of Narcotics and the BDAC into the Bureau of Narcotics and Dangerous Drugs (BNDD), transferring it from the Treasury to the Department of Justice, with a total of 600 agents. The next year 160 agents were added to the force.

Richard Nixon, elected the year before, knew better than to use the Vietnam War as a focal point of his campaign; the country was divided. The country was not divided over the war protesters, however: middle America found its bra-burning, free love and drug use appalling. Drug use. "As I look over the problems in this country, I see one that stands out particularly," Nixon bellowed to his supporters, "The problem of narcotics."

Under Nixon, Congress repealed virtually all prior drug legislation, including the Harrison Act and the Marijuana Tax Act of 1937 and replaced them with The Comprehensive Drug Abuse Prevention and Control Act of 1970. Taking its cue from the President's Advisory Council of 1962–63 and the findings of another Presidential Commission held in 1967, the Act codified drug laws into the framework of laws on the books today.

Unlike previous drug laws, where enforcement powers were spread among a number of police agencies, these specifically concentrated the bulk of newly-created powers to the Department of Justice and most specifically to the Attorney General. While the Attorney General today may think nothing of her dictatorial powers, it was a big deal in 1970.

Besides repealing the ban on international travel for drug users, the new raft of laws didn't do much else in the way of compassion or reason. It increased the number of BNDD agents from 760 to 1,150 in 1971. In 1973 President Nixon, declaring "an all-out global war on the drug menace," consolidated the BNDD, various agencies he'd created (including ODALE— a take-no-prisoners agency accused of beating and even murdering suspects), and the Customs Service Drug Investigations Unit into the Drug Enforcement Agency (DEA), which now had 2,000 agents and an operating budget of nearly half a billion dollars. The DEA closed 1998 with a budget of $1.2 billion and over 4,000 agents.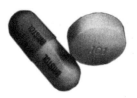

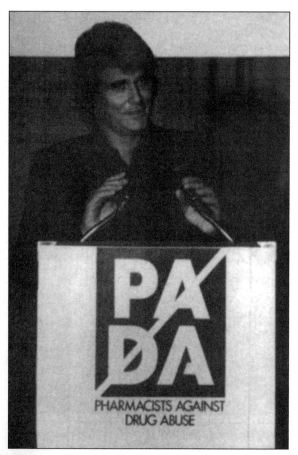

Michael Landon makes an anti-drug speech at the annual meeting of the National Accociation of Chain Drug Stores. According to one study, barbiturate abusers who started taking these drugs between the ages of 20 and 25 were most likely to have had their first exposure through legal prescriptions.

War on Drugs

In 1996 William F. Buckley, Jr.—advisor and voice of conservatives for decades—withdrew support for government restriction of drugs. He declared the drug war "Lost" on the cover of *The National Review*, the influential magazine he edits. "Kill it," he said, "Go for legalization." Like alcohol prohibition before it, the "cure" was far worse than any problem it may solve.

Speaking to the New York Bar Association in 1998, Buckley used the disease metaphor to describe what is behind the rapid destruction of U.S. society. The plague he cites is not drug addicts and illegal drug use, but drug enforcement—the whole drug war.

"We are speaking of a plague that consumes an estimated $75 billion per year of public money, exacts an estimated $70 billion from consumers, is responsible for nearly 50 percent of the Americans who are today in jail, occupies an estimated 50 percent of the trial time of our judiciary, and takes the time of 400,000 policemen—yet a plague for which no cure is at hand, nor in prospect."

Democrats are believed to be more lenient on law and order issues in general and drug enforcement in particular, but there is no evidence to support the belief. George Bush increased drug enforcement by an order of magnitude over Ronald Reagan's mind-boggling levels. Clinton has done the same. The 1994 Anti-Crime Bill jacks-up penalties for drug crimes, and invents even more. It pumps more resources to outfit the coast guard with new aircraft and radar balloons.

The propaganda effort needed to cajole and cow the population supporting the drug war's enormous burden periodically "discovers" new and more heinous drug than the one before it. Besides the ever-present threat of heroin, there is, at all times, another drug contending for the title of THE demon drug. Like pro-wrestling, the characters are garish and the action staged. There are more than three wings to the drug circus, and a "new" drug (like Rohypnol, say) makes a brief, cameo appearance to highlight the main act, the One Really Bad Drug, that is so manifestly evil that, the media covers it on a daily basis.

1941 Female sex hormones are discovered to be an effective treatment of prostate cancer. The fourth sulfa drug, sulfadiazine, is introduced.

1942 A vaccine to prevent yellow fever backfires when it causes hepatitis B in some of the thousands of U.S. Army troops inoculated with it. A new vaccine, which doesn't require human blood serum to produce, takes its place.

1943 Streptomycin is developed from a mold grown in soil. This new antibiotic kills negative bacteria making it effective against tuberculosis. All over the world, microbioligists are testing soil samples for antibiotics.

Scientist Dorothy Fennel discovers a potent new species of penicillin she calls Penicillium fennelliae.

1944 Benjamin Duggar and his troupe of co-workers discover Aureomycin, the first of the tetracyclines.

1948 Another antibiotic, called Nystatin, is discovered. Its applications include athlete's foot and the restoration of old books, eaten by mold.

1950 In Alberty Food Products Co. v. U.S., a court of appeals rules that medicine labels must include the purpose for which the drug is offered.

A chemical from Indian snake root, reserpine, is first used to treat high blood pressure. Two years later it is realized the drug is also a tranquilizer and is immediately put to use in mental hospitals.

1951 The Durham-Humphrey Amendment quietly springs the trap on pharmaceutical industry—using the innocuous "prescription drug" concept. The law now requires some drugs be sold "by prescription only" through a licensed medical practitioner. Prescriptions now become legal documents instead of formal medical instructions.

The Boggs Amendment to the Harrison Act ups penalties for all drug crimes. It outlines mandatory minimums, prohibits probation for all but the first violation and institutes a law mandating 10-20 years for three violations.

The very inventors of the fraudulent scare of "crack babies" were forced to discredit themselves when it came time to change the program. After years of moaning about the awfulness of supposedly irreversible brain-damage babies become teenagers. Soon they are mature enough to become prisoners and scapegoats. A few appearances on *Nightline* announced the spontaneous reversal of the disease's victim status.

The easy to make methamphetamine analogue, methcathinone, comes complete with mad scientist and a genie in the bottle. (In 1995,

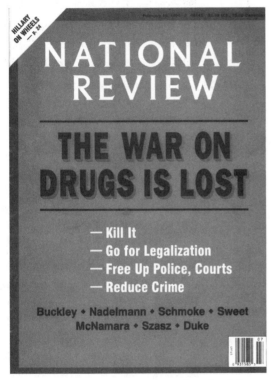

Spin magazine reports about cat, "Be afraid, be very afraid.") The story goes that in 1986, a college intern was supposed to burn the stuff, but he didn't. Instead, he unleashed another "plague" that fizzled so quickly, that almost no one but those convicted of cat crimes even noticed.

For the past few years, drug war propaganda has focused once again on methamphetamine. In the same scenario as always, meth perverts and destroys citizens by the townful. The stuff arrives from out of nowhere (until it is later discovered to have come from some evil foreign country), and it immediately seduces the salt of the earth, forcing the police to arrest and imprison them.

As 1998 marks a quarter-century of "excellence"

from the DEA, Clinton requests an additional 267 agents be added to the agency's payroll and 100,000 more police added across the country.

In June '98, President Clinton and drug Czar Barry McCaffrey unveiled a $17.1 billion plan to continue fighting those evil drugs, including a $1 billion advertising campaign featuring a teenage sexpot smashing up her kitchen with a frying pan in a heroin-induced rage. Despite accusations from the Republican House that his administration has been soft on drugs, Clinton has followed the map laid out by Reagan, shoveling two-thirds of the drug war's money to law enforcement and prison, constructing a federal death house in Terre Haute, Indiana to carry out the death penalty for drug offenders, and blacklisting countries like the Andean nations of South America.

Since at least 1996 the United States has been covertly spraying the hinterlands of coca country in Peru and Colombia with a genetically altered fungus, which is supposed to eat all the evil coca plants, so they can obediently become extinct. Needless to say, the simple organism had other plans for its species survival and has already diversified its palette. It now eats about anything but coca, bypassing the majority of the coca bushes it encounters.

Taken at face value, the War on Drugs is insane. If the self-appointed generals were truthful about their desire to "stamp out drugs" they would be gone. There are plenty of police to do the job and few legal limits on how they do this "job."

More than any other reason, the War on Drugs continues to exist because it is profitable. American workers have been forced to spend $150 billion in tax money since 1981 to finance attempts shilled them from cocaine, rape pills, heroin and now the "Nazi method" speed the workers themselves take to keep up the pace! The American gulag is a bonanza without peer. More than half the prisoners in 1990 were locked up for drug "crimes." Their caging cost the states $12 billion that year, money that is extracted from the incomes of the Drug War's future victims. Mind-control in the guise of "drug education" sucks up even more: $17 billion a year to pay for lessons teaching children how to snitch on their own parents. Twice that much money, however, is needed to police and prosecute their parents.

By 1991, seven years after Congress rewrote civil forfeiture law to allow seizure of "drug money" and "drug-related assets," the Justice Department collected more than $1.5 billion in illegal assets; in the next five years, the figure doubled.

The Legalization Movement and Pills

"Legalization" or "decriminalization" issues are problematic for pills, because most of them are already viewed as legal, though this is far from reality. Pills are harder to obtain than pot or heroin. Just try scoring a handful of Hydergine pills from the local "illegal" drug dealer. Heroin? Sure! Seldane? What might that be?

By being available only through the guiding hand of the proper state-approved, state-monitored authorities, pills are thought of as controlled substances and not illegal.

Up until recently, when methamphetamine was rotated to the front of the line of Threats to Society, the jail term for a person ingesting methamphetamine made by a "crank cook" was the same for the person whose illegal speed was made by Abbott Labs and simply diverted. Recent federal laws increase the penalties for "illegal" meth to those of crack cocaine.

Even Valium has jail terms associated with it and the only people who make diazepam are pharmaceutical companies! And countercultural types are among the first to swallow the hoax that pills need no "decriminalization," and almost never agitate for the liberation of penicillin, codeine, Prozac, or any of the thousands of prescription drugs that cannot be obtained without state permission.

This twilight world of quasi-legality means pills are seldom addressed during "drug legalization" debates. This same problem affects over-the-counter drugs, which are regularly banned ("illegalized") by administrative command. When diuretics, quinine pills, or stop-smoking chewing gum are outlawed, it is hardly mentioned in the news, even though the people's ability to self-medicate has been curtailed.

Anyone who doubts the manifest illegality of pharmaceuticals need only consider that "dangerous" or "recreational" drugs are not the only type

1954 Thorazine is introduced and begins the dramatic decline of the classic "insane asylum." Sometimes called a chemical straitjacket, thorazine is said to relieve patients of severe schizophrenia.

1956 Puerto Rican women line up for an enormous study of birth control pills.

The Narcotic Control Act continues to marginalize drug users by denying them passports.

Any further drug use ("relapse") results in further incarceration of convicted drug offenders.

Narcotics officers get permission to carry guns.

1959 The first new FDA district office opens in 24 years, in Detroit, Michigan, and is the first building designed for "scientific enforcement."

1960 Just before and during John Kennedy's presidency, drug abuse becomes a hot topic yet again with conservatives crying about dope fiends terrorizing the country. One of the biggest speed users around, Kennedy decries the indiscriminate use of amphetamines and appoints a presidential advisory committee which recommends of tight control of amphetamines.

1962 Pills take a beating this year. Thalidomide, a new sleeping pill, is found to cause birth defects in thousands of babies in Western Europe. An FDA medical officer, Dr. Frances Kelsey, who argus strenuously to keep the drug off the U.S. market, becomes a prototypical government hero. FDA milks the close call to make the case for stronger federal regulation of drugs.

The Kefauver Harris Amendments passed this same year requires drug manufacturers to prove effectiveness of their products before marketing them, and to include all possible side effects and contraindications in the drug's advertising. The Amendments are made retroactive for all drugs introduced after 1938, and are responsible for greatly lengthening and restricting the FDA drug approval process.

1965 Another FDA-directed law, the Drug Abuse Control Amendment of 1965, classifies barbiturates, amphetamines, LSD, and other medical wonders as "dangerous drugs."

of prescription drug under police control. Only about half of the medicines obtainable by "prescription only" contain controlled substances.

But all prescription drugs are policed by the armies of the state. And it's not a question of safety. The acetaminophen in your Vicodin might ruin your liver if you wash it down with some Chianti, but such health hazards are not the issue. The state's interest lies somewhere else—with the enforced separation between citizen and medicine.

While the government doesn't seem to care if you eat hemlock leaves or a handful of sawdust, it certainly does care if you come too close to the divine Host. There are also jail cells waiting for those who would blaspheme the state by possessing or transferring a bottle of erythromycin or Hydergine.

Even if you couldn't possibly be hurt or hurt anyone else with them, most pills are by prescription only. As a prescription drug, federal law prohibits damn near anything but full compliance with the parent/child relationship the government demands.

Few drugs are in as much demand as heroin. This may be because, in an illegal market, more potent drugs drive out weaker ones. This is the opposite of a legal environment where the trend is always toward "lite."

Most pills aren't strong enough to be smuggled or sold on the street. The exceptions, like amphetamines and Quaaludes, generally do something noticeable pretty quickly.

Social Control

One key feature of controlling drugs is the formidable power the government secures over even the most mundane aspects of everyone's daily life. The ability to forbid some things and to license others is the ability to regulate important aspects of society. The FDA has enormous power over the market in anything we eat or drink, since its imprimatur means life or death for any product in its realm. On a personal level, the ability to withhold or supply medicine means the agency assumes control of (but not responsibility for) sickness and health. Government bureaucrats now decide how much pain a citizen must endure—not the patient and not the physician. This power to regulate drugs can be as big a deal as life and death, and as small a deal as treatment of a hemorrhoid or a pimple.

Before the 1938 Food, Drug and Cosmetic Act was passed, only drugs containing certain narcotic or hypnotic preparations were required to be ordered by prescription. The Act mandated that the label bear the phrase, "Caution: May be Habit Forming," and made a tentative stab at restricting medications by outlining a classification of prescription drugs. But manufacturers would still determine each drug's prescription status. ("Is it safe? Of course! How long should you take it? For as long as you need it. Refills? Whenever you want. . . .")

With the Durham-Humphrey Amendment in 1951, that all changed, ostensibly to protect consumers from sliding into drug addiction and wanton, blasphemous self-medication. After all, the government knows what's best for you, not you or your doctor. The safety and habit-forming tendencies of drugs were used to formulate the first real law to enforce the idea of prescription medicine.

The Strange World of Prescription Medicine

Why is it that prescription drugs are harder to obtain outside the law than within it? That may seem a peculiar question but it seems odd a completely outlawed substance like heroin is almost as easy to find and buy as Preparation H.

It's not for lack of demand. There are literally millions of customers for scores of legal drugs—everything from Retin A to Zoloft. So why doesn't the black market provide them? (It's certainly not fear of breaking the law.)

Of the very profitable populations using any particular pill it's hard to imagine more than a few people would not gladly buy their pills over-the-counter. This is proven every time the FDA relents and permits a previously controlled drug to be sold without prescription. Few people prefer to depend on the doctor/pharmacist/government to get medications for them—or perhaps take them away. The benefits of a no-prescription policy are great, starting at the consumer level.

Being able to purchase medicine without going to a doctor first would lower the cost by at least as much as the perfunctory doctor's visit. This is why, for instance, Mexico and many other countries don't bother much with prescriptions. The dangers of not having medicine are greater than the dangers of self-medication.

Drug companies, too, would love to sell their pills directly to the consumer, as their markets would widen and profits increase (even if the price didn't). Proof of that is seen in Mexico, too, where all the drug companies sell their pills—often at lower prices.

Of course, prescription pills don't fit the typical "stronger sells better" profile of a black market drug. Compared to heroin, Prozac is definitely "lite." Then again, so is Sudafed, which is sold by the ton. So it's not lack of profit and it's not lack of demand that keeps prescription drugs behind the counter and off the black market.

There would be only one loser in the legalization scenario: the government. And therein lies the answer. As an illegal drug, heroin is the government's legal business only. Heroin and all other outlawed drugs are the source of a lot of revenue in seized assets and tax money stuffed into police pockets. Since we have allowed ourselves to become brainwashed and intimidated into giving the state the power over medicine this seems like an inevitable reality. But, should we ever stop playing along with this government-invented game, the crucial power of social control would disappear from the government's hands.

But don't count on anyone joining you if you buck the system.

As Dr. Thomas Szasz, author of *Our Right to Drugs*, says:

> The American people are scared to death of the freedom to have a free market in drugs.
>
> It comes from a one-hundred-year war on drugs, whose foundation is the prescription market; not the illegal market, not heroin. People are afraid of penicillin, of digitalis. That's what they are afraid of. They think they have to go to a doctor to get these drugs without informing themselves.
>
> You can be a professor of pharmacology at the local medical school and know more about drugs than nine out of ten physicians. But if your daughter has a sore throat, a strep throat, that professor of pharmacology cannot legally buy penicillin.
>
> And there is no interest in even discussing this. When people talk about a drug conference, they always talk about marijuana . . .

1965 Methamphetamine requires a prescription. Perhaps because it was most frequently called "desoxyephedrine," it didn't sound like an amphetamine. The famous "Valo Inhaler," which contains 150 mg of methamphetamine, disappears.

In a Seattle laboratory, an artificial sweetener called aspartame (aka NutraSweet) is invented.

1966 The FDA contracts with the National Academy of Sciences/National Research Council to evaluate the effectiveness of 4,000 drugs approved on the basis of safety alone between 1938 and 1962.

1967 LSD becomes illegal.

The introduction of the fertility drug clomiphene has the side effect of causing multiple births.

1968 The FBN becomes the Bureau of Narcotics and Dangerous Drugs, and moves from the Treasury Department to the Department of Justice.

1970 The Comprehensive Drug Abuse And Control Act of 1970 replaces all previous laws concerning narcotics and other dangerous drugs, and introduces Scheduling of controlled substances.

In Upjohn v. Finch, a Court of Appeals upholds enforcement of the 1962 drug effectiveness amendments and rules that widespread use by satisfied patients and doctors does not constitute substantial evidence of drug safety and efficacy. A number of drugs, used effectively for twenty years, are summarily pulled from the market.

1971 While the anti-cancer properties of Pacific Yew tree bark had been known for at least ten years, it wasn't until this year that scientists at the Research Triangle in North Carolina isolate the "active ingredient": taxol.

1972 President Nixon reorganizes the FBNDD to become The Drug Enforcement Agency.

Over-the-Counter review is begun to enhance the safety, effectiveness and appropriate labeling of drugs sold without prescription. Wyamine inhalers—the last source of decent OTC speed (mephentermine)—are pulled from the shelves.

Sneaky things go on behind the scenes in the pill world. We've got the FDA outlawing over-the-counter drugs by the bushel, Dan Quayle and George Bush acting as Eli Lilly trade reps, Hillary Clinton's naked attempt to take over pill manufacturing and dispensing . . . not to mention the government's ever-tightening grip over the use of prescription and non-prescription drugs by everybody in the country.

The government has even taken to sending in SWAT teams to terrorize people who dare to supplement their diets with "forbidden" nutrients.

Since 1991, the FDA has summarily banned hundreds of non-prescription items from chamomile to codeine from making any sort of claim. This trend started around 1989 when FDA Kommissar Frank E. Young banned the sale, possession and consumption of the amino acid tryptophan, even though he knew then and knows now that tryptophan is not dangerous at all. Tryptophan occurs naturally in cottage cheese, turkey and human flesh. It is, in fact, an essential nutrient the body cannot do without.

"We don't care whether no one was hurt by Dr. Wright and the so-called medicines he dispensed or treatments he gave," said the Headquarters Enforcement Staff FDA Insider. "He and his PR firm can submit all the testimonials they want from patients who claim he's given them back their health or made them well. What he is doing is injecting products into people and dispensing therapies that have not been approved or authorized by the FDA. That's against the law and we're going to put him out of business."

Compare this to the FDA's reaction to the discovery of syringes and other foreign objects in Pepsi cans. Within 24 hours of the first reports, the FDA's David Kessler was on *Nightline* declaring the discoveries to be hoaxes. He promised to investigate anyone who claimed to find foreign objects in a Pepsi can, bragging how some people were already on their way to five-year jail sentences.

He never pulled a single Pepsi from a single store.

Patenting Nature

Young's decision, though he used a freak poisoning of a batch of tryptophan made in Japan as his pretext, had little to do with public safety. The real reason is social control. This is made clear by what has happened since.

Since the banning of tryptophan—used by millions to promote sleep and improve mood —FDA cops have used battering rams and illegal police raids to halt its use. They have closed down entire chains of stores selling health food products and zeroed in on Dr. Jonathan Wright from Kent, Washington, who used naturopathic medicine more than the AMA thinks he should have. Dr. Wright also had some tryptophan. Pure tryptophan. One morning, a number of police agencies, including the FDA, burst guns drawn into Kent's offices, confiscated his files, ripped out his telephones and closed down his practice.

Since his arrest, Dr. Wright continues to be hassled by the authorities as he fights for the return of his property and practice. The FDA is quite candid about making an example of him.

Recently the FDA has been considering banning the use of guar gum—an inert filler—because it may constitute a "choking hazard." There has never been a single case of anyone choking on guar gum, but it is popular in OTC diet pills because it tends to expand in the stomach, producing a sense of fullness that deters some people from overeating.

Looking at these examples we see a common theme. The items most likely to be banned are not owned or patented by anyone.

Prune juice is a laxative and the FDA knows it. It also knows there are people out there who have paid good money to market a proprietary laxative who don't want competition. At the same time, companies that make and sell patented or trademarked laxatives know the hand that giveth can easily taketh away. It's not likely for drug manufacturers to squawk about the FDA, the government agency formed to protect the money players from underlings.

But if prescription drug makers had it their way, there would be far fewer barriers between customers and their product. A purely profit-motivated company would heed safety precautions to protect itself from lawsuits and dead or dissatisfied customers switching to competitive products (which is the same thing more or less).

The FDA's blatant use of a tainted batch of tryptophan to outlaw that amino acid has become emblematic of this trend. It's sickening that we must even argue about it. Tryptophan is not only safe—it's essential for human survival.

Still, the government gets certified experts to testify under oath that common substances should be regulated away from the hands of plain old citizens (whose only true function is to man the assembly lines, grow corn and shut up).

It is money that makes such people lie and conspire to make their fellow Americans miserable. No better example of the raw greed and deceitful intentions exist than one Dr. Richard Wurtman.

It's one thing to believe Bristol-Myers has a stake in the outcome of this or that tax bill, but it's quite another to find a single person who so clearly personifies the lying and malignant nature of today's government.

In an article by M. Greene and A. Byrd, which appeared in issue #13 of the excellent 'zine *Alter or Abolish,* the authors explain how business has a direct interest in the banning of non-patentable, naturally occurring substances. By obtaining "use-patents" on common items, jackasses hope to make money off something God gave us all. For now, "use-patents" fully explain the rationale behind the crazy crusade against natural dietary supplements. Yep, there's a method to this madness. Read on about one of the slimiest, lyingest elite bastards ever to elbow his way into your life:

> The king of "use-patents" has to be Dr. Richard Wurtman, a professor at the Massachusetts Institute of Technology. A recent search of U.S. patents revealed that Wurtman owns over twenty use patents on various medical applications of supplementary amino acids. Interestingly enough, he owns two use-patents on—you guessed it—L-Tryptophan: U.S. Patent #4,687,763 for increasing brain serotonin levels—to make you feel relaxed and good—and U.S. Patent

1972 The BNDD proposes restricting the use of barbiturates on the grounds that they are "more dangerous than heroin."

1973 The Supreme Court endorses FDA control over entire classes of products by administrative regulation. The ruling effectively prohibits any citizen from challenging FDA edict.

The FDA decertifies weight control claims for all amphetamines.

1976 The Vitamins and Minerals Amendments narrowly stops the FDA from regulating nutritional supplements as drugs.

The FDA bans the use of chloroform in all drugs and cosmetics as a suspected carcinogen.

1981 Nutrasweet is introduced into the U.S. Two years later it is approved for use in soft drinks.

A law signed by President Reagan nullifies the famous "Posse Comitatus" act, which forbids U.S. military to function against U.S. citizens on U.S. soil. Reagan orders the military to work with various civilian drug enforcement agencies.

1982 Tamper-Resistant Packaging Regulations are issued by the FDA as a result of deaths caused by cyanide-laced Tylenol capsules. The Federal Anti-Tampering Act passes in 1983, making it a federal crime to tamper with packaged consumer products.

1983 The Orphan Drug Act enables the FDA to promote research, approval and marketing of drugs needed for treating rare diseases, which otherwise would not be profitable to pharmaceutical companies.

The immunsuppressant drug, cyclosporine (isolated from a soil sample), is approved for use in the U.S.

1984 The Fines Enhancement Laws of 1984 (and 1987) amend the U.S. Code to greatly increase penalties. The maximum fine for individuals is now $100,000 for each offense and $250,000 if the violation is a felony or causes death.

Quaaludes are outlawed. Two years earlier they had gone from unrestricted to Schedule II.

#4,377,595 for reducing depression—to keep you from feeling tense and bad.

The ultimate hypocrisy is that Wurtman testified before the House Subcommittee last year on the side of the FDA. He stated that all amino acids are toxic and should be taken off the OTC market. He implored Congress to ban the sale of amino acids. He stated that "L-Tryptophan has nothing to do with nutrition." All the while he is secretly accumulating use patents. Unfortunately Wurtman is not the only greedy profiteer working on getting 'use patents' on nutritional supplements to benefit themselves at the expense of our health and well-being.

L-Tryptophan causes the body to produce serotonin, an important brain neurotransmitter. Serotonin is a natural pain killer, stress reducer and anti-depressant. L-Tryptophan is competitive with serotonin-affecting drugs like Prozac and Anafranil, two profitable, often dangerous drugs.

According to medical marketing media, neurological drugs that cause the production of serotonin are "hot." They are being used to treat migraine headaches, psychological problems, depression, insomnia and eating disorders. With natural L-Tryptophan out of the way, the drug companies have a free hand in the competition for serotonin-enhancing drugs and synthetic Tryptophan compounds. The winners could make billions of dollars in profits. But you and I would be the losers in this race for profit and we would pay for it with our health.

The FDA pharmocrats explained their ban of natural ingredients as "an effort to purge the nation's medicine chest of snake oil" (AP August 27, 1993). They insinuate they're doing nothing more than decertifying bizarre items like "dog grass" rather than effective medical ingredients.

But a gander at the recent list shows the FDA officially no longer considers codeine to be effective as a pain reliever. Nor does it consider aspirin to be helpful in relieving menstrual cramps. In fact, a look at this list shows a ton of things everyone knows are effective indeed. But, says the FDA, they have never been proven to be effective and therefore cannot make any claim. The Supreme Court ruled long ago that simple popularity and a history of successful use are of no value in determining anything about a drug. Therein lies the rub.

To certify a substance effective costs several million dollars at the very least. No company is going to shell out that kind of dough for anything non-patentable.

Which brings us back to herbs and vitamins and all the other stuff on the FDA's hitlist. Make no mistake about it, they mean to eradicate individuals' free access to the pharmacopoeia. For the FDA, the only good herb is a patented herb.

At the time this purge began, George Bush was boss and Eli Lilly (both ailing and American) had a virtual hotline to the president and all his men, but it strains credulity to believe this could be the work of one company. Then again, it strains credulity to believe the FDA would be so concerned with the public's use of dog grass, or aspirin.

In the meantime, we have now developed a keen interest in pill-independence and plan to provide as much "roll-your-own" information as possible on making your own medicines. This will have to include growing tips for plants like foxglove for home-production of digitalis. So, stock up on gelatin capsules and be ready. As much as we love store-bought pills, we must get back to our roots, so to speak.

The 1992 FDA List of "Unproven" Products

DIGESTIVE AID DRUG PRODUCTS
Alcohol, aluminum hydroxide, amylase, anise seed, aromatic powder, asafetida, aspergillus cryza enzymes, bacillus acidophilus, bean belladonna alkaloids, belladonna leaves (powdered extract), betaine HCl, bismuth subcarbonate, bismuth subgallate, black radish powder, buckthorn, calcium gluconate, capsicum, capsicum (fluid extract), carbon, cascara sagrada extract, catechu (tincture); catnip, chemomile flowers, charcoal (wood), chloroform, cinnamon oil, citrus pectin, onious benedictus (blessed thistle), diastase, diastase malt, dog grass, elecampane, ether, fennel acid, galega, ginger, cycline, hectorite, horsetail, huckleberry, hydrastis canadensis (golden seal), hydrastis fluid extract,

hydrochloric acid; iodine, iron ox bile, johnswort, juniper, kaolin (colloidal), knotgrass, lactic acid, lactose, lavender compound (tincture), linden, lipase, lysine HCl, mannitol, mycozyme, myrrh (fluid extract), nettle, nickel-pectin, nux vomica extract, orthophosphoric acid, papaya (natural), pectin, peppermint; peppermint spirit, phenacitin, potassium bicar-bonate, potassium carbonate, protease, prolase, rhubarb fluid extract, senna, sodium chloride, sodium salicylate, stem bromelain, strawberry, strychnine, tannic acid, trillium, woodruff.

TOPICAL ANTIFUNGAL DRUG PRODUCTS

1. *General use*—alum (potassium), aluminum sulfate, amyltricresols (secondary), basic fuchsin, benzethonium chloride, benzoic acid, benzoxiquine, boric acid, camphor, candicidin, chlorothymol, coal tar, dichlorophen, menthol, methylparaben, oxyquinoline, oxyquinoline sulfate, phenol, phenolate sodium, phenyl salicylate, propionic acid, propylbaraben, resorcinol, salicylic acid, sodium borate, sodium caprylate, sodium propionate, sulfur, tannic acid, thymol, tolindate, triacetin, zinc, caprylate, zinc propionate.
2. *Diaper rash products*—any ingredients for which antifungal claims are made.

EXTERNAL ANALGESIC DRUG PRODUCTS

1. *Diaper rash drug products*—any ingredients for which analgesic claims are made.
2. *Fever blister and cold sore treatment drug products*—allyl isothiocyanate, aspirin, bismuth sodium tartrate, camphor, capsaicin, capsicum, caposicum oleoresin, chloralhydrate, chlorobutanol, cyclomethy-caine sulfate, eucalyptus oil, eugenol, glycol salicylate, turpentine oil, zinc sulfate.
3. *Insect bite and sting drug products*—alcohol, alcohol (ethokylated alkyl), benzalkonium chloride, calamine, ergot fluid extract, ferric chloride, panthenol, peppermint oil, pyrilamine, maleate, sodium borate, trolamine salicylate, turpentine oil, zinc oxide, zirconium oxide.
4. *Poison ivy, poison oak and poison sumac drug products*—alcohol, aspirin, benzethonium chloride, benzocaine, (.5 to 1.25 percent), bithionol, calamine, cetalkonium chloride,

1984 The Drug Price Competition and Patent Term Restoration Act permits the FDA to approve applications to market generic versions of brand-name drugs without repeating the research done to prove them safe and effective. Brand-name companies can apply for a five-year extension on patent protection for new medicines to make up for time and money spent on the FDA's approval process.

1986 The Analog Substances Act makes it illegal to use or manufacture substances with effects and structures similar to existing illegal drugs. This outlaws substances not known to exist, but if they ever did exist, they would be illegal.

Ronald Reagan signs a Presidential "directive" designating drugs a matter of "national security." This does away with any Constitutional complaints citizens might have with drug enforcement operations.

1987 The Prescription Drug Marketing Act bans the diversion of prescription drugs from legitimate commercial channels.

The antidepressant fluoxetine (aka Prozac) is licensed for use in the U.S.

A Gallup poll reveals pharmacists are the most trusted among all professions.

1988 On November 18, Reagan signs the Anti-Drug Bill of 1988 to "reinvigorate" the DEA and creates the "Drug Czar," who becomes head of the entire federal drug enforcement budget.

Courts are permitted to deny drug offenders nearly all federal benefits for five to ten years. Death sentences are invoked against ill-defined drug "kingpins," as well as those convicted of "drug-related killings."

President Reagan sanctions countries involved in "money-laundering." And imposes further regulation of companies that sell chemicals which could be used to manufacture illicit drugs. The Bill authorises a "pilot program" in four states to require drug testing before allowing someone to obtain a driver's license. A positive test means loss of license for a year. This is the same law that mandates warning labels on alcoholic drinks. It also toughens child pornography laws and penalties.

chloralhydrate, chlorobutanol, chlorpheniramine maleate, creosote (beechwood); cyclomethycaine sulfate, dexpanehenol, diperodon HCl eucalyptus oil, eugenol, glycerin, clycol salicylate, hectorite hexylresorcinol, hydrogen peroxide, lead acetate, merbromin, mercuric chloride, methapyrilene HCl, panthenol, parethokycaine HCl, phenyltolokamine dihydrogen citrate, povidonevenylacetate copolymers, pyrilamine maleate, salicylamide, salicylic acid, simethicone, sulfur, tannic acid, thymol, trolamine, turpentine oil, zirconium oxide, zyloxin.

INTERNAL ANALGESIC DRUG PRODUCTS

Aminobenzoic acid, antipyrine, aspirin (aluminum), calcium salicylate, codeine, codeine phosphate, codeine sulfate, iodoantipyrine, lysine aspirin, methapyrilene fumarate, phenacetin, pheniramine maleate, pyrilamine maleate, quinine, salsalate sodium aminobenzoate.

As anyone can see, this list is bullshit. For instance, in the digestive aids section we find amylase and other enzymes produced by the body specifically to digest things. These digestive enzymes definitely do digest food. They will even do that outside of the body. Throw a piece of bread into a cup of water with a little enzyme medly (amylase and the others on the list for instance) and in a few hours, it will have been broken down into smaller units, including glucose.

And codeine doesn't treat pain?

The individual who controls chemicals through the medical policing role is the Food and Drug Administration Commissioner. The man who played the role through most the '90s was David Kessler, appointed to the job by Lilly stockholder George Bush. When Bill Clinton was elected, he kept Kessler in the plum position. Kessler decided to resign during Clinton's second term, and he replaced by Jane Henney in December, 1998. The last person we can think of to hold onto a politically-appointed office way past his bedtime was J. Edgar Hoover. And he did it through blackmail.

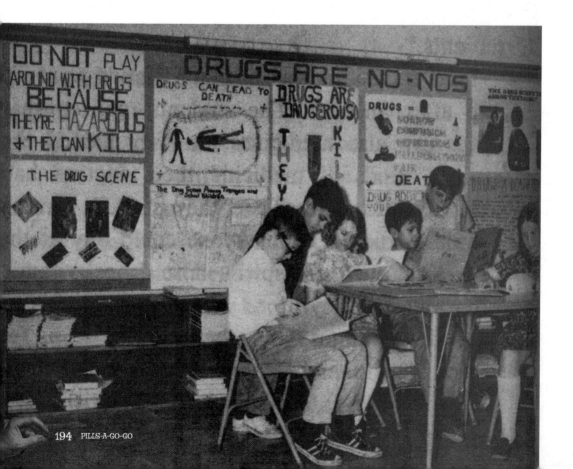

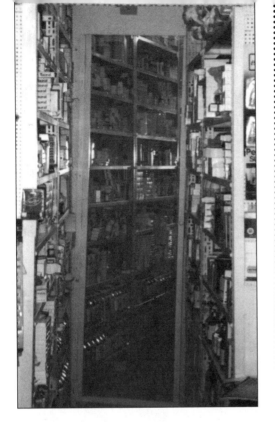

BREAKiNG iNTo A PHARMACY

Some drugstore cowboys post their dreams online. The following comes from an individual known as "Phreex."

I overheard two men talking, there conversion went something like this:

"It's not like we all haven't thought about it before . . . if one could frolic freely in a pharmacy it would be a wet-dream for the pharmie junkie . . . lets give some serious (hypothetical) thought to this. . . .

First, one would need to find a pharmacy to target . . . any big chain store (e.g., Eckards, Wallgreen) is OUT OF THE QUESTION! As an employee of a large pharmacy chain I can attest to one thing—the security is IMMACU-LATE! There's NO (practical) way in without alerting the authorities, and they respond FAST! So, it's obvious one would need to find a smaller "mom 'n' pop" place with slack security (keep in mind Eckards invested nearly $30,000 in their security for one store—that's more then mom 'n' pop can afford!

1988 The Food And Drug Administration Act of 1988 officially establishes the FDA as an agency of the Department of Health and Human Services with a Commissioner of Food and Drugs appointed by the President.

RU-486 (the abortion pill) is released on the French market. The two-pill treatment induces an abortion up to seven weeks after egg fertilization.

A battery-powered patch, developed by Drug Delivery Systems, uses a weak electric current to increase absorption of drugs in the skin beneath the gadget.

1988 The U.S. Department of Justice agrees to an out-of-court settlement with victims of its mind control experiments involving (among other things) unsuspecting citizens being dosed with various hallucinogens, then surveilled to observe their behavior. Some victims develop lifelong mental problems as a result of this treatment.

1992 The Generic Drug Enforcement Act imposes severe penalties for illegal acts involving approval of abbreviated drug applications.

The Prescription Drug User Fee Act of 1992 requires manufacturers to pay fees for drug and biologics applications and supplements. In addition, these firms must pay an annual establishment fee and annual product fees. The FDA will use these funds to hire more reviewers to assess applications.

The FDA approves the use of an effective migraine drug called sumatriptan (Imitrex).

1994 The Dietary Supplement Health And Education Act establishes specific labeling requirements to provide a regulatory framework, authorizing the FDA to promote good manufacturing practices for "dietary supplements" and "dietary ingredients," classifying them as food.

The Anti-Crime Bill of 1994 raises penalties for drug crimes even more, outfitting the coastguard to run new aircraft and more radar balloons to watch for illegal drug shipments.

Location is also important as you DON'T want anyone to have a clear view of you inside the store . . . you should also consider your escape—its best to park FAR AWAY and WALK as any car in the area could be an easy target for police! There should be other buildings around or SOMETHING to give you cover (woods, whatever). A nice residential neighborhood would be nice as you could hide in backyards or take a family hostage if need be!

Once you have a pharmacy, you need to case the outside, considering things such as:

- access to power meter
- access to the telephone network interface
- access to a window or door (for entry/exit)
- lighting
- external security such as cameras or alarms
- visibility to others

If all looks good outside, case the inside . . . consider things such as:

- motion detectors
- cameras
- physical security such as gates, bars, etc.
- location of entrance (e.g., will that back door take you into a stock room?)

- visibility from the outside (can people see you?)
- lasers
- battery back-up lights (more on this later)

Now, we have a target store . . . we can access everything we need to kill the alarm and we think we would have sufficient cover . . . we now need to find out WHERE the goodies are kept. Chances are the CII goodies will be either:

- hidden

or

- locked up

So, if you can go get yerself a script for some CII drug and go to the pharmacy weeks before you plan to do anything and OBSERVE where the pharmacist gets the drugs from: is it a drawer? a cabinet? Also keep in mind CII drugs might be moved after the store closes so look for anything like a safe!

For the truly paranoid, have someone else observe while the actual script holder wanders around doing something non-suspicious!

You now know what you need to watch for and where you need to go . . . let's (hypotheti-

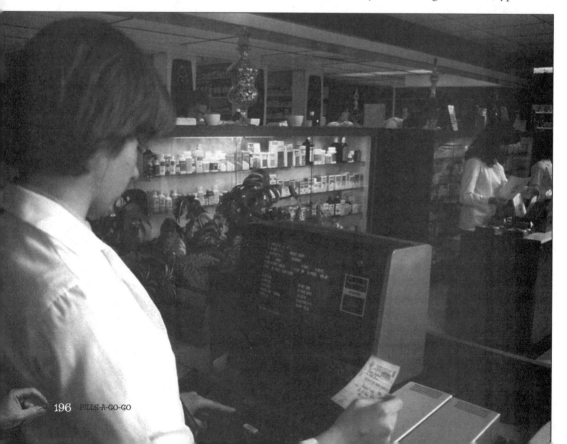

cally) think about what would be involved in the actual "getting in and getting the shit" process. . . .

Some tools are needed for this, here's an incomplete list:

- ✔ wirecutters for cutting the phone line and wire "lock" on power meter
- ✔ screwdriver [+/-] for opening telephone network interface. (NOTE: a "dyke" will have all of the above—GET ONE if you can!)
- ✔ pry-bar for opening locked drawers, doors, etc. also used for smashing stuff
- ✔ a flashlight

Fashion isn't essential but there are some things to keep in mind when choosing your apparel:

- ✔ gloves—LEATHER (latex won't help you)
- ✔ DARK jeans
- ✔ a LONG-SLEEVED dark shirt
- ✔ a mask of some sort
- ✔ a backpack, or better yet, "fag-bag" hip pack for carrying tools

Something else that I consider ESSENTIAL is a POLICE SCANNER . . . this way you will be able to listen to police and alarm company radio freq's and hear if anyone is dispatched. Of course you will want headphones for the scanner! A good scanner can be picked up Radio Shack for less then $80.

I also consider a second person a MUST, as you *NEED* a lookout!

So we have our store, we know where to go, and we have our tools . . . let's talk about security systems for a minute. . . .

There are a few types of alarm systems . . . the first type is a "no news is good news" system. Basically it's your typical alarm that, upon receiving a report of trouble (e.g., broken windows, motion detector) dials the alarm company and alerts them . . . this type of system can be defeated by CUTTING THE PHONE LINE! We MUST have this type of alarm!

The second type is a "no news is bad news" system. Same as the above but there is a STEADY signal to the alarm company via an open phone line. If there is any trouble, the

1994 Military equipment is provided to the BATF for its onslaught on the Branch Davidian compound in Waco as a result of a warrant that uses the misinformation that the religious sect was manufacturing methamphetamine.

1995 Michael Fortier informs on Oklahoma City Bomber Timothy McVeigh after the Department of Justice threatens him with methamphetamine drug charges.

1996 Asian herbal medications such as St. John's Wort become faddish cures for depression. The anti-depressant drug Prozac becomes a media cliché.

1997 The miracle anti-impotence pill, Viagra, is released to wide acclaim. But the weight-loss drug, Fen-Phen, is withdrawn from the drug market after users complain of complications.

1998 Methamphetamine is railed against by the government, who impose crack cocaine-type penalties against possession and sale of the drug.

1999 F. Hoffman-La Roche agrees to pay $500 million and BASF of Germany a total of $225 million in fines for conspiring to fix and inflate vitamin prices internationally in the '90s.

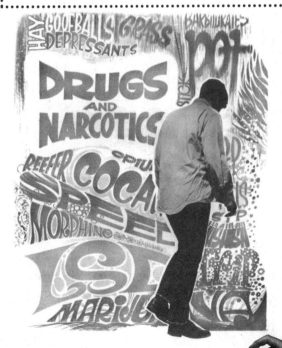

alarm company receives a signal . . . BUT if the phone line is cut (and the signal broken) then the alarm company is alerted and dispatched; we can't get around these as if we cut the phone line. We're fucked, and, of course, breaking into the store would set off the alarm. ALL the chain stores have these alarms but most mom 'n' pop places don't, as the monitoring cost is HIGH!

There are also cellular alarms that alert the alarm company via a cellular call but these seem to be rare. . . .

We want a "no news is good news" alarm and these are definitely the most common out there, also the cheapest for small-stores.

There really isn't any practical way to tell which system is in use. You could if you had a lineman's handset (aka "beige box") or use a line-voltage test meter. Even if you did, this is a risk as you could easily trip the alarm!

Its night time, about 1 am. You (and your accomplice) are at the location with tools . . . scanner tuned to the proper police frequency and you're ready to go . . . let's walk thru this the CAUTIOUS WAY!

First you need to make your way to the store (the back or some entrance where you can't be seen from the street); now its time to kill any lights. A pellet gun could come in handy but could also present a problem if any police came on the scene, so, first take out any external lights. With the lights out go for the telephone network interface—open it with a screwdriver and cut all the wires! Make sure you get the RED and GREEN wires first but cut ALL of them! With the wires cut, go ahead and close the box!

Now, listen to the scanner and HAUL ASS to a safe hiding place . . . just listen for any call of a break in; if you hear anything you know its a "no news is bad news" alarm and you need to GET THE HELL AWAY and do it fast!

If after a good HALF-HOUR you hear NOTHING and see NOTHING it's time to return to the store. The next order of business is the POWER, as those damn bells and lights can be annoying when you're trying to rob a place . . . You need to find the power meter . . . now, there might be a plastic/wire "lock" . . . if there is go ahead and break it off . . . the "face plate" of the meter will lift up . . . now, to cut the power, simply pull the meter (the glass bubble with the spinning things in it) towards you . . . careful, there's enough power in that thing to fry you! It should just be plugged in but it won't be held on with anything more then a screw, which might be holding a "collar" around it!

With the power cut, go ahead and break your entry! Whether it be breaking a window or breaking in through a door, now's the time to do it . . . again, listen to the scanner and haul ass back to somewhere where you can safely hide out for about a half-hour . . . again, we are doing this so if any law-enforcement type people would want to show up you wouldn't be there. After a good half-hour of waiting, make your approach . . . enter the store via whatever route of entry you prefer making sure no one can see you.

Now, we're inside the store . . . once I had a dream where I broke into a vet's office, in my dream (that never actually happened in real life since it would be illegal) I was surprised to find ALL the emergency lights on inside the vet. The alarm was killed but I was working under A LOT of light and anyone that drove by could have seen me . . . luckily for me I knew where the ketamine was, so it was a short stay inside the vet's office . . . in my dream, of course, that never really happened! So, be ready for something like this to (hypothetically) happen!

Once inside the store you want to get to the pharmacy as quick as you can! From here its a toss up as to what you do. Basically get to the drugs, get them, and get out . . . make sure you listen to your scanner the entire time. If you hear anything, then get out and make sure you don't leave anything behind!

Anyway, that's what I overheard two strangers talking about. . . .

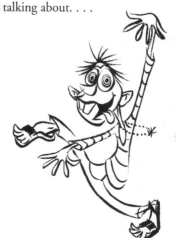

For a good three years, I had (note the past tense) the good fortune of having an almost constant supply of Vicodin and Xanax. As expected, I also had a never-ending supply of "best friends" more than willing to help me partake. Anyone who has been fortunate enough to have a good stock, be it pills, pot, or any other "illicit" material knows what I'm talking about. Freeloaders come in many forms; girls who flirt excessively, then hit you up for "just one . . . please?" Fakers stricken with whatever ailment you happen to have the pill for.

Actually, my favorite was when I was at school and this girl sitting in my group saw me slip (I thought covertly) a Vic to my friend (who happens to kick down when he's got it good). "Oooh," she squealed, "what's that? I want some, whatever it is!" She's fabulous, really. So now the whole table "wants some."

This raises the issue of drug/pill etiquette. I think that if one follows two basic rules, everyone is happy.

I like to think of pill protocol as just plain good manners, also known as the law of "do unto others." If you find yourself constantly on the receiving end of pills, something is fishy.

Conversely, if you are continually handing out your stash, you may also be known as a sucker.

While you may be racking up some good karma points (what goes around, comes around), here's a little (pointless) anecdote to illustrate; I gave out more Xanax to Nadia and Wenny than to be believed. I'm serious, I kept them medicated throughout our entire last year of college.

I mean, I figured I was getting, I may as well spread it around a little. They would take like four hits at a time, so my prescriptions would go pretty quick. Never did they bring me anything . . . I figured they didn't have a line to anything (except pot, and I don't smoke.) Well, up to Seattle these two piggies trotted to visit me. Of course they stayed with me. Hogged the Xanax and the TV. Come to find out, Wenny has a hotline to Soma and to Darvocet . . . but did she offer me any? You guess. I broke one of the rules of pill etiquette and asked her for a Darvocet. You'd think she'd have gotten the hint and given me a handful, but no . . . she kicked down ONE. Needless to say, I was much less generous from then on.

Basically, the first rule of thumb is equitability (I think I made this word up . . . you know what I mean). If you're constantly receiving, by all means, GIVE A LITTLE! IT WON'T KILL YA! If you have three pills, give one. If you have fifty, give five. It's cool . . . you get high and you spread the wealth. That's what it's all about. It's not even how much you give, per se, it's how generous you are.

The second rule (one I broke in the anecdote above) is DON'T ASK! People will give when they want to give. The chick I was talking about in the beginning asked all the time . . . and every time I told her to forget it. I really resented being placed that position. Jesus, if she wanted some, why didn't she just get her own? There was another girl, Judy, who found out that I dug/had Vic. Turns out she's a major pillhead, too, but of the worst kind. "Man, my head really hurts," she'd moan, always looking right at me. "Try some aspirin," I'd say, kind of cornered-like. She'd reply, "I did, but it's not helping. Hey, do you have, you know, anything?" "I, um, ran out, um, yesterday," I'd say.

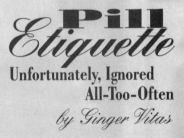

Pill Etiquette
Unfortunately, Ignored All-Too-Often
by Ginger Vitas

Then I'd have to spend the rest of the day hiding my own consumption. That really sucks. Generally, she'd hit up my friend Joker and ask him if he knew if I had "gone to the doctor lately." He'd cover for me, report back, and it would assure her not getting any. Once again, DON'T ASK! Sure, there are ways of hinting, but you have to be subtle, staying within the lines of good manners. If you want painkillers, mention a little pain. If you want speed, complain of being tired, but for god's sake, don't push it . . . even with friends. It's the surest way to end a friendship . . . and a good connection.

What about the practical aspects of pill etiquette? To be honest, there really are more than two.

1. Kick Down. I think this was covered well enough earlier. If you haven't got the idea by now, you probably never will.

2. Don't Ask. This was covered previously as well. I would like to make it clear(er) that this rule is based on subtlety. Take a good, close look at the nature of the relationship you have with your provider. Instinct (do not confuse with greed) should be a good guide.

3. If You're Gettin' It For Free, Don't Complain. Very few things are as irritating as giving away your last Vicodin (or Darvocet, or Xanax, etc.) and having the idiot you gave it to tell you that they "don't feel anything." Plenty of adjectives come to mind, including ungrateful, unthankful, wretched and inconsiderate. If you pay for something, by all means, expect your money's worth. But if it was a gift, be gracious. It was given to you with the best intentions.

4. Expect A Reasonable Return Rate. This one is tricky. What is gold to one person may be silver to another, but get real. Ten Xanax is not going to get you ten Percodan. Ten Xanax may get you two Percs, and that would be if your person is generous. Sometimes dealing is the best policy here. It can avoid hurt feelings and paranoia that you're being taken advantage of. Sometimes you win, sometimes you lose, but trades usually go smoother when terms have been discussed in advance.

5. If You Accept 'Em, Take 'Em. Otherwise don't accept them. You're only wasting the goods and depriving someone of a high (bad karma).

6. If You Accept 'Em, Don't Lose 'Em. Or if you do, don't tell. Butterfingers are butterfingers, but your generous friend doesn't need to know about them.

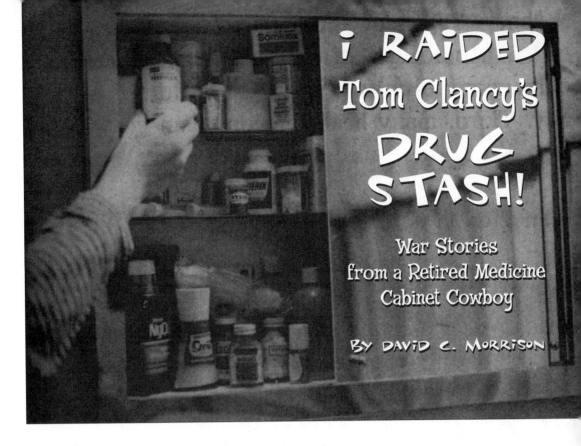

I RAIDED Tom Clancy's DRUG STASH!

War Stories from a Retired Medicine Cabinet Cowboy

BY DAVID C. MORRISON

A FEW YEARS BACK, in a rare fact-based story, *The Weekly World News* reported a news flash that came as no news to me—nor, I suspect, to any other red-blooded American pill freak. "A new study shows that two out of every five guests open medicine cabinets and snoop around in the bathrooms of homes they're visiting!" the easily shocked tabloid reported, citing the Bathroom Tissue Report, a "respected" annual survey conducted by the makers of Quilted Northern Toilet Paper. The ubiquitous Dr. Joyce Brothers, of course, was available for interview. "This confirms the basic human curiosity we all have about each other's secrets," she commented. "Guests are going to snoop."

Sorry, Dr. Joyce, but I think there's a lot more than that going on here. What the 1995 Bathroom Tissue Report really confirms is the basic human curiosity we all have about what kinds of free dope might be lurking in Grandma's medicine cabinet. The survey surely low-balls the ratio of guests cracking that cabinet door to scope out those beautiful brown prescription bottles. The Quilted Northern folks, moreover, seem utterly clueless as to the number of snoops who go on to help them-

selves to the good stuff. But you can bet that we are legion, we medicine cabinet cowboys.

Having used a little bit of everything and way too much of few things, I ran an ambitious program empirical psychopharmacological field research during an active drugging career spanning 28 years. Among other skills, I learned much about the safe, reliable and productive raiding of medicine cabinets. Advancing middle-age—and a currently drugless lifestyle—has left me feeling something of what wrinkled old Arapaho ladies must have felt around the turn of the century. Withered crones, their teeth worn down to stubs from a lifetime of gumming elk skins into silken softness, they boasted a rich harvest of obscure folkways and practical tips for surviving in a harsh and unforgiving environment—if only an indifferent new generation cared to listen to their garrulous babblings. Here, then, is my own bid to pass on some folkish wisdom of my own: How to reap the maximum take of free Percocet with the least amount of social embarrassment while inflicting the smallest amount of actual harm on your unwitting benefactors.

All of us inclined to do so learn the first things about medicine cabinet raiding where we learn the first things about most of life's mysteries: in the bosoms of our loving-or-not-so-loving-but-usually-well-medicated families. I first honed my own increasingly voracious and sophisticated appetite for pharmaceuticals swiping my mom's tiny 5 mg phenobarbital tablets and swapping regular aspirins for her Empirin 3s. Hitting the folks' stash is the perfect training ground for the novice pillhead: Because we live in a symbiotic relationship with the host organisms, we have unlimited access to their medicine cabinets and unlimited time in which to exploit that access.

Inevitably, though, the time comes to put away childish things and we move into the more challenging world at large. And what astonishing riches await in those uncharted medicine cabinets! Never is there any guarantee of what you might find. But, as with cruising for sex, half the true thrill lies in the tantalizing uncertainty of the hunt itself. In a lifetime of sneaking, peeking and taking, there's not many pills I've pondered in my dog-eared Physician's Desk Reference that I haven't eventually come across waiting patiently in some unassuming restroom: 10 mg Dolophines. 50 mg Demerols. 60 mg time-release morphine caplets. Percodans and Percocets and Roxicets and Tyloxes and all the other members of the justly acclaimed oxycodone family in numbers beyond counting. Not to mention pecks and quarts of hydrocodone bitartrate and, less interestingly, codeine phosphate, in all their many splendid forms: elixers, tablets and capsules. And, of course, depending on your tastes, the medicine cabinets of America afford the eager gleaner endless supplies of uppers (Ritalin, Dexedrine and the other attention-deficit drugs) and downers (most commonly such benzos as Valium, Xanax and so on and on and on), not to mention insulin syringes galore.

As those wizened Arapaho elders well knew, ours is a ruthless wolf-eat-wolf world. It should thus come as no surprise that the sick, the halt, the lame and the old are the best sources for the best drugs (especially if, like me, your pharmacological palate favors the drowsy, dreamy bouquet of opioid analgesics). Even better than the elderly ill are the newly dead of whatever age—especially when the loved one has passed beyond this vale of tears at home. Not only has the posthumous drug donor likely received the full brunt of modern medicine's chemical armamentarium, but he or she typically leaves behind an ample supply of Schedule II narcotics for which they no longer have any earthly use.

Unquestionably, the most astonishing find I ever stumbled across turned up at the wake for an old family friend who had just lost a lingering bout with cancer. While her surviving friends drank and talked in the living room, this medicine cabinet cowboy was scouting the bedroom/sickroom. There, waiting just for me, was a fresh prescription bottle with 130 yellow tablets, each containing 4 mg of hydromorphone, the famed "drug store heroin." Count 'em, and I did, again and again: one-hundred and thirty No. 4 Dilaudid, with a street value of upwards of $5,000.

In the end, this breathtaking windfall proved a mixed blessing. For one thing, I was "clean" at the time, and that stash of free dope provided the seeds for a killer habit I was unable to kick until nine near-ruinous months later. For another thing, the Dilaudid caper taught me how easy it can be to violate, even if wholly unintentionally, the first-do-no-harm principle that at must at all times guide the actions of the conscientious bathroom buccaneer.

One night when I was a teenage junkie, my friend Peter landed up on my doorstep with several tubes of water-soluble morphine tablets he had just liberated from his mother, then agonizingly dying in agony of ovarian cancer. How sharper than a 28-gauge needle is an ungrateful child; Peter had left the poor woman bereft of even a single grain of analgesic ease. I slammed more than my share of that morphine. But, even lulled in my deepest nod, I knew that my friend had done—by anyone's twisted morality—Something Wrong. When I was seeing my father through the final scenes of his own cancer drama many years later, I administered myself two units of morphine sulphate for every one that I gave him. But there was more than enough poppy juice to go around; Dad did not suffer unduly from my pharmaceutical parasitism.

Nor should anyone else suffer from yours. If

we medicine cabinet cowboys are to retain any shred of self-respect (we are, after all, among the pettiest of petty thieves) let us at least spare a milligram or two of consideration for our victims. Try, therefore, to know something about the current medical condition of host organism. Check the prescription date on the bottle to see whether those Percs have long since served their purpose and are simply being archived. In short, strive to discover whether your donor still needs the pills you covet.

If not, I strongly suggest that you take the whole damned bottle. Most people, frankly, are less likely to notice a vial that has gone wholly missing than they are one that has suddenly gone mysteriously half-empty. And the fact that they are so foolish as to keep desirable drugs in the medicine cabinet, where someone as singleminded as yourself might find them, suggests that your benefactors have no truly meaningful recreational interest in the substance in question. If you find yourself tossing the host's bedroom looking for the prescription cache—and I have—be aware that you are engaging in an entirely different order of thievery than mere misdemeanor medicine cabinet cowboyism. Besides —and I can't emphasize this firmly enough—by being as thorough as possible on the first pass and liberating all of a neglected 'script, you can avoid those ugly lingering regrets about the pills you left behind that assuredly will torment you once your immediate stash is consumed.

Conversely, if the prescription is still in active use, strive to be as conservative in your borrowings as your needs and desires can possibly allow. Foremost is the obvious humanitarian consideration: Why should anyone have to suffer discomfort just because you want to get loaded? In my cabinet cracking career, this ethical dilemma has presented itself in many and varied guises. On one occasion, while perusing the offerings in a friendly bathroom, I came across a dozen 5 mg tablets of pure hydrocodone, prescribed (inexplicably, it seemed to me) to their Bassett Hound, Ed. Being a dumb creature, Ed was unlikely to bitch and moan about the loss. So I took the lot. Later, upon confessing my sin, these friends explained that Ed had had to endure a nasty case of kennel cough, albeit uncomplain-

ingly, after his antitussives so oddly went missing. Ed forgives me, I'm sure. I still have nightmares of walking out of an Narcotics Anonymous meeting to be greeted by angry animal rights activists armed with picket signs: "Hycodan for Hounds, Not Hogs!"

There is a practical aspect to the first-do-no-harm principle, too: An excessive number of pills missing from a bottle being opened several times a day will be noticed. My experience has been that in many cases, civilians will be too embarrassed to confront the cowboy whose Rx rustling has come to their attention. But abuse the sickroom and the usual social graces will not protect you. Thus the recent anguished letter to Ann Landers from "Worried Sick in Newport Beach" whose idiotic greedhead sister, "Ellen," couldn't control her thoughtless gobbling up of Worried Sick's post-operative pain pills. (Ann, of course, recommended family confrontation and "professional help" for Ellen.)

Back to the great Dilaudid coup, the deceased no longer had any use for her treasure trove of hydromorphone. But her widowed husband did, it turns out. Many months later, after I had confessed my predations, he penned a tart letter saying he was "a bit pissed." The Ds were intended as "a handy suicide stash" should he ever find himself facing the same terminal pain his wife had suffered. "Now my sloppy inventory-keeping makes this next part awkward," he wrote. "There was a largish bottle of methadone tablets in that stash.... Did you cop the methadone the last time you were here?" Had I seen it, I surely would have, I wrote back, but someone else must have glommed onto the meth. I was able to ease my conscience a bit by pointing him to an equally largish bottle of Tylenol 3 I had stumbled across forgotten in an obscure corner of his kitchen. (By then, to paraphrase Cole Porter, I could get no kick from codeine, mere T-3s didn't thrill me at all.)

So much for the slippery ethical dimensions of riding the Rx range. Practical questions, too, abound. Fortunately, excretory logistics and social custom largely work in favor the medicine cabinet cowboy. Unwary civilians store their chemical treats in the bathroom. Nature, whenever She calls, conveniently provides us with a ready excuse not only for entering precisely that very room, but for locking the door firmly behind us. As any con artist will tell you, authenticity helps. Before visiting a home where there were likely to be goodies in the drug chest, I would avoid pissing beforehand so that a genuine need to use the facilities might present itself with some urgency upon my arrival. This stratagem also helps with providing realistic sound effects once you are closeted in the water closet.

Speaking of which—and here I'm addressing the male reader specifically—it is especially helpful if the drug cabinet is above or right next to the toilet so that the noise of your stream can cloak the creaking of the cabinet hinges as you pry the doors open for that first thrilling peek. (The Bathroom Tissue Report might one year explain why and how it is that four out of five medicine chests complain loudly when opened by interested strangers.) A wracking bout of faux coughing can also mask the sound of an opening cabinet, and a thorough-if-simulated handwashing with all the taps on full can cover up the telltale sound of pills rattling in bottles. Another Ann Landers column in the early 1990s struck horror through my dopefiend heart by suggesting that readers boobytrap recidivist bathroom snoops by filling the cabinet with loose marbles. Upon more mature reflection, I realized that this was more easily prescribed than accomplished. How could even the most vengeful host organism get the marbles in there in the first place?

That said, we must be as quiet as mice while ferreting out our chemical cheese. Do not, please, go hauling out pill vials by the fistful. Do not, in fact, take the bottles out of the cabinet at all, unless there are so many there you need to check the back rows. Do manipulate the bottles only as much as needed to scan the labels. Do return them to their original position so as to leave the cabinet looking just as you found it—minus, obviously, only those items you really need. Do accomplish these deeds as quickly as possible; extended stays in someone else's bathroom are sure to incite unwelcome commentary upon your red-faced return to the living room.

A studied knowledge of the *PDR* helps here. I also cannot recommend highly enough the encyclopedic *Drug Identification Bible*. Like any frontier scout, try to know what you're looking for as you survey the white tiled terrain before you. Just because a label makes reference to pain relief, for instance, don't assume that its contents are necessarily worth eating. Wholly worthless non-steroidal anti-inflammatory drugs and muscle relaxants, remember, are also prescribed for pain. If you roam much overseas, make it your business to know the offshore brand names of interesting pharmaceuticals. Eukodal is just Percocet by a German name. In the U.K., Pethedine is Demerol and Physeptone is methadone. (For the world traveler, I recommend the United Nation's excellent Multilingual Dictionary of Narcotic Drugs and Psychotropic Substances Under International Control.) Know your drugs and you'll surely find the drugs worth knowing.

Stealthily and silently, our prospector has hit pay dirt with that lovely slim brown vial containing, let's say, a couple of dozen hits of Vicodin. What now? If circumstances of the prescription are such that you can only take a few, nothing is simpler: Slip those Bad Boys into your mouth and carry on. Or slip them into a pocket for future reference. And, hey, why not wrap them first in toilet paper so the precious pills don't get lost, linty, cracked or chipped?

If you simply must have all of the pills, make sure to plug up the bottle with toilet paper. (Quilted Northern tissue would do quite adequately.) No need to have half-full bottles of someone else's medicine playing castanets in our pocket or sock for the rest of the evening. Sometimes, when opportunity knocks on the medicine cabinet door, we're not wearing clothing suited to concealing a prescription bottle. On such untoward occasions, I've been known to empty all of the pills into a pocket. Muffling the empty bottle thickly in a towel, I'd crush it under foot, secreting the shards in another pocket for disposal later. Speaking of which, never leave purloined prescription bottles laying around your base camp. At a minimum, once safely back at your own digs, peel off the labels and shred them. Better yet, crush the original containers and dump them into someone else's trash.

All of this grows vastly more complicated

when you're visiting a real house with several stories and multiple bathroom. As we've all learned to our rue, there's usually not much in those downstairs guest bathrooms save for those irritating little soap balls, even-more-irritatingly inadequate hand towels and that lone can of Comet cleanser. How to reach the Promised Land of the upstairs master bathroom?

Several opportunities commonly present themselves. If there are lots of guests, wait until the downstairs toilet is occupied and express an overriding interest in "shaking hands with the mayor." Any truly gracious host organism will promptly direct you to the upstairs convenience. Depending on the layout of the house, you might wait until all are seated at dinner before discretely announcing a need to commune with nature. While everyone else is clattering their cutlery, you are prowling your way upstairs to see what's what. This is a riskier approach, of course, and a tact so frankly sleazy that it cannot be recommended to any pill freak retaining more than a residual shred of self-respect. The social consequences of being caught pulling this stunt hardly bear contemplation. If nothing else, you are sure to see your name promptly crossed out of the Social Register.

Thankfully, there's always the I'm-dying-for-a-tour-of-your-lovely-home gambit. While you're being shown the upstairs precincts, you claim a burning need to piss and dive into the master bathroom. This threadbare tactic can actually be pulled off both graciously and believably and has stood me in good stead over the long, loaded years.

Bear in mind, though, that even the best laid plans of even the slyest mice and men oft go awry. Truly audacious medicine cabinet raiding is not for the uncommitted. If you can't stand the potential heat, stay the hell out of the bathroom! That said, having generally followed the rules and rituals laid out here, I can honestly say that I've never been badly caught, so to speak, with my pill-laden pants down. Except by my Mom. But, then, you know Moms—and my Mom sure knows me. She learned early on to hide her meds so professionally that, in time, it would take me well into the second day of a visit to find them.

In truth, though, the most crushing failure the prescription drug appropriator is likely to encounter is simply the disappointment of not finding anything worth taking. This all-too-common experience—our much-bemoaned "over-medicated society" is actually somewhat sadly under-prescribed—prompts one final war story. In this instance, a seemingly promising foray into celebrity medicine cabinet raiding resulted, anticlimactically, in crushing defeat.

Almost a decade back, I was contracted to write a profile of Tom Clancy, the superstar techno-thriller writer. After a lengthy interview under the vaulted ceiling of his cathedral-like study, I asked Clancy for a tour of his new mansion overlooking the Chesapeake Bay. Upon arriving, I'd been introduced to his then-wife (he's since traded her in for a "trophy" model, I understand). Wanda looked a bit peaked and none-too-pleased with her life—and who could really blame her? Were I married to Tom Clancy I'd be choking down all the damned Demerol and dexedrine I could get the docs to write for. I harbored high hopes for the Clancy's marital medicine cabinet. Alas, upon asking to use the john while being shown the master bedroom suite, I found nothing but the dreariest sort of over-the-counter cold-and-headache schwag. Tom being somewhat paranoid, maybe they had the good stuff stashed somewhere else. Maybe there was no good stuff. In any event, it was not mine to find.

This medicine cabinet cowboy has since hung up his chaps and spurs. Today, in fact, most of my friends are in "recovery." There is, believe me, no pharmacological wasteland more howlingly empty than those 12-step medicine cabinets. But, when visiting new and unscouted homes, I still have a hard time resisting poking the nose I'm keeping so clean into that mirror-fronted cabinet of wonders. For old time's sake, you know, and to satisfy that "basic human curiosity."

In 1905, at a time when so-called muckraking journalists were exposing corruption in business and government, Samuel Hopkins Adams, writing for *Collier's* magazine, set out on a crusade against the evils of patent medicines. Calling worthless and harmful nostrums "the great American fraud," Adams blamed the injury to the public not only on producers, but also on "advertising bunco men." He called the industry a "shameful trade," and he thundered: "Every man who trades in this market takes toll of blood."

Adams' articles appeared at the right moment; for years, Americans had been growing increasingly aware of the menace in fake remedies. In 1906 Congress passed the Pure Food and Drugs Act, which permitted the sale of narcotics as medicine but required the labeling of all dangerous ingredients. Even under this early, limited legislation, many nostrums were forced off the market; for the remainder, manufacturers either altered the formulas or rewrote the labels.

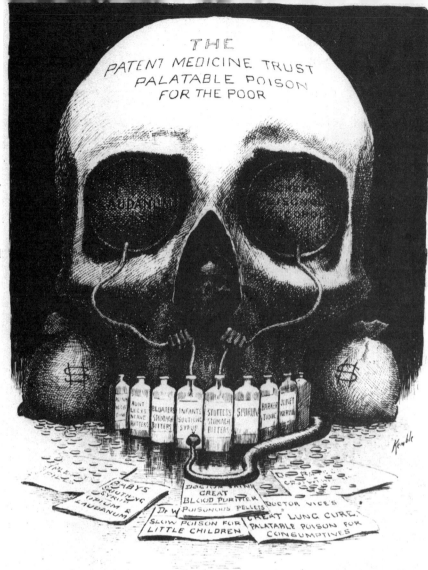

"Death's Laboratory," an advertising cartoon for *Collier's* magazine, promotes Samuel Adams' magazine articles on the patent-drug industry. In this medley of symbols, a grotesque skull leers malevolently, with barrels of alcohol and narcotics in its eyes and bottles of medicines forming its teeth. The shadowy creature filling the bottles is a bitter parody of the glamorous women featured in patent-medicine advertisements.

"Throughout history, the power that many psychoactive drugs have exerted over the behavior of human beings has been variously ascribed to gods or demons. We ascribe magical powers to substances, as if the joy is inside the bottle. Our culture has no sacred realm, so we've assigned a sacred power to these drugs. This is what [Alfred North] Whitehead would call 'the fallacy of misplaced concreteness.' We say, 'The good is in that Prozac powder,' or 'The evil is in that cocaine powder.' But evil and good are not attributes of molecules."

—Daniel Perrine, *The Chemistry of Mind-Altering Drugs*, quoted by Joshua Wolf Shenk in the May, 1999 issue of *Harper's*.

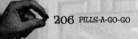

"New doc in town." The defrauder has his own script pads printed up; the office number listed on the pad is actually a phone booth. An accomplice takes the script in while a partner waits at the phone. When the pharm calls to verify, the con artist answer the phone, saying he's the doc, approving transaction.

Offender can call pharmacy and say he's a narc detective and there's a con man under surveilence about to approach the pharm w/bogus script. The "officer" tells the pharm to fill the script, explaining the police will then make an arrest. Of course, police never arrive . . .

A couple of bright thieves in Wisconsin managed to rip off a pharm by walking in during normal working hours, going into the adjacent room, and removing a few flimsy ceiling tiles and crawling up it, then making off with pharm cocaine, morphine, etc. Ten grand worth.

I've been dumpster-diving for Tussionex for awhile now, following chaos' advice, I got a script for 6 oz's Tues. night. I took about 3 oz's that night driving home from the pharmacy. After about an hour or so I wasn't that impressed, so I took 4 vikes and had a few vodka & grapefruit cocktails—finally caught a fair to midland buzz. The next day I took the other 3 oz's for breakfast on an empty stomach. After a few hours I still needed a few vikes for an appreciable buzz. Thanksgiving day, went to the rents house for food and leftovers, a few towns away. Thought I'd check a few new pharm dumpsters on the way home. The first one I almost didn't get out of the truck to check 'cause it looked empty. 1 bag, cut it open and gently dump the contents onto the floor of the dumpster. Out rolls a bottle of tuss, like a golden ray of light. The only way to get it out is to climb in, which I rarely do. The tuss bottle is capped, sides fully coated with ½ inch on the bottom. Since I was already inside, I did a thorough search of the contents of this one bag. Pulled out 3 more pint bottles, all capped. 1-hydrocodone and homatropine syrup (5 mg hydrocodone/tsp). 2-prometh w/codeine cough syrup (10 mg codeine phosphate/tsp). 3-acetaminophen and codeine oral solution (12 mg codeine phosphate/tsp). Said to myself,

Getting Pills

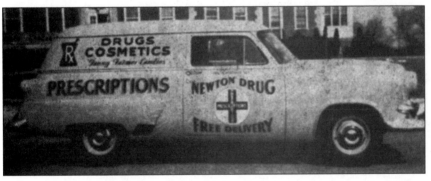

—from the Painkiller email Group

my work here is done. 1 for 1, not bad, headed home. I ran 6–8 oz's of vodka through the three non-tuss bottles, poured that into the tuss bottle & add grapefruit juice almost to top (leave room for vigorous agitation). Drank my cocktail, savoring every sip. Within an hour I'm exactly where I want to be. A pleasant and energetic place.

As far as scoring drugs right from the factory, a friend of mine told me a tale of a dope fiend he knew, someone whose pill jones would put most our habits to shame.

His pill of choice was percodan, although he always seemed to have half-gallon jugs full of Tussionex stashed and he would line up shot glasses for shooters before the guys went downtown Chicago to bar-hop. Somehow he had a massive connection for the stuff. . . .

He was always scamming: busting scripts from stolen script pads nicked from one of the many docs he had, rifling through the medicine cabinets of anyone . . . you get the drift.

One day he manages to get his mitts on a wholesale catalog from DuPont Pharma, the maker of his treasured percodan. So he sets up a fake mailing address at the post office as a new doctor, completes the paperwork and sends in an order for, like, 1,000 hits.

The only reason he wasn't arrested was the phone call he got from his postal worker friend informing him the feds were there waiting for him.

Importing Prescription Pharmaceuticals

While there may be one thousand and one ways of scamming meds in one's hometown, there are really only two methods that work elsewhere: travel extensively or find a way of getting foreigners to send you pills.

The average pillfiend knows that the laws in this country which govern the substances we may ingest, are insane—caught between the Drug War, a nit-picky, over obsessive FDA and pharmaceutical companies that charge us privileged Americans two or three times the usual cost for pills.

A new world opened up to pill takers of every stripe several years ago when laws relating to Americans and foreign pharmaceuticals were changed in two areas:

An international treaty was signed, allowing travelers to hold onto any meds obtained legally for legitimate reasons in another country. Few countries in the world have a medical system as regulated as the U.S., and what doctors prescribe without any sort of formal, written document in their country may be tightly controlled here. An American who was prescribed something abroad could no longer have their remaining supply confiscated upon re-entry to the U.S. ("importation"), provided, for instance, that they hadn't taped hundreds of sheets of diazepam tabs to their body, as did two women nabbed by Customs as they crossed the foot bridge at Laredo with 9000 hits of Valium, each taping 4,500 pills to their abdomens and asses in the attempt to look pregnant.

Since 1988, the FDA and US Customs allowed individuals to import foreign prescription drugs under the FDA Policy on Medication Importation. This very unusual move on the part of the FDA resulted from the agency's own realization that huge numbers of people with HIV/AIDS were dropping dead before the painfully long approval processes on break-through drugs were even close to over. How long an average? (I doubt the FDA would've moved a muscle, had it not been for AIDS activists.)

But macabre as it may be, AIDS-victims' pain was our gain. The FDA ruling was a pilot program and could be revoked at any time it considered the program "abused." It has allowed for all kinds of nonsense-by-mail.

These are the Rules

U.S. laws on the importation of medication are pretty hazy, and it's difficult to squeeze answers out of officials. Whether traveling abroad or importing via mail, there are a couple of very basic but important rules to follow.

The product must be purchased for personal use (same as coming back from Mexico). The number of pills allowed are a 90-day supply; and though Customs doesn't keep a booklet of numbers, such a supply is not hard to figure out.

Mexico, of course, remains a hot spot for pharmaceutical drug purchase, as does Canada. One reason is the ability to get drugs there over-the-counter for which one needs prescriptions in the States.

In Canada, for example, there are the cheap OTC "222s" (codeine/caffeine/aspirin or acetaminophen) tablets. The codeine pill hack section of this book tells you how to eliminate the liver-damaging acetaminophen that comes attached to it.

Another reason is cost. In 1992, a price study of 121 drugs found that 98 of them were significantly higher-priced, generally by 50% or more in the United States than over the border in Canada. At that time, for example, Xanax was 225% higher priced in the U.S., Zantac was 40% higher, and Premarin 190% more costly. Groups of Senior Citizens from Minnesota and other states close to Canada often rent buses for pill-buying tours to Canada. And the same thing happens to seniors in California, Arizona, New Mexico and Texas.

At the Mexican border, what do you think might be looked-out for, aside from weapons, fruit fly-tainted mangos and knock-off designer clothes?

Though it's true the vast majority of Customs' drug watch involves probing coke-laced oil tankers and heroin-packed Hispanic rectums, a chintzy box of foreign diazepam does seem to be worth their time.

"U.S. Customs seizes merchandise that a traveler or importer attempts to import in violation of U.S. on behalf of over 40 agencies (including the FDA and DEA)."

Mail Order Dos and Don'ts

Like shoplifting and a number of other illicit pastime activities, ordering pharmaceuticals through the mail used to be a piece of cake. Just as you used to be able to waltz out of even the largest department store with an ungodly amount of merchandise stuffed down your pants, it was just as easy to take advantage of the lax pharmaceutical laws of India, China and Thailand. But not any more.

There are many things U.S. Customs can and can't do with your package.

Customs is able to legally open any package without a search warrant, unless it appears to be correspondence, or they have an existing warrant, which allows them to rifle through your personal mail.

During a one year period encompassing most of 1997, Customs dogs sniffed out 303,380 pills and capsules which were seized by agents. This was before they began routinely opening personally-addressed packages entering the country sometime in mid-1998. Whether this unspoken new rule is a result of pressure from the DEA, Customs and/or the FDA, is

hard to say, but the order obviously came from somewhere.

On newsgroups, individuals have told about their experiences buying mail-order pharmaceuticals from overseas pharmacies. The ratio of seizures happens to be near one-third of all orders especially from well-known overseas companies, especially from Thailand, like International Pharmacy. But others have told about their good luck obtaining Valium (diazepam), codeine, Vicodin and other non-Schedule II drugs. Some posters have talked about getting a form in the mail from Customs, telling them their package has been seized, but they're welcome to visit Customs to talk about the problem. No one ever admitted going to Customs to try to talk them out of their supposedly illegitimate package.

The best way to obtain foreign mail order pharmaceuticals is to order your goods from a discreet and not-very-well known entity; if found broadly posted on the internet, it seems unlikely to be a safe place from which to order. If pharmacies were found posted in a book, that's also a sure indication of their material under watch by Customs or the Postmaster. That's why you won't see any posted in this book.

But it seems the worst thing that can happen in a foreign order for pills is that you lose your money, and that you're placed on some sort of DEA watch list. That doesn't seem so bad, and worse situations can happen to drug buyers.

Drugs like diazepam was once widely available in Los Angeles and New York in Mexican bakeries and even drug stores, but police crackdowns in 1998 have temporarily weaned them of this practice.

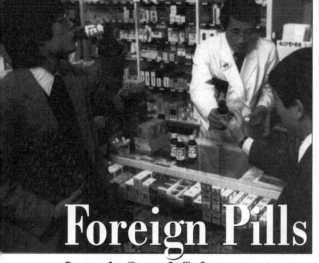

Foreign Pills

Japan's Speed Culture, "Fight in a bottle"

Japan—where test data was considered the quintessential example of sloppy and dangerous science until a couple years ago—has a pill culture all its own. Not only can you get some wild concoctions over-the-counter, something like half of a Japanese doctor's income comes from pills he sells directly to patients. Prescription drugs in Japan are less likely to have been extensively tested and consequentially, more pills are available. American companies are beginning to team up with Japanese pharmaceutical makers in droves. Will this bring more Japanese pills and Japanese pill culture our way? Or vice-versa?

Already some of our neatest pills (Pepcid and Noroxin are a couple) come from Japan. Japanese-American joint ventures and mutual trade compacts between firms in both countries suggest a lot of biotech drugs should be coming our way from Japan soon.

Japanese drive to business success has created a culture for a curious kind of "tonic" drink, called *eiyo*. Considered more than a soft drink and not quite a pharmaceutical, *eiyo* drinks occupy a special niche in the Japanese marketplace. More than a fourth of all pharmaceuticals sold in Japan are *eiyo* drinks.

Typically, tonic drinks are slugged down by slave/businessmen who work more than a 100-hour week and still manage to avoid a peculiar kind of Japanese

fate: *karoshi*, or "being worked to death." But the energy elixers are also consumed by cramming students, hangover sufferers, and presumably, partyers who need just one more ounce of strength to bop 'til they drop.

Named things like "Real Gold" (made and marketed by Coca-Cola) and "I am King," the drinks come in small brown bottles, each containing 50 to 100 mls of a special mixture of essential ingredients. While nearly all the tonic drinks have healthy doses of caffeine, ephedrine and nicotine (gets the old heart moving), each includes its own characteristic power ingredients. Various amino acids, ginseng, royal jelly, powdered deer antler, and viper extract are just some of the crucial ingredients found in *eiyo* drinks.

The first tonic drink was introduced in Japan in 1962 when a daring company abandoned pill-form nutritional supplements to market "Lipovitan D." It remains the leading *eiyo* drink in Japan, where the market is saturated and has begun to expand to other parts of Asia. Thais, for instance, drink more than 100,000 bottles of Lipovitan D a year and the company is aiming to take over Indonesia and Taiwan.

Eiyo drinks are tightly bound to ideas of endurance, success, and courage. They promise bursts of "fight" and the ability to "fight" for 24 hours straight. Some drinks are associated with blue collar workers while others are targeted at white collar "salarymen."

In fact, the drinking of the mostly lemon-flavored shots of adrenaline boosters has taken on subtle, ritualistic meaning to the Japanese. A cartoon depicts the abject shame of a balding salaryman as two co-workers remark that their colleague has never received a gift of Arinamin V from the big boss. One of the pencil-pushers brags that he's gotten a bottle from the boss two times already, putting him far above the "C-class salaryman" who has been ignored.

For the boss to give a bottle of crude speed to an underling is a sign of approval, that the boss considers him a valuable employee.

Pill Scandal Rocks Japan

While Americans remembered the December 7th sneak attack on Oahu, it was pills, not pearls, that grabbed the attention of the Japanese.

Yet another stampede of scandals rocking corruption-rife Japan hit the front pages on Pearl Harbor Day as Meiwa Industries, a distributor for Yamanouchi Pharmaceuticals, one of Japan's largest manufacturers of prescription medicines, was accused of re-routing some six million pills, capsules, and ampules specially priced for low-cost consumption in the People's Republic of China to the far more pricey Japanese domestic market. The Yomiuri newspaper reported that Meiwa and its Chinese partners reaped a windfall ¥650 million ($6.1M) from the illegal diversion of the ulcer-related medications. Both Yamanouchi and Meiwa have denied complicity and termed the incident "regrettable."

Pills have long been a substantial Japanese export item to China and southeast Asia. Until now, less affected than other industries by the devastating recession that hit Japan along with falling land prices and restricted lending since 1991, the pharmaceutical giants have maintained a steady flow of pills to the Asian mainland, backed by fat subsidies in the form of national health insurance and guaranteed Japanese government loans for research and development.

But peddling pills in Beijing is apparently not the way to turn a fast buck. The six million wayward pills from Yamanouchi that should have hit the shops at ¥23 (21 cents) in the People's Republic sold for a hefty ¥112 each ($1.05) in Japan, the normal domestic price.

Pills manufactured for export cannot be legally sold in Japan, but the enormous gap between domestic and export prices makes this commercial sleight-of-hand an attractive proposition. Export medicines reach their destinations unencumbered by local Japanese taxes or by cuts taken by middlemen in the Byzantine Japanese domestic distribution racket. Long-range business planning

also plays its part. Backed by the political muscle of the Health and Welfare Ministry and supported by loans from stockholding banks, the Osaka-based drug industry has long seen market share—not profit—as the grail of its southern and westward expansion. Pills bound for Asia are sold there at (or sometimes below) cost, partly in order to drive out admittedly inferior local products. Since development costs are not tacked onto government-produced pills in China, Japanese corporations have to cut their margins to near zero in order to muscle onto the shelves of thousands of Chinese hospitals and corner drug stores.

Pills sold at prices like these in Japan, however, would destroy price structures carefully erected there to sustain big manufacturers. The same drugs are therefore separated into those for sale overseas and those for domestic use, a situation that has existed openly, but quietly, for some time. Commenting on the situation, however, a spokesman for Yamanouchi declared that cheaper pills are sent to China "in order to contribute to medicine in the People's Republic."

So what does all this mean? Lots, if you're taking the pulse of Japan, because it involves pharmaceutical houses with impeccable financial credentials, the Meiwa/Yamanouchi case underscores the seriousness of the recession now ravaging Japan, Inc. Though fraud is no stranger to Japan, the distribution affiliates of Yamanouchi and other major drug houses would not have needed windfall profits, or the scams that produce them, some years ago. Friendly banks, seeing no point in devaluing their investments, rarely called in the loans of companies whose stocks they owned. From the banks' viewpoint, debt-heavy companies speculated—with borrowed money—in land. As long as land was going up faster than the interest rate, banks were more than willing to pour in more cash.

Hospitals, too, did well. Subsidized by the government's national health plan, and paid lucrative commis-

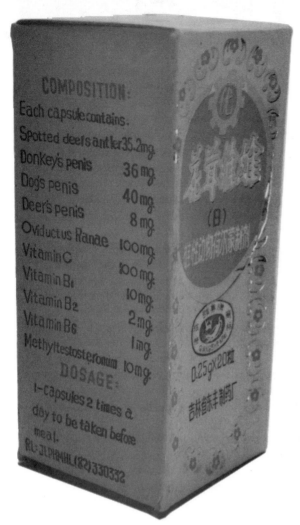

COMPOSITION:
Each capsule contains.
Spotted deer's antler 35.2mg.
Donkey's penis   36 mg.
Dog's penis   40 mg.
Deer's penis   8 mg.
Oviductus Ranae   100 mg.
Vitamin C   100 mg.
Vitamin B₁   10 mg.
Vitamin B₂   2 mg.
Vitamin B₆   1mg.
Methyltestosteronum 10mg.
DOSAGE:
1-capsules 2 times a.
day to be taken before
meal.

The Yamanouchi scandal does not signal a government crackdown on pill manufacturers. It was a major newspaper, not the public prosecutor's office, that investigated the scam and aired the charges, an unusual development for Japan.

In a country so awash in pills that books on how to take them reach best-seller status, it is unlikely that efforts to discredit or even reform such big buck-earners will be taken soon. But the episode does illustrate the depth of the economic problems now facing the country. Heavily in debt, even the once unassailable drug houses need cash, and need it quickly. Like the fleet its navy devastated in Hawaii long ago, Japan and its giant corporate pill-makers are slipping, wounded, out to sea, desperately seeking time and cover to regroup.

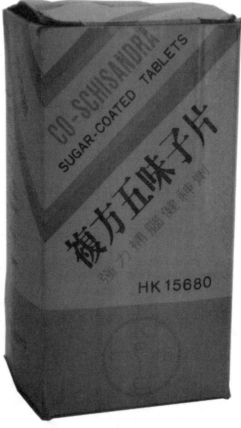

sions by manufacturers, doctors did (and still do) dispense more pills per patient than any country in the world. With doctors as their virtual sales reps and banks eager to provide the cash, Yamanouchi and other drug makers on Midosuji street in Osaka enjoyed the '80s the way Drexel, Burnham, Lambert enjoyed the Reagan years on Wall Street in New York.

Until, that is, the land price bubble burst. When that happened in late 1990, the collateral that Japan Inc. put up on all those loans began to shrink in value. More assets had to be hocked to cover previously borrowed money. Less money was there for drug development, new marketing campaigns, or diversification into other industries. Worse, new loans dried up as banks saw the value of collateral go south. With their fuel tanks nearing empty, Japanese companies put the brake on the rush for market share overseas and began what was unthinkable only five years before: layoffs.

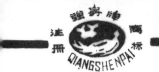

花茸维雄（B）

ANTLERVIRON(B)

雄是一种强力的雄性动物荷尔蒙制剂，由中国名贵产品梅□三种动物的鞭，还配伍哈士蟆油、多种维生素等，用科学方□而成。较其他单一补剂作用全面，经常服用功效显著，使人□增强荷尔蒙作用。

□茸在我国医学界早有记载，认为是不易获得的男性激素，尚□、碳酸钙、胶质等成份。其功用为助阳强筋骨。

□鞭、鹿鞭等属天然的生物雄性激素药品，与哈士蟆油、多种□服用，易被人体吸收，起着特殊的滋补营养作用。

□：
□丸内含：

□花鹿茸精	35.2毫克
□鞭	36毫克
□鞭	40毫克
□鞭	8毫克
□士蟆油	100毫克
□生素C	100毫克
□生素B₁	10毫克
□生素B₂	2毫克
□生素B₆	1毫克
□基睾丸素	10毫克

□：
□殖器发育不良、无睾症、先天性睾丸发育不全。

□经衰弱诸症：例如早泄、阳痿、性欲减退、以及腰膝酸痛。

□机体活力、心脏活动、消除心肌疲劳等作用。

□年男子衰老现象的预防与治疗。

□用于妇女更年期的一些妇科疾病。

每日二至三次，每次1粒。需要时可每次服2粒。
儿童忌服。

0.25克×20粒。

密闭于阴凉干燥处保存。

吉卫药准字 （83） 330332

吉林省东丰制药厂

Antlervi□on□is a′ strong animal androgen tonic elaborately preqared from spotted deer′s antler, a famous and valuab′e drug produced in China, together with three kinds of animal penes oviductus ranae and multivitamin, It has more benefits than other tonics. If taken regularly, this preparaton will increase one′s energy and improve the function of hormones.

Spotted deer′s antler has long been admitted in the early Chin ese medical history as arare male sexual hormone. Further moiet, it also contains calcium phosphate, calcium carbonate and coll oid, It can strengthen bone and muscles.

The penes of donkey, dog and deer contain natural male sexual hormones. When administered together with oviductus ranae and multivitamin, they′will be easily absorbed by human body ahd have special nutritional effect.

COMPOSITION:

Each capsule contains.

Autler extract	35.2mg.
Donkey′s penis extraet	36mg.
Dog′s penis extract	40mg.
Deer′s penis extract	8mg.
Oviducts Ranae	100mg.
vitamin C	100mg.
vitamin B₁	10mg.
vitamin B₂	2mg.
vitamin B₆	1mg.
Methyltestosteronum	10mg.

INDICATIONS:

1. Maldevelopment of sexual organs, eunuchism, conge. nital hypogenesis of testes.

2. Neurasthenia sexualis such as ejaculatio praecox, impotence, lack of sexual desire, aches in loin and knees.

3. Increasing vitality and cardiac activity, relieving myo ca′jial fatigus.

4. Prevention and treatment of premature senility in the middle.aged and old men.

5. Climacteric complaints in women.

ADMINISTRA TION AND DOSAGE:

1. capsule2-3 times a day.

2. capsules each time if neco ssary.

CONTRAINDICATION:

It should not be given to children.

PACKING:

In bottles of 0.25g×20pill

STORAGE:

Keep the bottl e will closed and storein a cool and dry place.

RL: JLPHPL(82)330332

THE PHAACEUTICA I FACTORY OF DONG FENG COUNTRY IN1 JILIN PROVINCE

Pharmaceuticals
in Thailand
by an109010@anon.penet.fi

I'**ve made a number of trips** to Thailand in recent years, and I was pleased to discover early on that it is very easy to purchase pharmaceuticals (as well as various other drugs) there.

It appears that most pharmaceuticals are available without prescriptions. In Thailand, someone who is sick would most likely go to the pharmacist instead of the doctor, describe his or her symptoms and buy medication over-the-counter.

Pharmacies are everywhere! You can hardly walk ten minutes in Bangkok without seeing one. They all look more or less the same—an open storefront with a glass counter along the right side of the store and glass-enclosed shelves along the walls. These displays are jam-packed with just about every medication imaginable. Usually, the glass enclosed shelf on the left (if you're facing the store) has things like cough drops, suntan lotion, etc. The counter contains things like hydrocortisone cream. It's on the shelves along the wall behind the counter that the good stuff is kept. Much of the good stuff is in big plastic bottles of 1,000 or more pills. Other things are in boxes or smaller bottles. The pharmacies almost always have a white sign with green letters hanging out front. This sign usually also displays a green cross.

As a dope-fiend, you can walk into one of these pharmacies and ask for just about any mid-level prescription drug, like Tylenol with codeine, Valium, Xanax, Prozac, etc. Sometimes they can tell that you are not purchasing for legitimate purposes and they'll tell you no. Other times they don't seem to care.

Over the years I have successfully purchased the following:

Tylenol w/Codeine (#2s w/15 mg Codeine)
Generic Acetaminophen w/Codeine
   (30 mg Codeine)
Tasty Green Apple Cough Drops with
   10 mg/Codeine (they had cherry, too!)
Phencodin/Codeine cough syrup. (Nice with a
   shot of Jaegermister!)
Cold medicine w/10 mg codeine per pill
Ethyl-amphetamine
Pseudo-amphetamine
Generic diazepam (Valium, 10/mg, blue)
Xanax (purple, 1 mg ?)
Halcion
Eunoctin (10 mg—not sure what this is)
Hydergine (4.5 mg)
Prozac
Bupenorphin (.2 mg—to be dissolved under
   the tongue. Very nice)
Lomotil

I have asked for things like Darvon, Percocet, Percodan, Dilaudid, Phenobarbital, etc. with no success. Apparently, stronger things are regulated more strictly.

Most of the pharmacists speak English. Those who don't will be able to read the generic names of drugs. Make sure you know the generic names of what you want. A lot of the better known drugs are marketed under completely different brand names in Thailand. Every pharmacy will have a book, which they can attempt to cross-reference a generic name to a local brand name.

The laws seem to be slowly changing to make these purchases a little more difficult. For example, in 1990 I purchased amphetamines OTC very easily. They were absolutely forbidden OTC in a subsequent trip in 1994. (Amphetamines are abundant in the black market in Thailand and used extensively by truck drivers and manual laborers. Amphetamines are generically referred to as Yaa-Maa horse medicine. I would not recommend trying to get hold of black-market amphetamines due to their high-illegality.

Many of the things I've purchased were stored in a back room or in a locked drawer or under-the-counter. One pharmacy that blatantly sells drugs to foreigners had some of the items (Halcion, bupenorphin and Eunoctin) hidden behind a secret hidden compartment. These items were apparently not supposed to be available OTC.

The prices varied widely—from 1 baht (U.S. $ .04) each for the Tasty Codeine Cough Drops to 65 baht ($2.40) for each Prozac.

Be careful bringing these back to your home country. I think that U.S. Customs officials are looking out for people bringing things like this back to the United States. During one thorough investigation of my bags by Customs, the officer discovered antacid that I bought (obviously OTC) as well as (non-codeine) cough drops. He was very interested and asked a number of questions about them.

Other Drugs—

Apparently pot is quietly available everywhere if you are looking for it. I'm not a pot-smoker so I never tried. There are some Thai meals that use pot as an ingredient—a special noodle soup in particular. I don't think this is something you can buy on the street or in a restaurant.

Opium smoking is usually available as part of the numerous "Hill Treks" available in the north of Thailand. I tried something called "Kratom," which is a leaf that is chewed—supposedly like the "Kat" or "Qat" they have in Somalia. I got really high the first time for about 15 minutes. Subsequent tries yielded little or nothing. The leaf is rather unpleasant tasting. Ask a trusted local if you want to try it.

Finally, there is a pharmacy in Bangkok on the 2nd (lesser) Soi (alley) at Patpong, right in the midst of prostitute bars and sex-shows and the like. It appears to sell antibiotics and narcotics exclusively. There are big letters in the windows that say "SEDATIVES/HYPNOTICS/NARCOTICS" in English. Both times I went there, the cute woman behind the counter was very helpful and between solicitous questions like, "Do you have a girlfriend in Bangkok?" she gave all sorts of advice on how to take what to achieve what kind of high. "Take the codeine and valium together for Percodan-like effect," she told me.

Making Hard Drugs Out of Mom's **Codeine Pills**

by Rhodium 980729

Codeine to Morphine Conversion

This text deals with four known methods of converting codeine to morphine by demethylation (codeine is morphine 3-methyl ether). Cleavage of aromatic ethers are commonly effected by reflux with concentrated HBr or HI. This relatively simple method can unfortunately not be used on codeine, as the oxygen bridge at the 9, 10 position on the morphinan carbon skeleton would also rupture, causing the rearrangement of the molecule to the very potent emetic apomorphine, completely devoid of opiate-like effects. The author takes no responsibility whatsoever of whatever the reader might do with the information contained in this document. Keep in mind that the procedures described herein are probably illegal to carry out in all civilized parts of the world. Please do not send any emails asking for tablet extraction help, or questions on where to obtain chemicals or codeine remedies.

Using Pyridine HCl

A mixture of 1.00 g of codeine and 3 g of pyridine hydrochloride was placed in a bath at 220°C and heated for six minutes in a nitrogen atmosphere, after which the reaction mixture was immediately cooled and dissolved in 20 ml of water, basified with 10 ml of 4 N sodium hydroxide, and the non-phenolic material was removed by extraction with four 15-ml portions of chloroform. The combined chloroform extracts were washed with 10 ml of 0.5 N sodium hydroxide and 10 ml of water, and the aqueous phase, after adding the washings, was adjusted to pH 9 and cooled thoroughly to precipitate phenolic material. After filtering and drying, this phenolic material was digested with 75 ml of methanol, the mixture was filtered hot and the filtrate was chromatographed on an alumina (Merck and Co., Inc.) column (120 × 11 mm) using 700 ml of methanol as eluent. The residue after evaporation of the methanol was dissolved in 10 ml of 0.2 N sodium hydroxide, filtered, and the filtrate was adjusted to pH 9, precipitating the crude morphine. After drying, this crude morphine was sublimed (180–190°C (0.1 mm)), and the sublimate was crystallized from absolute ethanol. There was thus obtained a total of 210 mg (22%) of morphine, m.p. 254–255°C.

The Homebake Method

This is excerpted from a report dealing with clandestine manufacture of morphine and heroin from OTC codeine remedies, in so-called "homebake" laboratories in New Zealand. The method used is the same as the one introduced by Rapoport in 1951, using pyridine hydrochloride. The authors report some perp's claims of 50% conversion from the codeine, but say they obtained 30% typically, and further state that this is about what one would expect from Rapoport's paper. Purity of up to 92% with a more typical purity in the 80% range was reported by the forensic chemists evaluating the method.

The following is the actual procedure used in the clandestine labs, with some elaboration:

1. Crush sufficient pills to yield 2 g of codeine and mix with distilled water. Filter with a vacuum funnel to remove insolubles and add to a separatory funnel. Add NaOH solution to make the solution pH 12.

Extract twice with chloroform (2 × 25 mL). This will be the bottom layer. Discard the water layer, which contains the aspirin or acetominophen) and evaporate the chloroform layer to dryness under gentle heat. The result is codeine base, a white crystalline powder.

2. Combine 20 mL pyridine and 25 mL conc. HCl in a beaker and heat strongly to 190°C to drive off any water. Cover and cool rapidly to obtain a white waxy material. This should be stored in a sealed container in the freezer if not to be used immediately.

3. The reaction is carried out in a glass boiling tube (here one could use a large ignition type test tube) which is sealed on one end. This should be oven dried before use. Then 3.5 g of the pyridine salt is added to the tube and this is then heated until it melts and for a few minutes more to drive off any moisture. Add 1.5 g of the base and seal the tube with a rubber stopper covered with a filter paper. Heat until the mixture begins to fume and continue until the mixture develops a reddish-orange color and becomes noticeably more viscous, typically 6–12 minutes.

4. Pour this into a 500 mL sep funnel and make the volume up to 100 mL with distilled water. Add 10% NaOH until strongly basic. The contents will become milky brown and then clear brown as the solution is made basic. When this point is reached, extract with 20 mL chloroform. This will contain any unreacted codeine (up to 70%) and may be saved for recovery if desired. The morphine is in the water layer.

5. Put the water layer in a beaker and carefully adjust the pH with HCl to pH 9 using a narrow range pHydronium paper. This is critical. Rapidly filter using two layers of paper (here one could use a paper designed for very fine crystals) and a vacuum flask/funnel as in step 1. A very fine brown powder will collect on the paper. This is unwanted byproducts and should be discarded.

6. Pour the filtrate into a clean beaker and, while carefully adjusting the pH to 8.5, vigorously rubbing the inside of the beaker with a "seeding stick" (here the authors mention that a split wooden peg is sometimes used in the home labs in NZ; a glass stirring rod would be preferable). Crystals should begin to form. These are allowed to settle for at least 5 minutes and then are recovered by vacuum filtering to recover the morphine as a beige to dark brown product.

Using Boron Tribromide

A solution of 2.99g (10 mmol) of anhydrous codeine in 25 ml of $CHCl_3$ was added during 2 minute to a well-stirred solution of 15g (59.9 mmol) of BBr_3 in 175 ml of $CHCl_3$ maintained in the range 23–26°C. A 10 ml portion of $CHCl_3$, which was used to rinse the addition funnel, was added to the reaction mixture and stirring was continued for 15 minute at 23–26°C. The reaction mixture was then poured into a well-stirred mixture of 80g ice and 20 ml of concentrated (28–30%) ammonia. The two-phase system was kept at -5°C to 0°C for 0.5h (continuous stirring) and filtered. The resulting crystalline material was washed thoroughly with small portions of cold $CHCl_3$ and H_2O and dried to give 2.67g (88.1%) of slightly off-white morphine hydrate, mp 252.5–254°C.

Using Sodium Propylmercaptide

A solution of 3.00 grams (10 mmol) of codeine in 60 ml of dry dimethylformamide was degassed under nitrogen by repeatedly stirring under vacuum, followed by inletting nitrogen. Following the addition of 3.00 grams (26.7 mmol) of potassium tert-butoxide, the degassing process was repeated, and 3.0 ml (32.7 mmol) of n-propanethiol was injected by syringe. The mixture was stirred at 125°C under nitrogen for 45 minute (similar results at 110°C for 3h), cooled, and quenched with 3.0 ml of acetic acid. The solvent was removed under high vacuum, and the residue dissolved in 30 ml of 1N hydrochloric acid. The acid solution was washed with several portions of ether, treated with 5ml of 20% sodium bisulfite, and alkalized to pH 9 with ammonium hydroxide. The precipitated solid was collected, washed with water, and dried in vacuo (100°C) to leave 2.30g (80%) of morphine as tan crystals.

Using L-Selectride (Lithium tri-sec-butyl Hydride)

482 mg (1.6 mmol) of codeine was dissolved in 4 ml of an 1 M solution of L-selectride in THF (4.0 mmol) and was refluxed for 3.5h. The reaction was quenched with water (5 ml), followed by 2ml of 15% NaOH solution and removal of the THF. The resulting mixture was washed twice with CH2Cl2, cooled to 0–5°C and acidified to pH 1 with 10% HCl. After basification with ammonium hydroxide to pH 9, the mixture was extracted into CHCl3, the organic phase was washed with brine and dried over Na2SO4. Removal of the solvent, followed by recrystallization from water gave 355mg (73%) of morphine hydrate. Unreacted codeine was recovered from the non-phenolic extracts, and after purification by recrystallization from water, it amounted to 71mg (14%).

References

1. H. Rapoport, *The Preparation of Morphine-N-Methyl-C14,* J. Am. Chem. Soc., 73, 5900 (1951)

2. H. Rapoport, *Delta-7-Desoxymorphine,* J. Am. Chem. Soc., 73, 5485 (1951)

3. K. Bedford, *Illicit Preparation of Morphine from Codeine in NZ,* Forensic Sci. Int., 34(3), 197–204 (1987)

4. K.C. Rice, *A Rapid, High-Yield Conversion of Codeine to Morphine,* J. Med. Chem., 20(1), 164 (1977)

5. J.A. Lawson, *An Improved Method for O-Demethylation of Codeine,* J. Med. Chem., 20(1), 165 (1977)

6. A. Coop, *L-selectride for the O-Demethylation of Opium Alkaloids,* J. Org. Chem., 63, 4392–96 (1998)

7. G. Majetisch, *Hydride-Promoted Demethylation of Methyl Phenyl Ethers,* Tet. Lett. 35(47), 8727–8730 (1994)

7-chloro-1-methyl-5-phenyl-3H-1, 4-benzodiazepin-2(1H)-one

Hacking Valium (Diazepam)

Raw Materials: 2-amino-5-chlorbenzophenone-ß-oxime, chloroacetyl chloride, phosphorus trichloride, sodium hydroxide, diazomethane

Manufacturing Process: Into a stirred, cooled (10°–15°C) solution of 26.2 g (0.1mol) of 2-amino-5-chlorpbenzophenone-ß-oxime in 150 ml of dioxane were introduced in small portions12.4 g (0.11 mol) of chloroacetyl chloride and an equivalent amount of 3 N NaOH. The chloroacetyl chloride and NaOH were introduced alternately at such a rate so as to keep the temperature below 15°C ansd the mixture neutral or slightly alkaline. The reaction was completed after 30 minutes. The mixture was slightly acidified with HCl, diluted with water and extracted with ether. The ether extract was dried and concentrated in vacuo. Upon the addition of ether to the oily residue, the product, 2-chloroactetamido-5-chlorobenzophenone ß-oxime crystallized in colorless prisms melting at 161°–162°C.

20 ml of 1 N NaOH were added to a solution of 6.4 g (20 mmol) of 2-chloroactetamido-5-chlorobenzophenone ß-oxime. After 15 hours the mixture was diluted with ice cold 1 N NaOH and extracted with ether. The ether extract was discarded. The alkaline solution was acidified with HCl and extracted with methylene chloride. The methylen chloride solution was concentrated to a small volume and then diluted with petroleum ether to obtain 7-chloro-5-phenyl-3H-1,4-benzodiazepin-2(1H)one 4-oxide.

To a stirred suspension of 10 grams (35 mmol) of 7-chloro-5-phenyl-3H-1,4-benzodiazepin-2(1H)one 4-oxide in approximately 150 ml methanol was added in portions an excess of diazomethane in ether. After about one hour, almost complete solution had occurred and the reaction mixture was filtered. The filtrate was concentrated in vacuo to a small volume and diluted with ether and petroleum ether. The reaction product, 7-chloro-1-methyl-5-phenyl-3H-1,4-benzodiazepin-2(1H)one 4-oxide, crystallized in colorless prisms. The product was filtered off and recrystallized from acetone, MP 188°–189°C.

A mixture of 3 grams (0.01 mol) of 7-chloro-1-methyl-5-phenyl-3H-1,4-benzodiazepin-2(1H)one 4-oxide, 30 ml of chloroform and 1 ml of phosphorus trichloride was refluxed for 1 hour. The reaction mixture was then poured on ice and stirred with an excess of 40% NaOH solution. The chloroform was then separated, dried with sodium sulfate, filtered and concentrated in vacuo. The residue was dissolved in methylene chloride and crystallized by the addition of petroleum ether. The product, 7-chloro-1-methyl-5-phenyl-3H-1,4-benzodiazepin-2(1H)one, was recrystallized from a mixture of acetone and petroleum ether forming colorless plates melting at 125°–126°C.

FROM U.S. PAT. 3,136,815

Home Chemists Discuss Making a **New Quaalude Online**

For some months people have been talking about the synthesis of methaqualone analogues. I have never been fortunate enough to try these wacky downers but knowing a fair number of junkies, you get to know what pills give the best buzz. For the record, the hardcore smoke 'ludes on a bong! Check out South Africa, that is their MAIN drug problem.

Anyway, the reason you are reading this is to find a BETTER 'lude, right? The drug is "Clomethiazol," which you can read up the synthesis of in U.S. patent number 5648498. This drug is like a mixture of E and valium, wicked high! The legal form comes in a similar format to soft-gel capsules of temazepan. The hardcore shoot the caps and lose their mind. I saw it done and It made H look like baby food! These guys were FUCKED UP.

A friend gave me a good bit of advice . . . "Don't try and be clever and take two. You will just wake up six hours later, confused."

Anyway, back to the plot. You just read that patent and realized that the thing is a bitch to synthesize. But wait! Please direct yourself to the structure of vitamin B1. Do you see any sort of similarity? Oh look, cleavage with HCl gets the target drug . . . Or so I am told. No details, but I should think you bright fellows can work it out. Clomethiazole was used as one of the intermediates MAKING B1, by the way.

P.S. I don't think you can get this drug in the U.S. The U.K. trade name is "Heminevrin" made by Astra. One (slightly) interesting fact is that the dosage is 192 mg 192? Why not 200, what a weird figure. Then I sussed it out. It's such an old product (Keith Moon killed himself with them) that the weight was in Grains. So this is 5 grains of clomethiazole . . .

—*Piglet*

This stuff is STRONGER than 'ludes. The only side-effect is that it causes conjunctivitis. You get sort of hay-fever effects (not too bad) so those in the know take an antihistamine first. Choose the right one for an even bigger buzz . . .

—*Jamex*

Another note for you folks, this stuff isn't illegal to possess ANYWHERE as far as I can tell. It's used to help alcoholics and these winos are usually up for selling them. I paid £2.50 each In Leeds earlier this year. Leeds, ay, first place in the U.K. with 24 hour pubs! (That must sound crazy to all you non-U.K. bees but it's new to us).

I couldn't resist! I smoke . . . so I dumped the tobacco and mixed it with you-know-what put it back and lit up.

Taste like crap, smells like crap but hooooweee. I may never go back to capsules again. That stuff hit fast and strong. I gotta go now and find a girl. Any girl. Hell, maybe anything female! Lock up your daughters and dogs!!!!

http://www.vrp.com

100 gm powder—$16.95

—*Piglet*

Anybody know ANYTHING about ethchlorvynol? This downer is controlled and is indeed still in use. The only thing I know is that it has a "mint-like" aftertaste and can cause facial numbness. Cool, huh? I have often thought that drugs that are good from an abuse viewpoint but had some side-effect that prevented them being more common. Like Hemi causing hay-fever symptoms. It's supposed to be safer than most other downers, but it's only used to get alky's off the booze . . .
—*beagle boy*

Ethchlorvynol = Placydyl in the US. Had a girlfriend that was given it once in the hospital as a hypnotic. She liked it VERY much. I saw a synth for it once, but it looked like too much hassle. However ethinimate (sp) looks like it might be quite similar in effect and much easier to syn.

For those of you interested in the practical aspects of clomethiazole synthesis, I submit to you a dandy excerpt. This article, JACS, 57, 1935, 536-537, describes the degradation of vitamin B1 into the starting material for our chlorinated friend. Enjoy.

"1,000 grams of vitamin was dissolved in 15 cc of sodium sulfite solution containing sufficient excess sulfurous acid to bring the pH to 4.8–5.0. The total sulfite content was 2.6 N. After standing overnight at room temperature the liquid had deposited copious amounts of the sparingly soluble acidic cleavage product in crystalline form. After standing for several days, the crystalline product was collected, washed and dried; weight 535.8 mg.

"The mother liquor and washings were brought to pH 10 with strong sodium hydroxide and the alkaline solution extracted seven times with 50 cc. Of chloroform each time. The combined chloroform extracts were extracted with dilute hydrochloric acids, the acid aqueous extract was evaporated in vacuo, and the residue was extracted with absolute alcohol. The alcoholic solution on evaporation left a residue of 518.8 mg of the crystalline hydrochloride of the basic cleavage product, the purity of which was demonstrated by analysis; yield 97.4%. The recrystallization of this material is effected by dissolving in a minimum amount of absolute alcohol, adding an excess of dioxane and allowing to stand."

You're welcome,
—*drone #342*

From Micromedix Drug Evaluation Monographs

5-0(2-chloroethyl)-4-methyl-1,3-thiazole (533-45-9), aka Distraneurin, Distraneurine, Hemineurin, Heminervin. It is a colorless to slightly yellow-brown liquid w/a characteristic odor. slightly sol in H2O, miscible w/ether and CHCl3.

Chlormethiazole dose: 500–1,000 mg oral dose for sedation. 1,000 mg every four hour for delirium tremens or opiate withdrawal, 32mg/minutes IV bolus w/8mg/minutes continuous IV infusion for seizures or as a hypnotic. ½ life = 4–6 hours in healthy adults, 8.9 hours in cirrhotic patients. Used extensively in alcohol withdrawal in europe. Gaining wide acceptance for geriatric patients because of relative lack of adverse effects, compared to benzos. Onset is 20–30 minutes as the oral syrup, 2 hrs as the capsule. Duration of the syrup is 1–4 hours! Peak plasma conc. After 500 mg tablet is 35 minutes.

Exact mech of action is unclear, but appears to enhance transmission of GABA (gamma-amino-butyric acid) in the CNS. This enhanced transmission appears to be mediated through Ca dependent Cl ion channels and differs significantly from benzos and barbs mech.
—*Piglet*

222 or AC&C

by Tim Johnson

AC&C Tablets—known as "222s"

in Canada (that's just a brand name for these pills) are a lively and brilliant concoction of three fine ingredients—aspirin, codeine, and caffeine. Not only do they do a bang-up job of destroying headaches (especially hangover headaches) they are cheap. Buy an off-brand of about 200 hits and pay less than five bucks American. I say American, because the bad news is, these pills are available in Canada only. The good news is they're over-the-counter! That's right, all you gotta do is ask the pharmacist and she'll hand 'em to you without so much as a dirty look.

It's hard to get anything more than a mild buzz off these things as each tablet contains just 8 mgs of codeine along with the standard 325 mgs of aspirin or acetaminophen and 15 mgs of caffeine. (But elsewhere this book tells how to get a buzz by removing the liver-damaging acetaminophen.)

In Canada, the law says codeine can only be sold without a prescription if it's combined with at least two other ingredients—hence, it's hard to get codeine cough syrup without also getting antihistamines and deconges-tants, too. But in this case the caffeine is quite useful for offsetting the sedative effects of codeine, and aspirin is just unsurpassed as a general tonic anyway. Best of all, these three ingredients are time-tested and derived from natural sources. So dump that ibuprofen and take a day-trip to Canada.

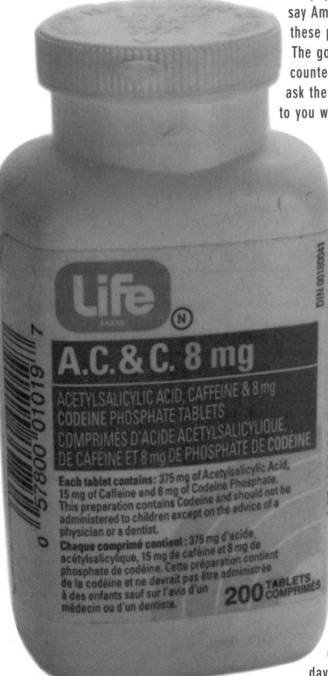

Life ℕ

A.C.&C. 8 mg

ACETYLSALICYLIC ACID, CAFFEINE & 8 mg
CODEINE PHOSPHATE TABLETS
COMPRIMES D'ACIDE ACÉTYLSALICYLIQUE,
DE CAFEINE ET 8 mg DE PHOSPHATE DE CODÉINE

Each tablet contains: 375 mg of Acetylsalicylic Acid, 15 mg of Caffeine and 8 mg of Codeine Phosphate. This preparation contains Codeine and should not be administered to children except on the advice of a physician or a dentist.

Chaque comprimé contient: 375 mg d'acide acétylsalicylique, 15 mg de caféine et 8 mg de phosphate de codéine. Cette préparation contient de la codéine et ne devrait pas être administrée à des enfants sauf sur l'avis d'un médecin ou d'un dentiste.

200 TABLETS COMPRIMÉS

DIN 00180041

0 57800 01019 7

The Codeine Pill Hack

Sooner or later every fan of "T-3s," Canadian 222s and the like, is going to start hankering for an easy way to get away from that liver-bustin' acetaminophen all mixed up in there with the drug you *really* want. Getting pills that have aspirin instead much better—you might get a bleeding ulcer from the severe inflammation aspirin can cause . . . to say nothing of the kidney damage and ringing ears!

First off, the procedure that's called for here is some kind of separation—look at all the variables of the different ingredients in the pill and create an environment to break up this relationship. A quick and dirty separation technique that'll serve the pillhound well is called "extraction."

If you know how to make coffee, then you know how to do an extraction. In the case of coffee, you want the good-tasting stuff, you don't want the indigestible parts, you've come to like the coloring and above all, you want the caffeine.

Pills can be like coffee beans at times. You take the chunks of whatever has your target substance in it, grind it up and pour a solvent through the stuff to collect the target-laden solvent afterward.

Of course there are variables right where you'd expect them to be. Your solvent choice is one, solvent temperature is another. How long to keep the reaction going (how long to steep the tea . . .) is still another. Sometimes you've got to let the raw material "stew." In coffee-making this is called "percolation." In chemistry it's called "reflux."

Find out as much as you can about the pill and its constituents, then figure out how to rescue your favorite(s). To that end, the single most important tool to have handy is a *Merck Index*. This tome has got all kinds of physical data about thousands and thousands of chemicals and products, with particular emphasis on pharmaceuticals. Along with solubility information, boiling points, molecular weights and more, it gives brief information on how the compound is made (with cites to lead you to more extensive stuff) and what it's used for.

In the U.S., they gotta put everything on the label. So reading the label we find Canadian 222 tablets contain: 325 mgs of aspirin or acetaminophen, 15 mgs of caffeine, and 8 mgs of codeine phosphate. These numbers are related to each other by the two most common systems of weighing drugs: grains and grams. Be ready to convert the information so it's more uniform. A grain is approx. 64 mgs (1,000 mgs to a gram).

Our *Merck Index* tells us that both A/A (aspirin and acetaminophen) aren't very soluble in 21c water, and even less soluble as the temperature drops. One very quick & dirty way to remove most of the junk in AC&C pills is to simply mix the mashed up pills in, say, a tablespoon or so of distilled water (the cleaner the water the better you're extraction) and cool it. Or just use cold water in the first place.

The unwanted sludge sinks to the bottom. You can remove the water layer (which contains almost every bit of the codeine and caffeine and trace amounts of the aspirin/acetaminophen) by decanting it off (pouring it off in such a way that the solids remain behind), or better, use a filter. A coffee filter is adequate but use two layers since coffee filters are pretty porous.

You can also use a syringe or a straw to draw off the liquid part. If you don't mind the 150 mgs of caffeine in the stuff (like drinking a cup and a half of coffee) then slug this down. It should be noted that doing a number of small extractions is better than one big extraction. This is one of the differences between "paper chemistry" and what really occurs in the lab. Cutting your solvent volume in half and doing two extractions yields more product. It may not be a lot more, but it is more.

The basic procedure to get at the codeine and remove the aspirin or acetaminophen in Canadian OTC codeine pills is this.

1. Double-check the ingredients. The easiest pills to deal with in my experience are generic 222s called Life Brand AC&C tablets.
2. Measure out a quantity of pills according to however much codeine you want to obtain and how much calculating you want to do. Ten pills gives you 80 mgs of codeine (just shy of three Tylenol 3s) or eight pills gives you 64 mgs—about one grain.

Remember, you will NOT get 100% of it. A perfect score is impossible in all chemical reactions. Usually, a 50% yield in an organic synthesis is considered pretty good. Sometimes 25% or 30% is good. In this extraction, though, you should be able to recover about 90% of the codeine. You might want to add a couple extra pills for good measure.

Measure out some nice hot water, use approx. 40 ml/20 tablets or more if needed. I would suggest you don't go over 50 ml for 20 tablets. I don't know if the use of boiling water would destroy any of the codeine but your best bet is not to use it. Use hot water but not boiling. Make sure the tablets dissolve completely. Some dissolve on contact with water while others need some help dissolving by crushing them. Note: not all of the tablet will dissolve, there are water-insoluble fillers in the tablet and not all of the A/A will dissolve either (which is what we want).

Place the solution in a cold bath, I just use some ice cubes in a container of water. Stir the mixture occasionally until the solution drops to about 15°C or lower. You won't need a thermometer to measure the temperature, just make sure it's "cold." This will take about 30 minutes. If you wish to speed this up, you can use less water to dissolve the tablets, and add ice chips to cool the mixture faster. Just make sure you don't add so much ice that you drastically increase the volume of the mixture.

Filter the solution using whatever you have. Coffee filters work well, but lab filters work the best. Just make sure you don't end up with obvious solids in the filtered solution. This will take about one hour. You may also want to rinse the solids left over in the filter with some ice water to extract any remaining codeine.

Drink and enjoy! The solution will be very bitter, so I mix a little Kool-Aid powder into the solution. The taste isn't really bad but it's similar to sucking on a lemon.

Sit back and wait for the effects. Because the codeine is already in solution it only needs to be absorbed, while codeine in the tablet form must dissolve before being absorbed. Because of this, the effects will probably become noticeable within 15 minutes.

NOTE: I don't suggest you evaporate the mixture unless you are willing to wait a while. The *Merck Index* warns that codeine is sensitive to heat and light. For that reason if you wish to evaporate the mixture, do it without heat, and shield the solution from light.

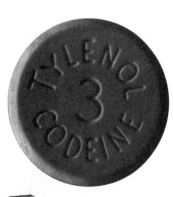

Active Ingredient The specific chemical in a drug or plant that is responsible for the drug action ascribed to the entire preparation.

Agonist Drug that mimics the action of a normally present biological compound, such as a neurotransmitter or hormone.

Analgesic Drug that produces an insensitivity to pain without loss of consciousness.

Anesthetic Drug that causes loss of sensation or feeling, especially pain, by its depressant effect on the nervous system.

Antagonist Drug that opposes or counteracts the action of a normally present biological compound, such as a neurotransmitter or hormone, or of another drug, such as a narcotic antagonist.

Anticholinergic A drug that (by blocking certain impulses) blocks bodily secretions. These drugs are used in cough, cold and diarrhea medicines, and although ineffective for this use, are also contained in some medicines for hemorrhoids.

Antiemetc Drug or substance which prevents vomiting or relieves nausea.

Anti-inflammatory Drug that reduces inflammation, like cortisone.

Antihistamine Medications that relieve the symptoms of allergies or colds by blocking the production of histamines.

Antipsychotic (neuroleptic) Drugs that produce an effect of emotional quieting and relative indifference to one's surrounding; also called major tranquilizers.

Antitussive Substances that act to inhibit an uncontrollable, dry or unproductive cough.

Anxiolytics Anti-anxiety drugs

Ataraxic Any drug that creates a feeling of calmness; the tranquilizers.

Benzodiazepine A class of drug that relieves anxiety and insomnia. Like Valium.

Contraindication A reason not to use a given medication in a given situation; for example, many drugs are contraindicated during pregnancy.

Cross-dependence Different drugs, like barbiturates and alcohol, may cause physical dependence because of their similar pharmacological activity and can be used interchangeably to prevent withdrawal symptoms.

Cross-tolerance A condition of tolerance to one or more drugs caused by the body's tolerance to another drug.

Depressant Any of several drugs that sedate by acting on the central nervous system; medical uses include the treatment of anxiety, tension and high blood pressure.

Dosage Form The physical state in which a drug is dispensed for use. For example: a frequent dosage form of procaine is a sterile solution. The most frequent dosage form of aspirin is a tablet.

Dose The quantity of drug, or dosage form, administered to a subject at a given time; for example, the usual dose of aspirin for relief of pain in an adult is 300-600 milligrams. Dose may be expressed in terms appropriate to a specific dosage form, i.e., one teaspoonful of a liquid medication, rather than the weight of drug in the teaspoonful.

Drug interaction When a drug action is modified by another substance, it may (1) add to, (2) inhibit, or (3) be inhanced; see also Potentiation.

Endogenous drugs Drugs produced within the body.

Enteral Refers to a drug that is taken orally.

Enteric coated Covered or coated with a special substance that prevents dissolving until the intestine is reached; used for drugs that would upset the stomach.

Ethical Drugs Those drugs advertised only to doctors and pharmacists.

Expectorant Compounds that enhance the removal of respiratory tract fluids by coughing.

Glossary

Generic drug Drug formulations of identical composition with respect to the active ingredient a drug that is no longer patented. Drug dosage forms considered "generically equivalent" are more properly considered "chemically equivalent" in that they contain a designated quantity of drug chemical in specified stable condition and meet pharmacopoeial requirements for chemical and physical properties. A number of preparations of a given drug entity may carry a different "proprietary name" or "trademark" registered with the U.S. Patent Office. All such preparations—identical with respect to content and specification of active ingredient—may be viewed as comprising a "genus"; they are generically equivalent and are generic drugs.

Habituation The psychological craving for effects produced by the administration of a drug.

Half-life The time (usually expressed in hours) required for half the dose of a drug to be secreted from the body. (This is an important consideration for determining the amount and frequency of drug dosage.)

Hypnotic A central nervous system depressant that induces sleep; see also **Sedative**.

Idiosyncratic Response A qualitatively abnormal or unusual response to a drug which is unique, or virtually so, to the individual who manifests the response.

IND (Investigational New Drug) number An FDA-assigned code number used during human clinical tests of a new drug prior to the granting of permission to market it.

IU International Unit. Used to measure doses of drugs or biologicals.

Lethal Dose, or LD The dosage that will kill; LD-50 means that this dose would be lethal to 50% of the test animals.

Main Effect A drug's desired effect; no known drug has only a main effect; see also side effect.

Margin of safety Dosage range between an ineffective (threshold) amount and a lethal amount of a drug; see therapeutic index.

MOAIs Abbreviation for monoamine oxidase inhibitors; a group of antidepressants that promotes an elevation of levels of amine messengers in the emotional regions of the brain.

Molecular Structure The architecture of a compound. By making small changes in the molecular structure of a drug, analogues are produced and the pharmacological effects of the original substance may be altered.

Narcotic Numbness producer; this term has two definitions. Medically, a narcotic is any drug that produces sleep or stupor and also relieves pain; legally, a narcotic means any drug regulated under the Harrison Act and other federal narcotic laws.

Neuroleptic Antipsychotic major tranquilizer.

NF Refers to a drug compounded according to the National Formulary, a semi-official directory of drug standards and specifications, issued every five years by the American Pharmaceutical Association (also USP).

Nostrum A medicine recommended by its maker, but without any scientific proof of its value or effectiveness.

NSAIDs Non-steroidal anti-inflammatory drugs used in the treatment of arthritis, to reduce fevers, and pain.

Opiate Drug that contain opium of a derivative; also used to indicate a drug acting as a sedative or narcotic.

Opiate agonist Drugs that bind with opiate receptors and thereby produce their characteristic effects.

Opiate antagonist Drug that, when administered, prevents an opiate from producing its characteristic effect.

Over-the-Counter (OTC) drug Pharmaceutical substance that can be purchased without a prescription, as can, for example, aspirin; claims for its effectiveness are regulated by the FDA; compare to Prescription Drug.

Pharmacodynamic tolerance The increasing tolerance of the nervous system to a drug, or the state in which a drug's target tissue, such as the brain, has adapted to the drug gradually, over a period of weeks to months, by an unknown mechanism, so that the same concentration of drug produces a decreased response.

Pharmacology (Gr. Pharmakon-drug, and Logos-word) is the study of drugs in all their aspects. Pharmacy, although often confused with pharmacology, is, in fact, an independent discipline concerned with the art and science of the preparation, compounding, and dispensing of drugs. Pharmacognosy is a branch of pharmacy which deals with the identification and analysis of the plant and animal tissues from which drugs may be extracted. Pharmacodynamics, which in common usage is usually termed "pharmacology," is concerned with the study of drug effects and how they are produced. The pharmacodynamicist, or pharmacologist, identifies the effects produced by drugs, and determines the sites and mechanisms of their action in the body. The pharmacologist studies the physiological or biochemical mechanisms by which drug actions are produced. The pharmacologist also investigates those factors which modify the effects of drugs, i.e. the routes of administration, influence of rates of absorption, differential distribution, and the body's mechanisms of excretion and detoxification, on the total effect of a drug.

Physical Dependence Physiological adaptation of the body to the presence of the drug and has a continuing need for the drug. Once such dependence has been established, the body reacts with predictable symptoms if the drug is abruptly withdrawn.

Placebo An inert substance, such as a sugar tablet or injection of sterile water, given as if it were a real medication; also, an ineffective dose of an active drug. Can be highly effective, psychologically.

Polypharmacy The lethal interaction of several drugs; also, the giving of more than one drug concurrently.

Potency The absolute amount of a drug required to produce a given pharmacological effect; see also **Therapeutic index**.

Potentiation A special case of synergy (q.v.) in which the simultaneous effects of two or more drugs is greater than the sum of the independent effects of these drugs.

Precursor Refers to (1) a chemical substance that is converted to another chemical substance (flurazepam is the precursor of its long-lived metabolite); or (2) a previously-existing disorder that leads to a disease.

Prescription drug Pharmaceutical substance whose prescription order is regulated by law to a licensed person, such as a physician; classified in one of Schedules II-IV of Controlled Substances.

Proprietary drugs Drugs advertised directly to the public, produced by licensed drug manufacturers and dispensed by licensed physicians or other medical personnel, or sold in pharmacies by licensed druggists.

Psychoactive (psychotropic) drug One that affects mood and/or consciousness; may be a prescription (Valium) or a non-prescription (marijuana) drug.

Psychotoxic Drugs, including therapeutic and abused, that can produce 1. psychosis, 2. mood change, or 3. anxiety. The psychotogenic drugs can produce euphoria in low doses but, in high doses, a psychotic state...

Receptor site Specialized cells in a body tissue to which a drug or chemical attaches to exert its pharmacological effect.

Sedative Psychoactive drug that decreases excitability and anxiety as part of its general depressant action; higher doses may be hypnotic (sleep inducing).

Semisynthetic drugs Drugs created by chemists from materials found in nature.

Side effect An expected or predictable action of a drug that accompanies the main, desired effect. Side effects are usually but not always undesirable.

Stimulant Any of several drugs that act on the central nervous system to produce excitation, alertness, and wakefulness.

Sublingual Under the tongue.

Synergy (potentiation) The combined action of two or more drugs is greater than the sum of the effects of each drug taken alone.

Synthetic drugs Created by chemists in labs, as opposed to endogenous drugs or semisynthetic drugs.

Tachycardia Rapid heartbeat as a result of stress or stimulant drugs.

Teratogen A drug or agent capable of causing birth defects by its action upon the embryo or fetus.

Therapeutic equivalent A drug that can be substituted for another without loss of efficacy.

Therapeutic index Relative margin of safety of a drug; the dose required to produce toxic effects divided by the dose required to produce therapeutic effects.

Tolerance Where dosage is increased to maintain the same effect.

Tranquilizers, major Drugs used to relieve severe psychosis (Thorazine).

Tranquilizers, minor Psychoactive drugs with sedative and antianxiety effects; also used as anticonvulsants, muscle relaxants (Valium) and to relieve emotional stress associated with organic disease.

USP Refers to the United States Pharmacopeia, a semiofficial pharmacological directory of drug standards and specifications, issued every five years by a national committee of physicians, pharmacists, and academicians.

Vasodilator Causing the blood vessels to dilate.

Pill-Related
INTERNET SITES
&NEWSGROUPS

The ultimate pill site is being constructed by Jim Hogshire, friends and fiends.
www.pagg.com

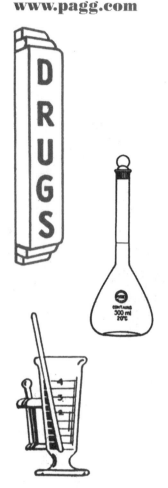

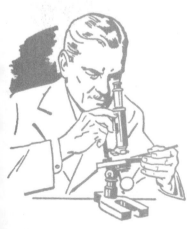

http://www.druginfonet.com/ "Drug InfoNet is your one-stop www site for all your healthcare needs. We provide both information and links to areas on the web concerning healthcare and pharmaceutical-related topics."

http://www.fairlite.com/ocd/articles/ser90.shtml Here's the article, "Serotonin: The Neurotransmitter for the '90s," by Ronald F. Borne, Ph.D., Department of Medicinal Chemistry, School of Pharmacy, University of Mississippi.

http://www.virtualdrugstore.com/ "The Virtual Drugstore database for cutting-edge information including the drug's use, how the drug works, its side effects and interactions and instructions on how best to use it. References to research articles are also included to provide you with more information."

http://www.cmhc.com/guide/pro22.htm Primary Psychopharmacology site, with info on drugs by name, drug references and databases, newsgroups, mailing lists, journals, publications and research papers, professional organizations and centers.

http://www.nlm.nih.gov/ National Library of Medicine. Biggest repository of medical and pharmaceutical information. Many things accessible online.

http://www.pharmacy.org/
Mirror Sites:
http://vlib.stanford.edu/Home.html
huttp://www.ugems.psu.edu/~owens/VL/
Practically everything on things pharmaceutical, including Pharmacy Schools, Companies, Journals, Books, Databases, Conferences, Databases, Listserves, News Gropus, Government sites.

pain killers:
http://www.egroups.com/list/pain-killers/ Method to join pain-killers email group.

http://www.ncpa.org/health/pdh/mar98t.html Article on Adverse Drug Reaction death overreaction from the infamous Journal of the American Medical Association.

http://www.lycaeum.org/~rhodium/chemistry/opium.html Perhaps the only place to find a remarkable government (DEA/DOJ) article on how to farm opiates.

Subject: heroin extraction directions
http://www.lycaeum.org/~rhodium/chemistry/heroinmfg.txt
http://www.medec.com/html/products/pharmacy/pharmacyframe.html
Where the various *PDR* publications and leading pharmaceutical magazine, Drug Topics, hawks their products.

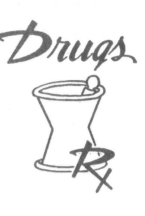

http://www.pnc.com.au/~cafmr/online/medical/index.html
Articles and book excerpts on medical/pharmaceutical conspiracy.

http://www.geocities.com/CapeCanaveral/3861/russian1.htm
A Russian flouts his ideas for weird pill dispensers.

http://micro.magnet.fsu.edu/pharmaceuticals/index.html
Optical microscopy of many different pills, including Viagra and
Valium. Very colorful, psychedelic looks at pills.

http://www.mdconsult.com. MD Consult is the most comprehensive
online medical information service. This is a charging website, but it
offers a ten day free trial period.

http://rxlist.com/ Internet drug index that also offers hundreds of
online monographs and is beginning an alternative drug search.

http://www.the-revolution.org/platform.shtml R.U. Sirius' yippie-
like entry into terrorism for peace, especially against against the War
on Drugs.

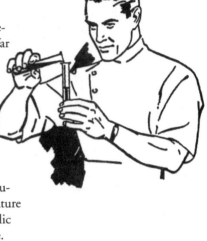

http://www.drcnet.org/ Drug Reform Coordination Network
archive. Anti-Drug War. Pro drug.

http://www.druglibrary.org/schaffer/index.HTM Remarkable
research site on drugs and drug policy.

http://www.lindesmith.org/ Features a searchable database of thousands of library documents from both academic and popular literature
focusing on drug policy from economic, criminal justice, and public
health perspectives, and a subject index of full-text material online.

Slanted Government Resources
http://www.fda.gov/default.htm The Food and Drug Administration
shows its public face. It even has, like the CIA site, a little kiddie corner.

http://www.usp.org/index.htm The U.S. Pharmacopeia is yet
another strange interaction of the government and business. They
even sound confused explaining who they are on their home page:
"From a technical, legal perspective, USP (United States Pharmacopeia)
is a nonprofit corporation. In reality, however, it functions as a quasi-
public institution, responsible for developing public standards and
information in an open manner. Because of its unusual character, it
often is difficult to explain the many facets of the organization."

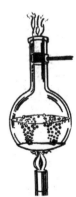

http://www.usdoj.gov/dea/
The Drug Enforcement Administration (DEA) site.

http://www.whitehousedrugpolicy.gov
The Office of National Drug Control Policy (ONDCP) site.

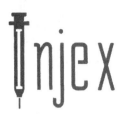

Injex

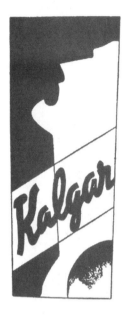

http://www.nida.nih.gov
The National Institute on Drug Abuse (NIDA) site.

http://www.undcp.org/index.html
The United Nations International Drug Control Policy (UNDCP) site.

Newsgroups

rec.drugs.misc: general discussion of drugs, emphasis on recreational use.

rec.drugs.announce: moderated newsgroup for high SNR traffic.

rec.drugs.chemistry: synthesis, extractions, etc.

rec.drugs.smart: smart drugs/drinks and nootropics.

alt.drugs: general discussion of drugs, emphasis on recreational use.

alt.drugs.chemistry: synthesis, extractions, etc.

talk.politics.drugs: political discussion of drugs only.

sci.med.pharmacy: medical discussion of pharmaceuticals.

sci.med.psychobiology: medical psychoactives (antidepressants, neuroleptics, etc.).

Pharmaceutical
MANUFACTURERS'
WEBSITES

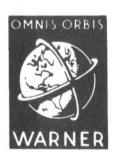

Stock quotes, breaking news about various diseases, company histories, and even job listings from the major pharmaceutical empires.

Abbott Laboratories **http://www.abbottrenalcare.com/**

Astra Merck **http://www.astramerck.com/**

Bayer Corporation **http://www.bayer.com/bayer/index_e.htm**

Boehringer Ingelheim Pharmaceuticals, Inc.
http://www.boehringer-ingelheim.com/

Bristol-Myers Squibb Company **http://www.bms.com/**

CibaGeneva Pharmaceuticals **http://www.ciba.com**

Dista Products **http://www.dista.com/**

DuPont Merck Pharmaceutical http://www.dupontmerck.com/

Glaxo Wellcome Inc. http://www.glaxowellcome.com/

Hoechst Marion Roussel Pharmaceuticals Inc. http://www.hmri.com/

Johnson & Johnson http://www.jnj.com/

Eli Lilly and Company http://www.lilly.com/

Merck and Company, Inc.
http://www.merck.com/

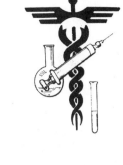

Parke-Davis http://www.parke-davis.com/

Pfizer, Inc. http://www.pfizer.com/

Roche Laboratories http://www.roche.com/

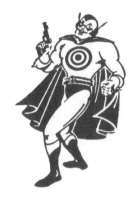

Sandoz Pharmaceuticals http://www.novartis.com/

Schering-Plough Corp. http://www.sch-plough.com/

Searle & Company,G.D. http://www.searlehealthnet.com/

SmithKline Beecham http://www.sb.com/

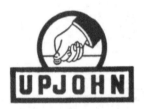

The Upjohn Company (Pharmacia and Upjohn)
http://www.pnu.com/

Wyeth-Ayerst Laboratories http://www.ahp.com/wyeth.htm

Zeneca Pharmaceuticals http://www.zeneca.com/

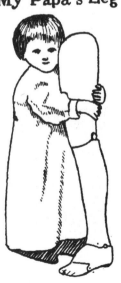

My Papa's Leg

It's a
"Universal"

KING OF PAIN

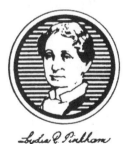

Lydia E. Pinkham

More PILL RESOURCES

Smart Drugs

Cognitive Enhancement Research Institute
PO Box 4029
Menlo Park, CA 94026

Organizations

The American Institute of the
History of Pharmacy
425 North Charter Street
Madison, WI 53706-1508
(608) 262-5378

"The mission of the American Institute of the History of Pharmacy is to contribute to the understanding of the development of civilization by fostering the creation, preservation, and dissemination of knowledge concerning the history and related humanistic aspects of the pharmaceutical field." Memberships and AIHP-published pamphlets, books, prints and slide shows dissecting all kinds of pharmaco minutiae.

Drug and Medicine Special Collections
Philadelphia College of Pharmacy and Science
Joseph W. England Library
42nd Street and Woodland Avenue
Philadelphia, PA 19104
(215) 596-8960

Holds 56,000 volumes, 35,000 microforms, 24 vertical file drawers, and audiovisual programs on pharmacology, chemistry, and toxicology. Includes special collection on the history of the pharmacy.

U.S. Food and Drug Administration Center
for Drugs and Biologics
Medical Library/HFN-98
5600 Fishers Lane, Room 11B-07
Rockville, MD 20857
(301) 443-3180

Pharmacology, pharmacy, and pharmaceutical technology are main subjects; repository for FDA archives and U.S./foreign drug compilations.

University of Houston
College of Pharmacy Library
Houston, TX 77204-5511
(713) 749-1566

Holds references on pharmacy and pharmacology, toxicology and general chemistry, with a special history of pharmacy collection. 14,000 volumes.

University of Iowa
College of Pharmacy
Iowa Drug Information Service
Westlawn, Box 330
Iowa City, IA 52242
(319) 335-8913

Holds 24,000 articles on microfilm on drugs and drug therapy.

University of Mississippi
John Davis Williams Library
Austin A. Dodge Pharmacy Library
215A Fraser Hall
University, MS 38677
(601)232-7381

Subjects include pharmacy, organic chemistry, botany, and related subjects. Holds 28,000 volumes.

University of Wisconsin, Madison
F.B. Power Pharmaceutical Library
School of Pharmacy
425 North Chater Street
Madison, WI 53706
(608) 262-2894

Covers pharmacy and related subjects. Special collections include catalogs of drugs and pharmaceutical equipment, 1860 to present. Holds more than 12,000 books plus other research materials.

Pharmacists seem pretty keen on preserving their occupation's past—building period recreations of apothecary shops from coast to coast. Is it simple nostalgia for an age that treated pharmacists as men of science?

Notable PHARMACY MUSEUMS

Yale Medical Library
333 Cedar Street
New Haven, CT 06510
(203) 785-4354
European and American pharmaceutical paraphernalia dating from the 1500s are housed in the Yale med school and the Yale Medical Library alongside a large collection of medical instruments, periodicals and artifacts.

Blackberry Historical Farm Village
R.R. 3 Box 591 Galena Blvd. and Barnes Road
Aurora, IL 60506
(708) 892-5664
"Early Streets of Aurora" museum features storefronts and turn-of-the-century merchandise including an Apothecary Shop with over 2,000 objects in the collection.

University of Illinois College of Pharmacy
833 South Wood Street
Chicago, IL 60680
(312) 996-7190
Objects from the late 19th century donated by Illinois pharmacists or their heirs, including prescriptions dating to the 1840s, before the founding of the Chicago College of Pharmacy in 1859.

Hooks' Historical Drug Store
and Pharmacy Museum
Indiana State Fairgrounds
1202 East 38th Street
Indianapolis, IN 46205
(317) 924-1503
A vast collection of American pharmacy artifacts plus early wares from England, France and Germany, and a working 1880 Lippincott soda fountain.

Eli Lilly Center Exhibition and Archives
893 South Delaware Street
Indianapolis, IN 46206
Seven major exhibitions the company's "diversified" interests in pharmaceuticals, corporate archival displays, a room devoted to mementos and the history of the Lilly family, and the discovery and production of the company's medications.

The New Orleans Pharmacy Museum
514 Rue Chartres, Vieux Carre,
New Orleans, LA 70130
(504) 565-8027
Founded in 1950, the museum is located in the heart of the French Quarter. It consists of an apothecary shop constructed in 1823 for Louis Dufilho, Jr., the nation's first licensed pharmacist. Handmade drug jars, gris gris potions used by voodoo practitioners, Civil War-era surgical instruments and cosmetics, rare patent medicines, and a collection dating to 1880, containing a prescription file as well as the chemicals and tools used to compound them. Also a rare 1855 Italian black and rose marble soda fountain.

Grand Rapids Public Museum
54 Jefferson Avenue, S.E.
Grand Rapids, MI 45903
Over 15,000 items represent a complete display of an early-1900s American pharmacy.

Albany College of Pharmacy
Union University
106 New Scotland Avenue
Albany, NY 12208
(518) 445-7211/7253
The contents of a New York drug store originally opened in 1800 were moved to the College of Pharmacy in 1936.

Museum and Pharmaceutical Exhibits

The Philadelphia College of Pharmacy
and Science
43rd Street and Kingsessing Avenue
Philadelphia, PA 19104
(215) 386-5800
Exhibits at the first pharmacy school in
the country includes a general pharmacy
museum, the George Glenworth Pharmacy
shop (opened in 1812), the Bohlander
Drugstore, and the Joseph England Library
collections.

Wall Drug Apothecary Shoppe and
Pharmacy Museum
510 Main Street
Wall, SD 57790
Fashioned after the original drug store
which was located across the street from
the present location and founded in 1931, it
contains over 400 pharmaceutical artifacts.

Hugh Mercer Apothecary Shop
1020 Caroline Street
Fredericksburg, VA 22401
(703) 373-3362
This is the oldest known original building
in America to house an apothecary shop.
It has been meticulously restored to its
original 1764 appearance and became a
pharmacy museum in 1928. Prescription
orders, pharmacy equipment and archival
materials (including accounts written by
George Washington, a frequent patron) are
on display. The original owner, Dr. Hugh
Mercer, died on the battlefield during
the Revolutionary War.

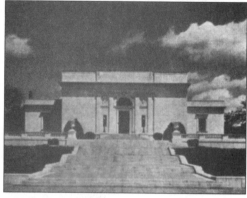

National Museum of American History
Smithsonian Institution
12th and Constitution Avenue, N.W.
Washington, D.C. 20560
(202) 357-2145
Three types of exhibits are housed in the
Hall of Pharmaceutical History: the development of machines, and equipment used
in the manufacture of dosage form preparations from the 19th century; the evolution
of the drug jar, mortars and pestles, and
other apothecary tools; and two pharmacy
restorations on loan—an 18th century
German "Muenster Apotheke" and 1890
American drugstore.

Wisconsin State Historical Society
Stonefield at the Nelson Dewey State Park
Complex
Cassville, WI 53806
(608) 725-5210
This pharmacy recreation from the late
19th century is part of a period Wisconsin
village. Fixtures and artifacts were shipped
from Wisconsin pharmacies. Shelves are
stocked with medicinal ingredients, and the
exhibition includes a cigar maker, an 1890
operational pill-making machine, drug
mixing and ice cream making equipment.
There is also a re-creation of a physician's
office, circa 1880.

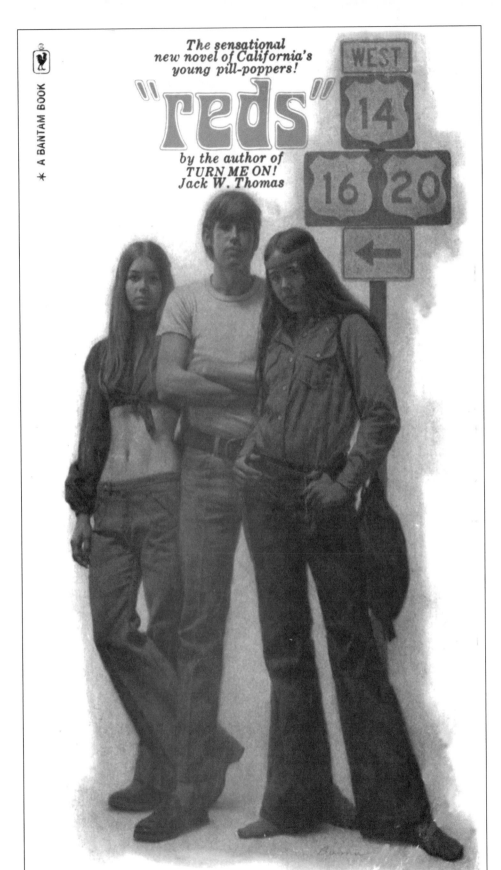

The sensational
new novel of California's
young pill-poppers!

"reds"

by the author of
TURN ME ON!
Jack W. Thomas

WEST
U.S. 14
U.S. 16   U.S. 20
←

A BANTAM BOOK

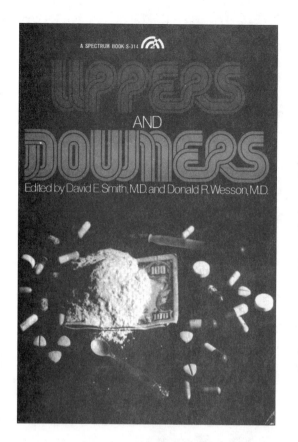

AND

Edited by David E. Smith, M.D. and Donald R. Wesson, M.D.

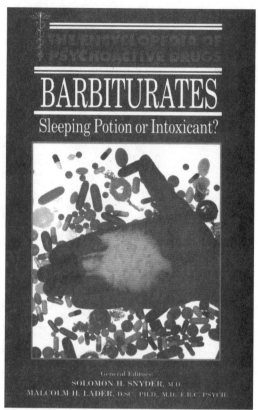

THE ENCYCLOPEDIA OF PSYCHOACTIVE DRUGS

BARBITURATES
Sleeping Potion or Intoxicant?

General Editors:
SOLOMON H. SNYDER, M.D.
MALCOLM H. LADER, D.SC., PH.D., M.D., F.R.C. PSYCH.

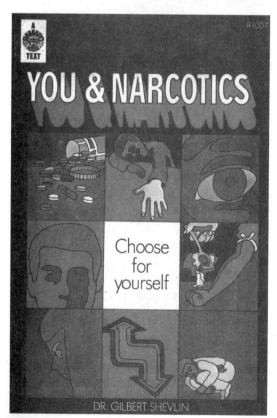

TEXT

YOU & NARCOTICS

Choose
for
yourself

DR. GILBERT SHEVLIN

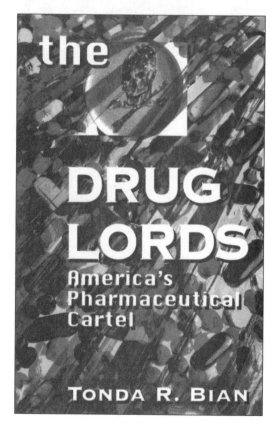

the

DRUG
LORDS
America's Pharmaceutical Cartel

TONDA R. BIAN

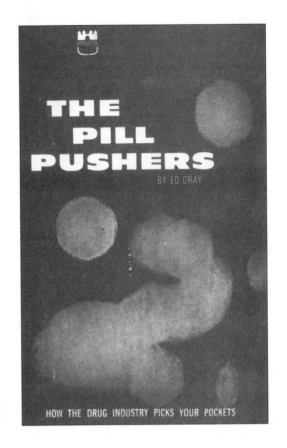

FAMILY CONCERNS

PILLS POPPERS & CAFFEINE

Addiction and Your Family

DAVID PARTINGTON

THE PILL PUSHERS

BY ED CRAY

HOW THE DRUG INDUSTRY PICKS YOUR POCKETS

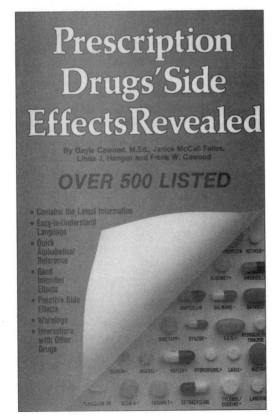

Prescription Drugs' Side Effects Revealed

By Gayle Cawood, M.Ed., Janice McCall Failes, Linda J. Hangen and Frank W. Cawood

OVER 500 LISTED

- Contains the Latest Information
- Easy-to-Understand Language
- Quick Alphabetical Reference
- Good Intended Effects
- Possible Side Effects
- Warnings
- Interactions with Other Drugs

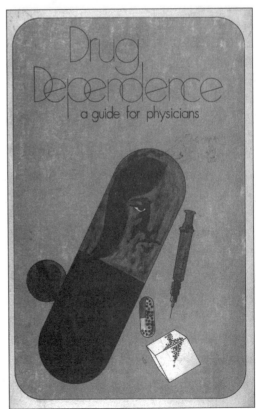

Drug Dependence
a guide for physicians

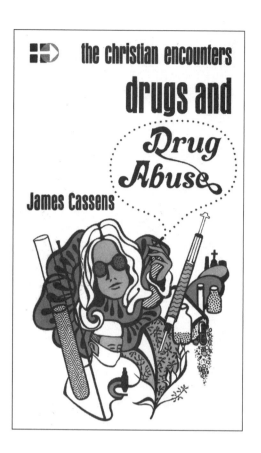

the christian encounters
drugs and
Drug Abuse

James Cassens

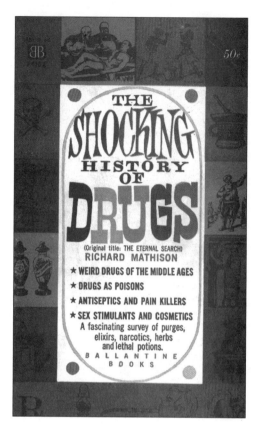

50¢

THE SHOCKING HISTORY OF DRUGS

(Original title: THE ETERNAL SEARCH)
RICHARD MATHISON

★ WEIRD DRUGS OF THE MIDDLE AGES
★ DRUGS AS POISONS
★ ANTISEPTICS AND PAIN KILLERS
★ SEX STIMULANTS AND COSMETICS

A fascinating survey of purges, elixirs, narcotics, herbs and lethal potions.

BALLANTINE BOOKS

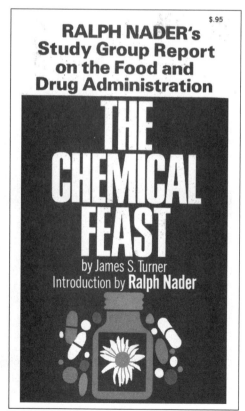

$.95

RALPH NADER's Study Group Report on the Food and Drug Administration

THE CHEMICAL FEAST

by James S. Turner
Introduction by **Ralph Nader**

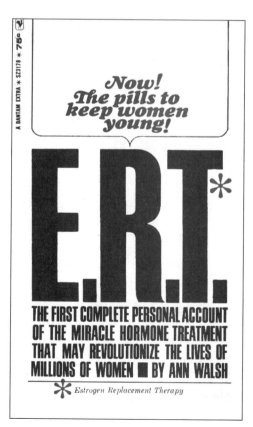

A BANTAM EXTRA ★ SZ3178 ★ 75¢

Now! The pills to keep women young!

E.R.T.*

THE FIRST COMPLETE PERSONAL ACCOUNT OF THE MIRACLE HORMONE TREATMENT THAT MAY REVOLUTIONIZE THE LIVES OF MILLIONS OF WOMEN ■ BY ANN WALSH

✳ *Estrogen Replacement Therapy*

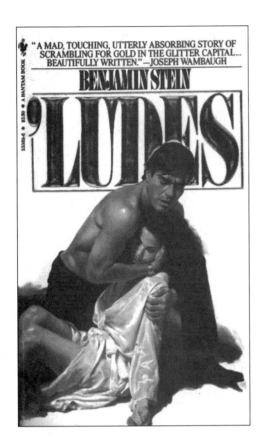

"A MAD, TOUCHING, UTTERLY ABSORBING STORY OF SCRAMBLING FOR GOLD IN THE GLITTER CAPITAL... BEAUTIFULLY WRITTEN."—JOSEPH WAMBAUGH

BENJAMIN STEIN

'LUDES

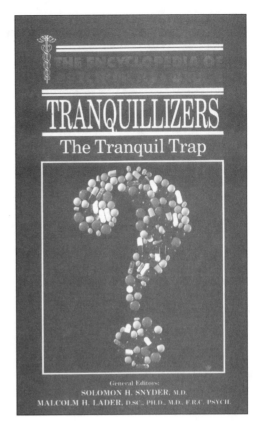

THE ENCYCLOPEDIA OF

TRANQUILLIZERS

The Tranquil Trap

General Editors:
SOLOMON H. SNYDER, M.D.
MALCOLM H. LADER, D.SC., PH.D., M.D., F.R.C. PSYCH.

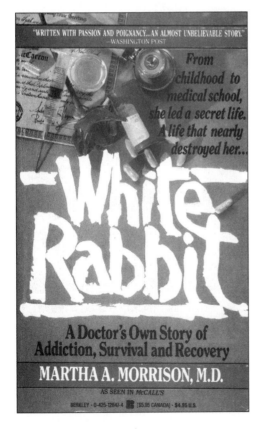

"WRITTEN WITH PASSION AND POIGNANCY...AN ALMOST UNBELIEVABLE STORY."
—WASHINGTON POST

From childhood to medical school, she led a secret life. A life that nearly destroyed her...

White Rabbit

A Doctor's Own Story of Addiction, Survival and Recovery

MARTHA A. MORRISON, M.D.

AS SEEN IN McCALL'S

BERKLEY · 0-425-12647-4 ■ [$5.95 CANADA] · $4.95 U.S.

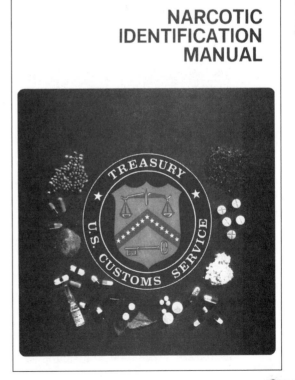

NARCOTIC
IDENTIFICATION
MANUAL

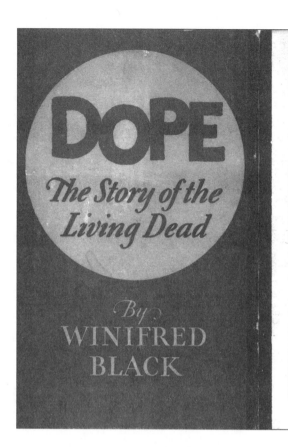

DOPE
The Story of the Living Dead

By
WINIFRED BLACK

DOPE
by
Winifred Black

IN trenchant style Winifred Black gives here the result of her investigation into one of the urgent social problems of the day—that of the increase in narcotic addiction. This growing menace of the drug habit is spreading like a virulent disease in this country among all classes. It threatens the youth of both sexes; it is making criminals and crowding jails and prisons; it is sapping the vitality and wrecking the happiness of innocent millions, who become its victims through ignorance.

The effects of the evil sisterhood of Dope—opium, cocain, morphin, heroin, marihuana—are reviewed in turn and illustrated by tragic human stories; and the enlightened plans most recently devised for coping with the situation are ably explained in this vivid "Story of the Living Dead."

Price $1.00

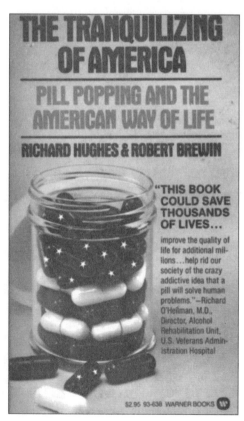

THE TRANQUILIZING OF AMERICA
PILL POPPING AND THE AMERICAN WAY OF LIFE

RICHARD HUGHES & ROBERT BREWIN

"THIS BOOK COULD SAVE THOUSANDS OF LIVES...

improve the quality of life for additional millions...help rid our society of the crazy addictive idea that a pill will solve human problems."—Richard O'Heilman, M.D., Director, Alcohol Rehabilitation Unit, U.S. Veterans Administration Hospital

$2.95 93-638 WARNER BOOKS

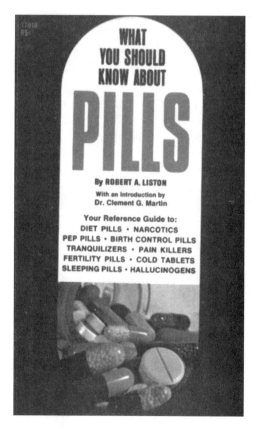

WHAT YOU SHOULD KNOW ABOUT PILLS

By ROBERT A. LISTON

With an Introduction by
Dr. Clement G. Martin

Your Reference Guide to:
DIET PILLS · NARCOTICS
PEP PILLS · BIRTH CONTROL PILLS
TRANQUILIZERS · PAIN KILLERS
FERTILITY PILLS · COLD TABLETS
SLEEPING PILLS · HALLUCINOGENS

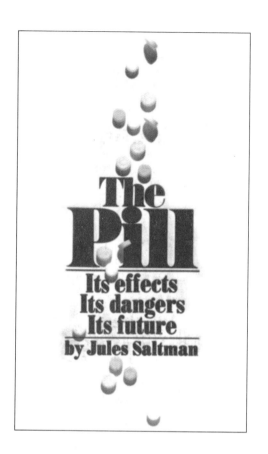

The Pill
Its effects
Its dangers
Its future
by Jules Saltman

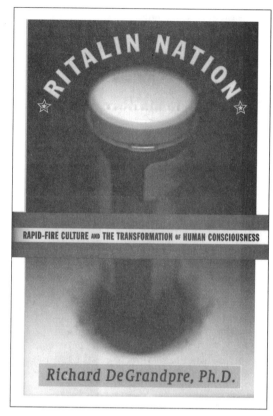

RITALIN NATION

RAPID-FIRE CULTURE AND THE TRANSFORMATION OF HUMAN CONSCIOUSNESS

Richard DeGrandpre, Ph.D.

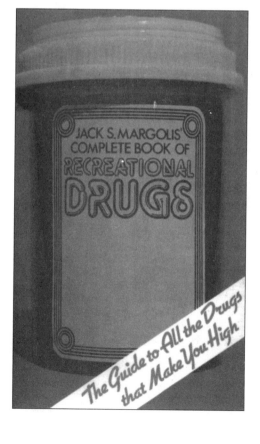

JACK S. MARGOLIS'
COMPLETE BOOK OF
RECREATIONAL
DRUGS

The Guide to All the Drugs that Make You High

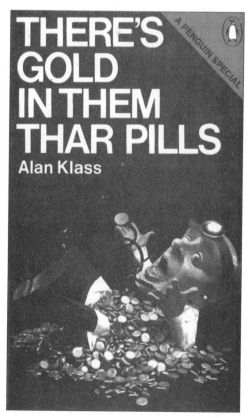

A PENGUIN SPECIAL

THERE'S
GOLD
IN THEM
THAR PILLS
Alan Klass

Bibliography

Abbott Alkaloidal Co., 1913–14 *Pharmaceutical and Biologic Products of The Abbott Laboratories*, 33rd Edition (Second Printing), Ravenswood: Abbott Alkaloidal Co.

Bargmann, Eve, *Stopping Valium*. Public Citizen's Health Research Group, 1982.

Baum, Dan, *Smoke and Mirrors: The War on Drugs and the Politics of Failure*. New York: Little Brown, 1996.

Bealle, Morris A., *Dangerous Doses: Patent Medicine Industry's False Advertising Gimmicks*, Washington, D.C.: Columbia Publishing Company, 1964.

Benowicz, Robert J., *Non-Prescription Drugs and Their Side Effects*, New York: Grosset & Dunlap, 1977.

Bentley, Arthur Owen, *A Text-Book of Pharmaceutics*, London: Bailliere, Tindall and Cox, 1933.

Bian, Tonda R., *The Drug Lords: America's Pharmaceutical Cartel*. Kalamazoo: No Barriers Publishing, 1995.

Black, Winifred, *Dope: The Story of the Living Dead*, New York: Star Company, 1928.

Blakeslee, Alton, *What You Should Know About Drugs and Narcotics*, The Associated Press, 1969.

Blum, Kenneth, *Handbook of Abusable Drugs*, New York: Gardner Press, 1984.

Brecher, Edward M. and the editors of Consumer Reports, *Licit and Illicit Drugs: The Consumers Union Report*, Boston: Little, Brown and Co., 1972.

Breton, Nina, *Marihuana, LSD y Otras Hierbas*, Guatemala: Ediciones Interamericanas, 1970.

Burback, Richard, *The Handbook of Prescription Drugs: Official Names, Prices and Sources for Patient and Doctor*, New York: Pantheon Press, 1967.

Burlingham, Robert, *The Odyssey of Modern Drug Research*, Kalamazoo: The Upjohn Company, 1951.

Byer, Curtis O., Jones, Kenneth L., Shainberg, Louis W., *Drugs: Substance Abuse*, San Francisco: Canfield Press, 1975.

Carey, James T., *The College Drug Scene*, Englewood Cliffs: Prentice-Hall, Inc., 1968.

Cassens, James, *The Christian Encounters Drugs and Drug Abuse*, St. Louis: Concordia House, 1970.

Cawood, Gayle, Falles, Janice Mc Call, Hangen, Linda J., Cawood, Frank W., *Prescription Drugs' Side Effects Revealed*, Peachtree City: F, C & A Publishing, 1984.

Cerio, Steven, *Steven Cerio's ABC Book: A Drug Primer*, New York: Gates of Heck, 1998.

Charley, Michael Francis and others from pharmaceutical companies, *A Primer of Public Relations For The Pharmaceutical Industry*, New York: The American Pharmaceutical Manufacturers Association, 1953.

Clayman, Charles B., ed. *The American Medical Association Guide to Prescription and Over the Counter Drugs*, New York: Random House, 1988.

Colvin, Rod, *Prescription Drug Abuse: The Hidden Epidemic*, Omaha: Addicus Books, 1995.

Consumer Report Books, *The Medicine Show: Consumers Union's Practical Guide to Some Everyday Health Problems and Health Products*, Mount Vernon: Consumers Union, 1983.

Cook, James, *Remedies and Rackets: The Truth About the Patent Medicines Today*, New York: W. W. Norton and Co., 1958.

Cray, Ed, *The Pill Pushers: How the Drug Industry Picks Your Pockets*, North Hollywood: Brandon House, 1966.

Cuadroz, Elias Taxa, *Drogas Y Hippies: Dramatico Problema Mundial*, 1976.

Curtis, Lindsay R., *Let's Talk About Goofballs and Pep Pills (Including Tranquilizers and LSD)*, General Military Training and Support Division, 1967.

DeGrandpre, Richard, *Ritalin Nation: Rapid-fire Culture and the Transformation of Human Consciousness*, New York: W. W. Norton & Company, 1999.

Department of the Treasury, *Narcotic Identification Manual*, U.S. Customs Service, circa 1989.

Duke, Steven B. and Gross, Albert C., *America's Longest War: Rethinking Our Tragic Crusade Against Drugs*, New York: Tarcher/Putnam, 1993.

Eli Lilly and Company, *The Story of the Lilly Laboratories*, circa 1954.

Felter, Harvey Wickes and Lloyd, Uri John, *King's American Dispensatory, "Entirely Rewritten and Enlarged,"* 18th Edition, Third Revision. In Two Volumes. Republished by Eclectic Medical Publications, 1983.

Fry, T. C., *The Myth of Medicine,* published by Life Science, circa 1969.

Gannon, Frank, *Drugs: What They Are, How They Look, What They Do,* New York: Warner Books, 1975.

Gray, M. *M. Gray's Pharmaceutical Quiz Compend.* Chicago: M. M. Gray and Co., 1905.

Hughes, Richard and Brewin, Robert. *The Tranquilizing of America: Pill Popping and the American Way of Life,* New York: Warner Books, 1980.

Hull, William H. *Public Relations for the Pharmacist,* Philadelphia: J. B. Lippincott, 1955.

Humphry, Derek. *Final Exit: The Practicalities of Self-Deliverance and Assisted Suicide for the Dying,* Eugene: The Hemlock Society, 1991.

Illich, Ivan, *Medical Nemesis,* New York: Bantam Book, 1976.

Inaba, Darryl S. and Cohen, William E. *Uppers, Downers, All Arounders,* Ashland: CNS Productions, Inc., 1991. "In co-operation with the Haight-Ashbury Detox Clinic."

Kehrer, James P., and Kehrer, Daniel M. *Pills and Potions,* New York: Arco, 1984.

Klass, Alan, *There's Gold in Them Thar Pills: An Inquiry Into the Medical-Industrial Complex,* Middlesex: Penguin Books, 1975.

Knowlton, Calvin H. and Penna, Richard P., eds. *Pharmaceutical Care,* New York: Chapman and Hill, 1995. (quoted essay-Higby, Gregory, "From Compounding to Caring: An Abridged History of American Pharmacy.")

Kondratas, Ramunas, *A Salute to Pharmacy: The Community Pharmacy in History,* Booklet 1, New York: Ayest Laboratories.

Kondratas, Ramunas, *A Salute to Pharmacy: Pills and Other Solid Dosage Forms,* Booklet 5, New York: Ayest Laboratories.

Kreig, Margaret, *Black Market Medicine,* Englewood Cliffs: Prentice-Hall, 1967.

Kuhn, Cynthia, Swartzwelder, Scott, and Wilson, Wilkie, *Buzzed: The Straight Facts About the Most Used and Abused Drugs From Alcohol to Ecstasy,* New York: W. W. Norton and Company, 1998.

Kunkin, Art, *Los Angeles Free Press,* "Narcotics Agents Listed" issue, August 8-14, 1969.

Lader, Malcolm, *Introduction to Psychopharmacology,* Kalamazoo, Upjohn Company, 1983.

Lenson, David, *On Drugs,* Minneapolis: University of Minnesota Press, 1995.

Liebenau, Jonathan, *Medical Science and Medical Industry: The Formation of the American Pharmaceutical Industry,* Baltimore: Johns Hopkins University Press, 1987.

Lieberman, M. Laurence, *The Essential Guide to Generic Drugs,* New York: Harper and Row, 1986.

Madison, Arnold, *Drugs and You,* New York: Pocket Books, 1972.

Mahoney, Tom, *The Merchants of Life: The Story of the Pharmaceutical Industry, Its Research and Its Life-Saving Discoveries in the War Against Disease,* New York: Harpers and Brothers, 1959.

Margolis, Jack S. *Jack S. Margolis' Complete Book of Recreational Drugs,* Los Angeles: Cliff House Books, 1978.

Marsa, Linda, *Prescription for Profits: How the Pharmaceutical Industry Bankrolled the Unholy Marriage Between Science and Business,* New York: Scribner, 1997.

Mason, David and Dyller, Fran, *Pharmaceutical Dictionary & Reference For Prescription Drugs,* New York: Playboy Paperbacks, 1981.

Mathison, Richard, *The Shocking History of Drugs,* New York: Ballantine Books, 1958.

Meier, Kenneth J. *The Politics of Sin: Drugs, Alcohol, and Public Policy,* New York: M.E. Sharpe.

Mendelson, Wallace B., *The Use and Misuse of Sleeping Pills: A Clinical Guide,* New York: Plenum Publishing, 1980.

Miller, Richard Lawrence. *Drug Warriors and the Prey: From Police Power to Police State,* Westport, Conn.: Praeger Publishers, 1996.

Mintz, Morton, *The Therapeutic Nightmare,* Boston: Houghton Mifflin, 1965.

Morgan, H. Wayne. *Drugs in America, a Social History,* Syracuse University Press, 1991.

Morrison, Martha A., *White Rabbit: A Doctor's Own Story of Addiction, Survival and Recovery,* New York: Berkley Books, 1989.

Newman, Joseph, ed., *What Everyone Needs to Know About Drugs,* Washington, D.C.: U.S. News and World Report, 1970.

Nowlis, Helen H., *Drugs on the College Campus,* Garden City: Anchor Books, 1969.

Page, Irvine H., ed., *Modern Medicine: The Journal of Diagnosis and Treatment,* Minneapolis: Modern Medicine Publications, July, 1964.

Partington, David, Pills, *Poppers & Caffeine: Addiction and Your Family,* London: Hodder and Stoughton, 1996.

Partridge, Eric, *A Dictionary of the Underworld,* New York: Bonanza Books, 1961.

Pekkanen, John, *The American Connection: Profiteering and Politicking in the "Ethical" Drug Industry,* Chicago: Follett Publishing Company, 1973.

Pettey, Geo. G., *The Narcotic Drug Diseases and Allied Ailments: Pathology, Pathogenesis and Treatment,* Philadelphia: F. A. Davis Company, 1913.

Philips, Peter and Project Censored. *Censored 1998: The News That Didn't Make the News, The Year's Top 25 Censored Stories,* New York: Seven Stories Press, 1998.

Physicians' Desk Reference, 51st Edition, 1997.

Physicians' Desk Reference for NonPrescription Drugs, 16th Edition, 1995.

Pitchess, Peter J., *Narcotics and Dangerous Drugs,* Sheriff's Department, Los Angeles County, circa 1966.

Proger, Samuel, ed. *The Medicated Society,* New York: Macmillan, 1968.

Rayburn, William F., Zuspan, Frederick P., Fitzgerald, Jeanne T., *Every Woman's Pharmacy: An Invaluable Guide For All Women About the Prescription and Over-the-Counter Drugs They Take and Their Side Effects,* Garden City: Doubleday, 1984

Reader's Digest, *Prescription & Over-the-Counter Drugs,* Pleasantville: The Reader's Digest Association, Inc., 1998.

Remington's Pharmaceutical Sciences, 17th Edition, Easton: Mack, 1985.

Ross, David, *Pissing Away the American Dream: How the War on Drugs is Destroying the Bill of Rights,* Norcross: The Digit Press, 1991.

Saltman, Jules, *The Pill: Its Effects, Its Dangers, Its Future,* New York: Grosset and Dunlap, 1970.

Sandoz, *It's All In Your Head* (Headache Art Book), Sandoz Pharmaceutical Company, 1991.

Scoville, Wilbur. *The Art of Compounding: A Text Book for Students and a Reference Book for Pharmacists at the Prescription Counter.* Philadelphia: P. Blakiston's Son and Co., 1914.

Shevlin, Dr. Gilbert, *You and Narcotics,* New York: Ramapo House, 1971.

Silverman, Harold M., *The Pill Book,* New York: Bantam Books, 1996.

Silverman, Milton, etc. *Bad Medicine: The Prescription Drug Industry in the Third World,* Stanford: Stanford University Press, 1992.

Silverman, Milton, *The Drugging of the Americas: How Multinational Drug Companies Say One Thing About Their Products to Physicians in the United States, and Another Thing To Physicians in Latin America,* Berkeley: University of California Press, 1976.

Silverman, Milton, *Magic in a Bottle,* New York: Macmillan, 1942.

Silverman, Milton and Lee, Philip R., *Pills, Profits and Politics,* Berkeley: University of California Press, 1974.

Smith, David and Wesson, Donald, eds. *Uppers and Downers.* Englewood Cliffs, N.J.: Prentice-Hall, 1973.

Smith, Mickey C. *Small Comfort: A History of the Minor Tranquilizers.* New York: Praeger, 1985.

Smith Kline & French Laboratories: *Ten Years Experience with Thorazine: 1954–1964, Tranquilizer, Potentiator, Antiemetic,* Philadelphia: SmithKline & French, 1964.

Smith Kline & French: *Drug Abuse: A Manual for Law Enforcement Officers,* Philadelphia: SmithKline & French Laboratories, Revised Third Edition, 1968.

Smith Kline & French, *Drug Abuse: Game Without Winners, A Basic Handbook for Commanders,* Washington, D.C.: U.S. Government Printing Office, 1968.

Smith, Warren, and Olson, *Eugene: The Menace of Pep Pills,* Chicago: Camerarts Publishing, 1965.

Snyder, Solomon, ed. *The Encyclopedia of Psychoactive Drugs: Barbiturates: Sleeping*

Potion or Intoxicant?, New York: Burke Publishing Company, Ltd. 1988.

Stein, Benjamin, *'Ludes,* New York: Bantam, 1983.

Stern, Edward L., *Prescription Drugs and Their Side Effects,* New York: Perigree Books, 1987.

Szasz, T. S. *Ceremonial Chemistry: The Ritual Perscution of Drugs, Addicts and Pushers.* Rev. ed., Holmes Beach, FL: Learning Publications, 1985.

Szasz, T. S., *Our Right to Drugs: The Case for a Free Market.* Syracuse University Press, 1992.

Tanner, Ogden, *The Prudent Use of Medicines,* Alexandria: Time-Life Books, 1981.

Taylor, Norman, *Narcotics: Nature's Dangerous Gifts,* New York: Dell, 1976.

Truax, Greene & Co., *Physicians' and Hospital Supplies, Price List of Chemical and Pharmaceutical Products,* Chicago: 1906.

Turner, James S., *The Chemical Feast: Ralph Nader's Study Group Report on the Food and Drug Administration,* New York: Grossman, 1970.

University Medical Research Publishers, *Amazing Medicines The Drug Companies Don't Want You To Discover,* Tempe: University Medical Research, 1993.

Urdang, George. *Pharmacy's Part in Society.* Madison, Wisconsin: American Institutue of the History of Pharmacy, 1946. Limited to 1500 copies.

Vermes, Jean C., *Pot Is Rot* (And Other Horrible Facts About Bad Things), New York: Association Press, 1970.

Wakefield, Dan, ed., *The Addict,* Greenwich, Conn: Fawcett Publications, 1969.

Walsh, Ann, *E.R.T.: The First Complete Personal Account of the Miracle Hormone Treatment That May Revolutionize the Lives of Millions of Women,* New York: Bantam Books, 1965.

Wigder, H. Neil, Dr. Wigder's *Guide to Over-The-Counter Drugs: A Consumer's Reference Guide to Over 850 Nonprescription Brand-name Drugs,* New York: Delta Books, 1979.

Wisotsky, Steven. *Beyond the War on Drugs: Overcoming a Failed Public Policy,* Buffalo, New York: Prometheus Books,

Witters, Weldon and Jones-Witters, Patricia, *Drugs and Society: A Biological Perspective,* Ohio University, Wadsworth Health Sciences, 1983.

Wohl, Stanley, *The Medical Industrial Complex,* New York: Harmony Books, 1984.

Wolfe, Sidney M., and Coley, Christopher M., *Pills That Don't Work: A Consumers' and Doctors' Guide to 610 Prescription Drugs That Lack Evidence of Effectiveness,* Washington, D.C.: Public Citizen's Health Research Group, 1980.

Wolman, Walter, ed., *Drug Dependence: A Guide for Physicians,* Chicago: American Medical Association, 1969.

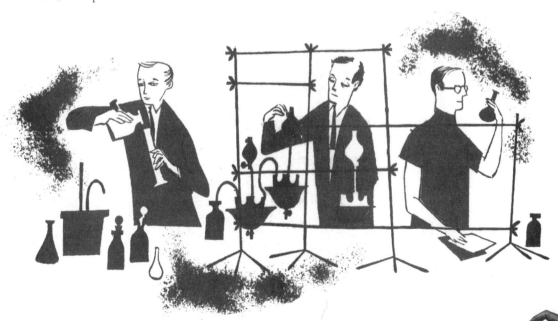

Notes

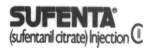

LORTAB® 7.5/500℃

7.5 mg hydrocodone bitartrate (Warning: May be habit forming)
and 500 mg acetaminophen

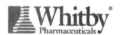

Whitby
Pharmaceuticals

SUFENTA®
(sufentanil citrate) Injection ℃

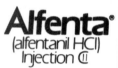

Alfenta®
(alfentanil HCl)
Injection ℃

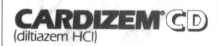

For The Long And Short Of It

CARDIZEM® CD
(diltiazem HCl)

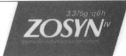

ZOSYN™
3.375g q6h
piperacillin sodium/tazobactam sodium

3.375g
q6h

Please see enclosed full Prescribing Information, including
WARNINGS, ADVERSE EFFECTS, and CONTRAINDICATIONS.

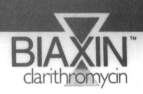

BIAXIN™
clarithromycin

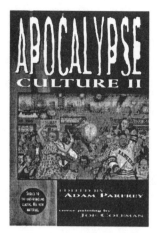
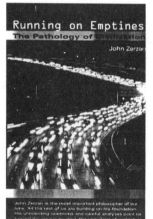
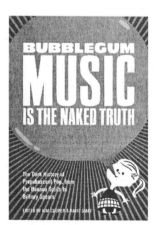